Indian Ethnic Rhinoplasty

Virendra Ghaisas

Indian Ethnic Rhinoplasty

A Surgical Guide

Springer

Virendra Ghaisas
Ghaisas ENT Hospital, MIMER Medical college
Pune, Maharashtra
India

ISBN 978-981-16-2477-3 ISBN 978-981-16-2478-0 (eBook)
https://doi.org/10.1007/978-981-16-2478-0

This Springer imprint is published by the registered company Springer Nature Singapore Pte Ltd.
The registered company address is: 152 Beach Road, #21-01/04 Gateway East, Singapore 189721, Singapore

Foreword

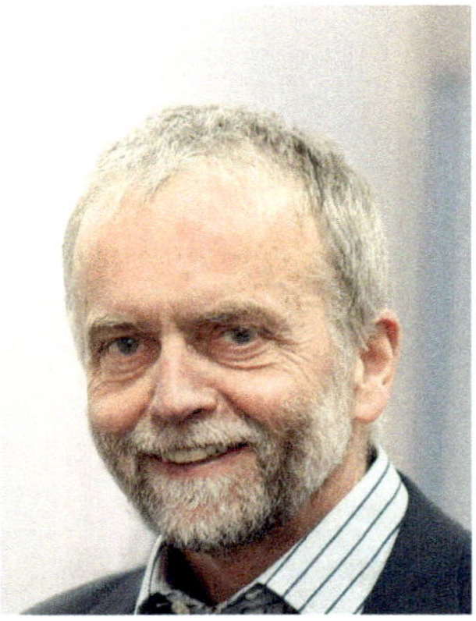

There are already many books out there, dealing specifically with Indian noses, but this one is the latest version. The book is incorporating the most recent techniques which have been developed during the last years and extended the armamentarium of rhinoplasty surgeons.

Dr. V. Ghaisas enlightens all aspects of this challenging topic and emphasizes the need to respect the wide variety of Indian skin for getting a good final outcome.

Having guided many rhinoplasty courses in India myself I know that traumatic deformities are quite common and mostly need a sophisticated septal work to achieve a good long-term result. Therefore it is very helpful that Dr. V. Ghaisas discusses this problem in detail and also shows very good cases, which demonstrate not only his precise analysis, but also the clear concept and the skillful performance by which he achieved good functional and aesthetic results. The balance of these two issues is essential for a successful rhinoplasty.

Therefore I hope that this well-written book combined with all the very good photos will cause great insights to all colleagues who are interested in this difficult and challenging field. This book can definitely lead to new ideas about modern concepts in rhinoplasty and improvements of results and therefore many happy patients.

Stuttgart, Germany — Wolfgang Gubisch

Contents

About the Author

Dr. Virendra Ghaisas has attained primary schooling and college in Pune. He did his MBBS from KIMS, Karad in 1996 and obtained his post-graduate degree (MS) from J. N. Medical College, Belagavi in 2001.

With an acquired interest in rhinoplasty, he pursued his training in rhinoplasty at Stuttgart, Germany under renowned surgeon Professor Dr. Wolfgang Gubisch in 2004. He has work experience as a specialist in the field of ENT and as a rhinoplasty surgeon for 18 years in Pune, India. He is a senior consultant surgeon at Ghaisas ENT centre. He also holds a position as Director of MIMER Medical College, Talegaon, Pune.

Having worked with various ENT and rhinoplasty surgeons and with a caseload of about 100–150 rhinoplasty procedures per year and having conducted multiple regional, national and international hands-on surgical and cadaveric workshops across India from Kashmir to Tamil Nadu and in the Middle East and Sri Lanka has helped him develop a plethora of surgical skills in the field of ENT and rhinoplasty.

He has a wide experience of more than 2000 rhinoplasties till today with all varieties of noses.

My Journey

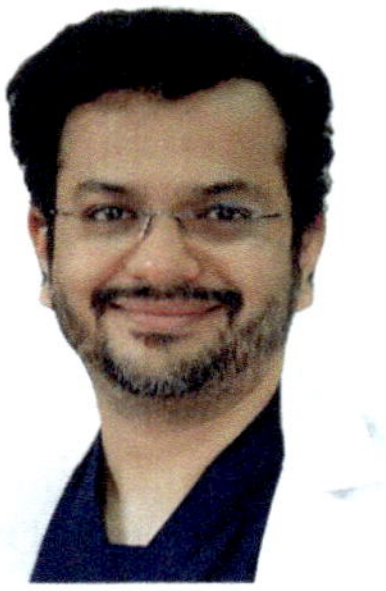

After my MBBS, I did my masters in ENT & HNS in JNMC, Belgaum. I had observed Dr. Ashutosh Pusalkar from my undergraduate days operating at our hospital along with my father. He is a great personality and excellent surgeon. He has influenced me in my career in ENT and as a personality in a big way. My father Dr. Suresh Ghaisas, I do not have to words to describe as to how much he has inflenced me. He has given me a platform of MIMER Medical College, ENT educational and hospital setup and has shown me how to be humble and down to earth.

I was fortunate to have great teachers at JNMC Belgaum, in specific, Dr. R N Patil, Dr. Bagewadi and Dr. Belaldawar. As a person and as teachers, all were in different phases of my life and I have learnt from everyone in the department from teachers to my senior co PGs.

I was fortunate enough to observe rhinoplasty during my postgraduation days along with Dr. R N Patil. He is a perfectionist and has a lot of patience which has formed a base in my career of rhinoplasty. After passing, I had joined ENT Hospital in Fort, a wonderful Municipal Hospital in South Mumbai under Dr. Ashutosh Pusalkar. I got to learn a lot of otology and ENT surgeries there. I had liking towards rhinoplasty but it increased when I started practising in Pune. I noticed that very few doctors are doing a perfect rhinoplasty job and many ENT surgeons are doing only septoplasty for deviated nose are keeping internal nasal valve obstruction and giving half-hearted aesthetic results to patients. Similarly, plastic surgeons with good aesthetic result are not doing a great septoplasty work and again giving half-hearted functional results. So I was convinced that rhinoplasty is the field I should focus as my long-term goal. I contacted Dr. Pusalkar and instantly he wrote to Professor Wolfgang Gubisch about my visit in Stuttgart. I was fortunate enough and Professor Gubisch immediately accepted my request and I went there for 3 months in 2004. He is my mentor and I dedicate my entire Rhinoplasty career along with this book to him. I met Dr. Sebastein Haack, he was a young junior chap who had just joined the department. I never thought that he will become a close friend of mine and now he is a head of the department of the same facial aesthetic centre in Stuttgart.

After coming back, the main task was to apply the rhinoplasty skills which I had learnt in the European setup to Indian patients. Indian patients are different from European patients in many ways. To apply this in the Indian setup with Indian patients was a major task. Cadaveric dissections, live surgical workshops, free hand of surgeries by Prof Gopal sir and free surgical camps were key factors help of departmental colleagues Dr. Mubarak Khan, Dr. Ganesh Pentewar and many more helped me in this. Arranging international workshops is a part of my rhinoplasty career, entire MIMER Medical staff with Dr. Suchitra Nangre has been helping me in that. I should also thank my colleagues Dr. Nilesh Madkikar, Dr. Manjusha Vispute, and Dr. Sapna Parab for supporting me and helping me in my learning curve of rhinoplasty, special mention of Dr. Ajit Agashe, anaesthetist, he is with me from day one of my career giving me excellent field and keeping patience in my learning phase. Also thankful to Dr. Kshitij Patil, Dr. Vikas Kulkarni, Dr. Santosh Patil, Dr. Hina Baxi, Dr. Suhasini, Dr. Shailesh Pandey and Dr. Ajay doiphode by teaching them rhinoplasty I have learnt so many things from them and I really believe that they these people have enriched my personality. With everyone's help, we all have founded Association of Rhinoplasty Surgeons of India (ARSI). Special thanks to Dr. Kshitij Patil and Dr. Vikas for letting me use intraop photos from their OT. Dr. B P Belaldawar for constant support in writing and allowing to use cadaveric photos. I thank Dr. Kshitij Patil and Dr. Hina Baxi to have co-authored the chapters Deviated noses and Cleft nose deformity respectively. It was Dr. Suhasini and Dr. Neeta Ghates constant help and support with which I could finish this effort in rhinoplasty in book form. Mrs. Nilofer has amazing skills of drawing diagrams and her illustrations have made this book beautiful and easier to explain. Words cant be enough to thank Dr. Suhasini who through her unparalleled dedication and passion for Rhinoplasty, had a pivotal role for compiling this work. I thank photographer artist Mr. Kumar Gokhale for the cover image.

My wife Ashwini is my strong support and she is a beautiful photographer too. She had come to OT for intraoperative photography and helped to get good illustrative photos. My elder son Soham was just 6 months old when she allowed me to go to Germany to learn and practice. She single-handedly carried responsibilities on family background and without her support I could not have achieved whatever I have done it till now.

Indian nose is different in all sense. We get to see a variety from Kashmir to Northeast to the middle part of India to South India. Luckily, I got a chance to operate all over India in my 15 years of rhinoplasty experience. This I am putting forth because juniors should learn from my journey so that they can reduce a learning curve in rhinoplasty. Please remember, rhinoplasty journey is never-ending.

How to Start Journey of Rhinoplasty for Beginners

1

Beginners in rhinoplasty do not mean that you should start learning at young age only; you can start learning rhinoplasty at any stage of your surgical career. If you are a ENT surgeon, then you are good at septoplasty, but the aesthetic sense is never taught in ENT curriculum. If you are a plastic surgeon, then you are aware of the aesthetic sense of face, but the functional surgeries like septoplasty/turbinoplasty are not taught during plastic surgery training curriculum. Hence, whoever wants to master the technique of rhinoplasty should make an effort to learn the aesthetic sense and the functionality of the nose both equally.

With different experience of operating all over India over so many years, I am of conclusion that we should simplify rhinoplasty according to region where you are operating. It should be a combination of mathematics of deformity, aesthetic sense of surgeon and patient, appropriate nasal functionality and ethnicity of that region. These should be the main pillars in operative planning. I have made an effort to simplify it so anyone interested in rhinoplasty can follow. One should master open approach basic fundamental rhinoplasty surgery first. This can be applicable to maximum nasal deformities. There are 5% difficult deformities which can be done by surgeon after his 3 or 5 years of rhinoplasty journey.

As far as rhinoplasty is concerned, I am influenced by Professor Dr. Wolfgang Gubisch from Germany and his clarity of thoughts, finesse in surgery and hunger to learn new and influenced me in my professional and personal career. The book which has influenced me in mastering rhinoplasty is by Dr. Rollin Daniel:

- *Learning* rhinoplasty is not all about attending workshop or two and directly starting with performing surgeries. It is a combined philosophy which is influenced by aesthetic vision and functional results. You should begin to follow one school of thought and pursue it at least for 3 years.
- *Why 3 years*? One should master basic fundamentals of open approach surgery. Once you operate, the final result is after 1 year. After a critical review of 1-year post-op photos and patient's nose, even then patient is happy, you will come to know drawbacks of techniques used. You will correct or add other methods in the next patient, and again it will take 1 year to analyse. After 2 years, you will start developing confidence and will start getting predicted results, so ultimately it takes around 3 years to master technique to treat 95% of cases.
- Then, subsequently one can start adding up finer points, and then difficult cases can be tackled. It will take another 2 years to master these difficult cases. Therefore, it's a journey of 5 years to master all kind of deformities. It's 5 years of continuous learning with one school of thought, and then eventually one can see the other surgeon's techniques from other school of thoughts and can start adding new techniques in your armaments. Following many surgeons at the inception of this journey

V. Ghaisas, *Indian Ethnic Rhinoplasty*, https://doi.org/10.1007/978-981-16-2478-0_1

may confuse you more and can affect the results. Hence, it's always better to follow one school of thought at least for 5 years and then change or modify according to your surgical results and comfort zone.

- Aesthetic sense. Start observing good-looking faces and good-shaped noses, and analyse why they are good and what are the positive factors in them which make that particular face attractive. One must develop aesthetic sense. Aesthetic sense varies from generation to generation, and with social media trend, it changes, and we must be aware of it. Start subscribing movie magazines to see new trends of attractive faces.
- What is a must is to buy good sharp surgical instruments. Maintenance of osteotomes, scissors and drills and adding new gadgets like Piezo are arts of journey towards excellence. It is essential and you should use the headlight with a loop.
- Good hypotensive anaesthesia is essential, and a good tuning with anaesthetist is very important. If the field is too bloody, then it becomes difficult to do many finer steps; also it affects post-op healing.
- To start with, analyse the pre-operative pictures. Write down the operative plan. Write down the deformity assessing different angles with photographic analysis. Discuss this with the patient and don't hesitate to share it with your teachers and mentor. 3D software is an excellent tool and to be used to calculate different angles.
- Intraoperative videography and photography are not only helpful to publish paper and for presentation, but they are useful in analysing your own surgery. Many times watching your own videos will teach you a lot and will often realise why I am doing this now. You will realise many things by watching your own surgery.
- Post-operative visit every month with patient's actual or virtual consultation is important. For both the patient and doctor, understanding the healing is important. Post-op photo documentation is a must.
- Preoperative judgement, intraoperative findings and post op analysis helps you become a perfectionist.

Books to Read

- ***Fundamentals of Rhinoplasty* by Dr. Rollin Daniel**
- ***Mastering Advanced Rhinoplasty* by Dr. Wolfgang Gubisch**

2 An Overview of the Anthropological Perspective of Indian Noses and Its Implications for Rhinoplasty

Main

In a systematic review, Doddi and Eccles discussed the origin of anthropometric measurements. They have noted that in the seventeenth and eighteenth centuries, anthropologists proposed various systems for classification of human race on the basis of observable characteristics such as skin colour, hair type, body proportions and skull measurements. Detailed measurements of human skulls to categorise race by anthropologists led to the beginning of craniofacial anthropometry.

By the twentieth century, Topinard et al. defined the 'anthropological nasal index' for racial differentiation. Facial proportions evidently vary between races. It has been proposed that the different nasal shapes and sizes were an evolutionary adaptation to the climate, especially the broad noses.

2.1 Effect of Migration

The present-day population of the Indian subcontinent has been derived from six main racial groups as described by Dr. B. S. Guha:

- The Negrito
- The Proto-Australoids
- The Mongoloids
- The Mediterranean or Dravidian
- The Western Brachycephals
- The Nordic

India's population structure is quite complex. Currently, our present population is a result of a very long process of historical immigration which has resulted in diversity of various traits among people of different regions of our country. For the ease of understanding these, racial types can be reduced to three basic types—the Indo-Aryan, the Mongolian and the Dravidian.

The Mongolians and Dravidians account for the racial composition of tribal India.

2.2 Effect of Climate

The geographic subdivisions of India are classified on the basis of similar climatic conditions (Fig. 2.1):

- **North India**: Jammu and Kashmir, Punjab, Haryana, Delhi and Himachal Pradesh
- **Central India**: Uttar Pradesh, Madhya Pradesh, Bihar, Chhattisgarh and Jharkhand
- **South India**: Karnataka, Tamil Nadu, Kerala, Andhra Pradesh and Telangana.
- **Western India**: Rajasthan, Maharashtra and Gujarat
- **North-East Himalayan**: Assam, Arunachal Pradesh, Meghalaya, Manipur, Sikkim, Nagaland, Tripura, Uttarakhand, Leh and Darjeeling

North Indians inhabit a cooler region. So, people here are very light complexed and have

V. Ghaisas, *Indian Ethnic Rhinoplasty*, https://doi.org/10.1007/978-981-16-2478-0_2

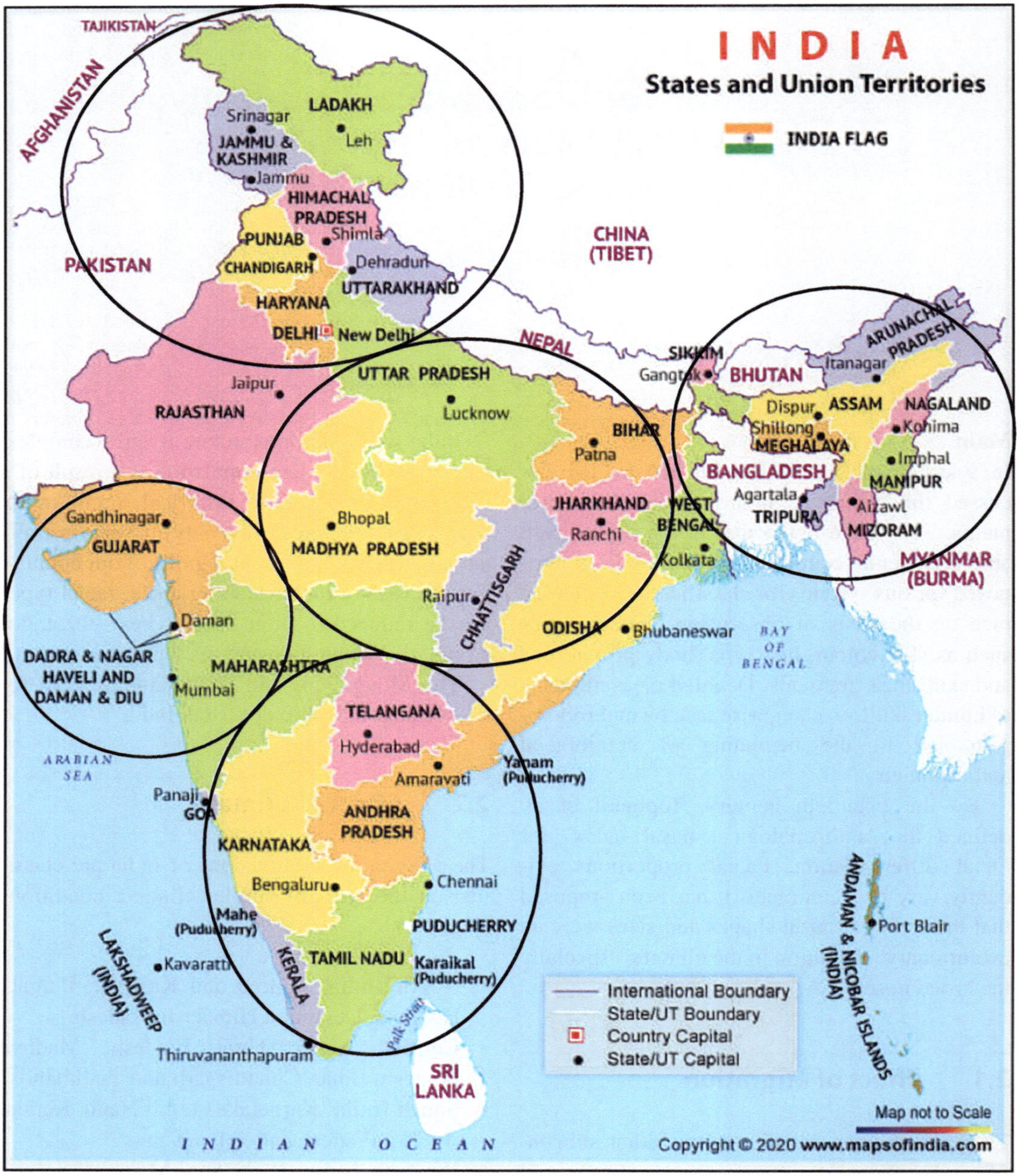

Fig. 2.1 Indian map - regions are circled and categorised north west central north east and south

Caucasoid-Aryan look. Populations inhabiting Central and Western India have a medium to light complexion owing to tropical heat in these regions. South Indians are Dravidians who mostly have thick skin with brown or dark complexion with fewer light complexion thin-skinned individuals. North-East Indians are fair with thin skin and have modified Mongoloid features.

Populations adapted to dry environments tend to have large, protruding external noses, downwardly directed nostrils and narrower skeletal apertures which induce turbulence to nasal airflow, thereby maximising filtration and humidification of air within nasal passages.

Populations living in humid environments have a relatively smaller, flatter external nares, more anteriorly directed nares and shorter pyriform apertures. These structures make the nose better adapted to humid environments.

In one of the largest studies on anthropometric evaluation of Indian noses, Mehta and Srivastava (2017) analysed 1000 noses from 5 regions—North, Central, West, South and the Himalayan regions—to determine differences in nasal variations and regional variations. The study also established that most of the Indian populations have a mesorrhine (asian) nose. Regional differences showed North Indians had the longest nose with Caucasoid features with mean height of 50.48 mm and width of 36.59 mm, whereas South Indians had the broadest nose (width), and those from the Himalayan region had the shortest nose (length). With respect to the substantial regional variations in the architecture, the Indian nose should be considered a different entity as compared to the nose of Caucasian, Oriental and African population.

Indians in general have non-Caucasian nose features—i.e, shorter nasal bones with weaker alar cartilages and lack of a sizeable septal cartilage. This results in a wide dorsum with poor anterior projection (nasofacial angle less than 30 degrees). The pyriform aperture is wide.

The skin is often thick with a prominent subcutaneous fibro-fatty pad. This contributes to a poorly projected tip with lack of definition.

The nasal alae tend to be wider than the intercanthal distance and flared, with more horizontally oriented nostrils.

The premaxillary area is often hypoplastic.

2.3 Interregional Variations of Some Nasal Parameters

1. *Nasal Height* (Fig. 2.2)

Nasal height is described as the length from the nasion (nasal root) to the nasal base (subnasale).

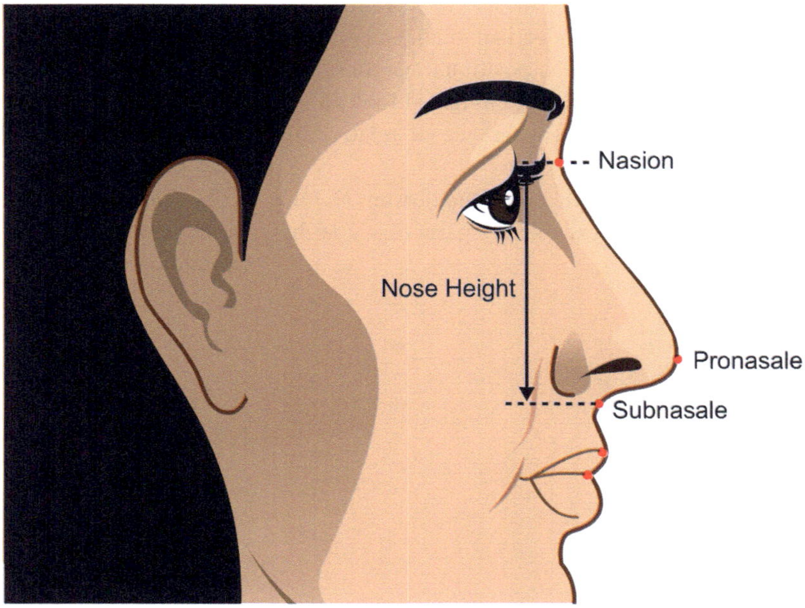

Fig. 2.2 Nasal height—nasion to subnasale

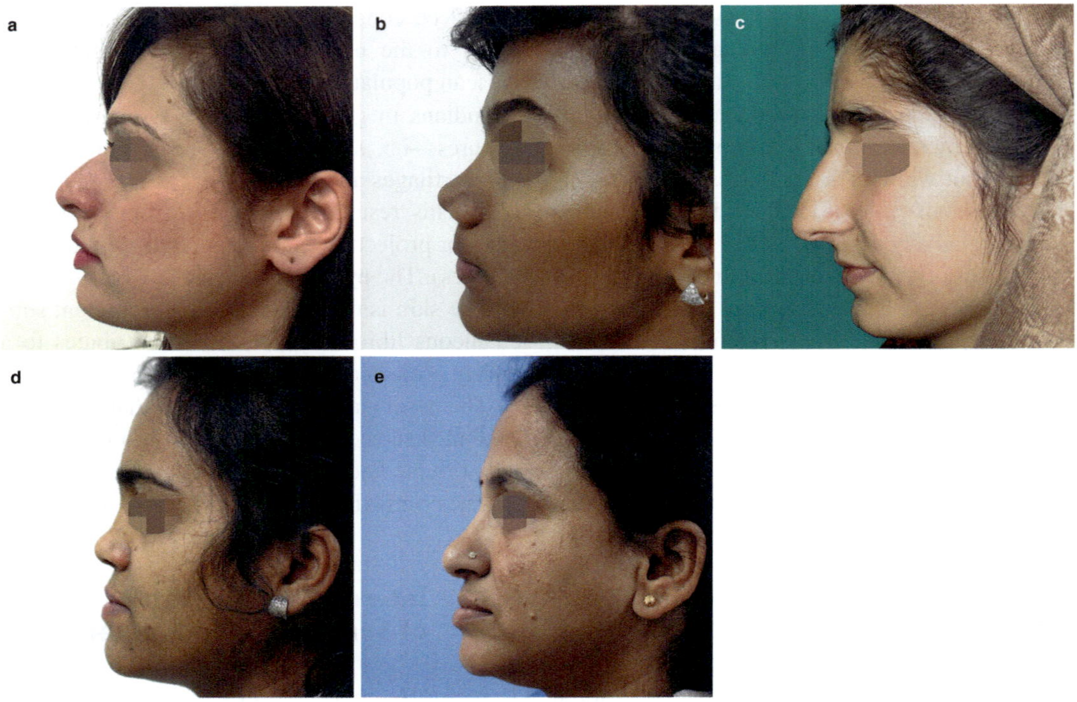

Fig. 2.3 (**a**) Central, (**b**) North-East, (**c**) North, (**d**) South, (**e**) West

The height of the nose is important when assessing the profile of individuals. Although the profile of Indians has varied appearance, the nasal height is almost identical in all. Only dorsal augmentation moves the positional height of the radix upward and gives an elongated look to the nose, and an alleged appearance of relative tip deprojection.

For a better tip projection, the dorsum should not be augmented excessively particularly at the radix (Fig. 2.3a–e).

2. *Nasal Length* (Fig. 2.4)

The nasal length is the length between the soft tissue nasion to pronasale.

Patients from Rajasthan have large external noses. Patients from north-east region have flatter noses with more anteriorly directed nares and shorter nasal apertures (Figs. 2.5, 2.6, 2.7, 2.8 and 2.9).

To lengthen the nasal bridge dimension, dorsal augmentation or tip de-rotation technique is commonly employed in rhinoplasty.

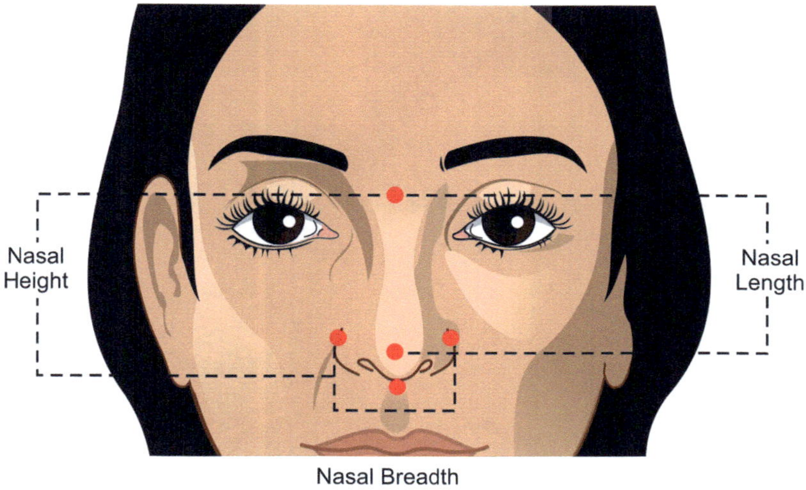

Fig. 2.4 Nasal length—nasion to pronasale

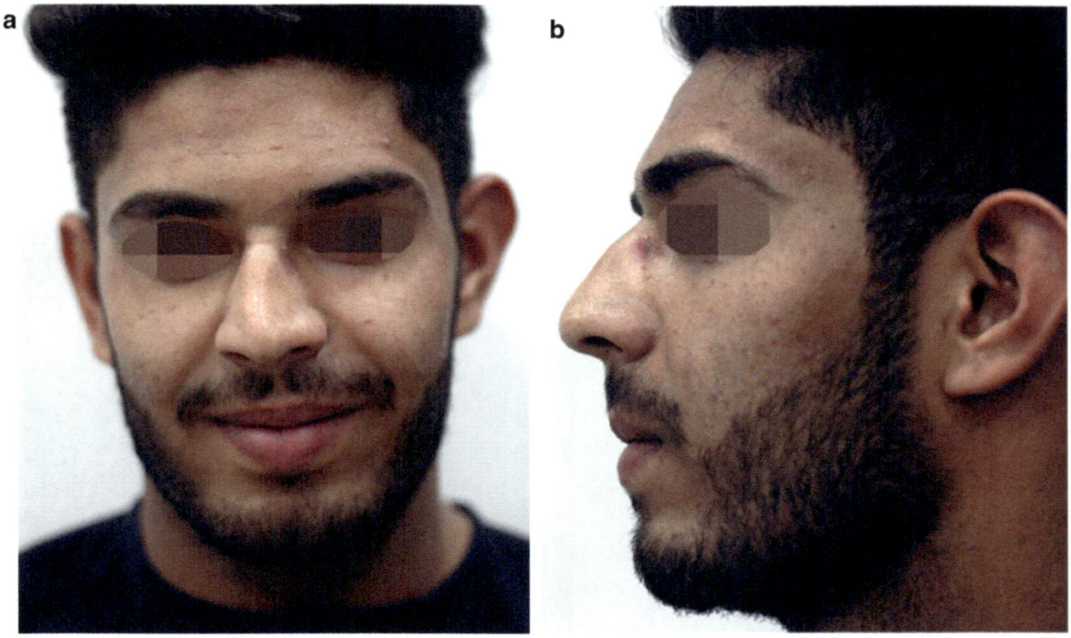

Fig. 2.5 Central

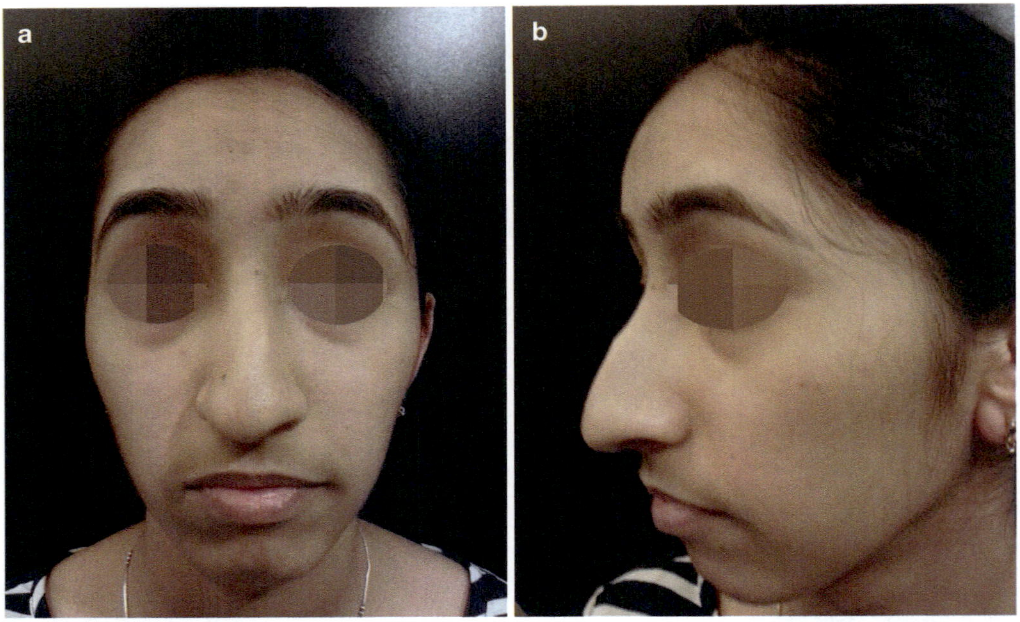

Fig. 2.6 North

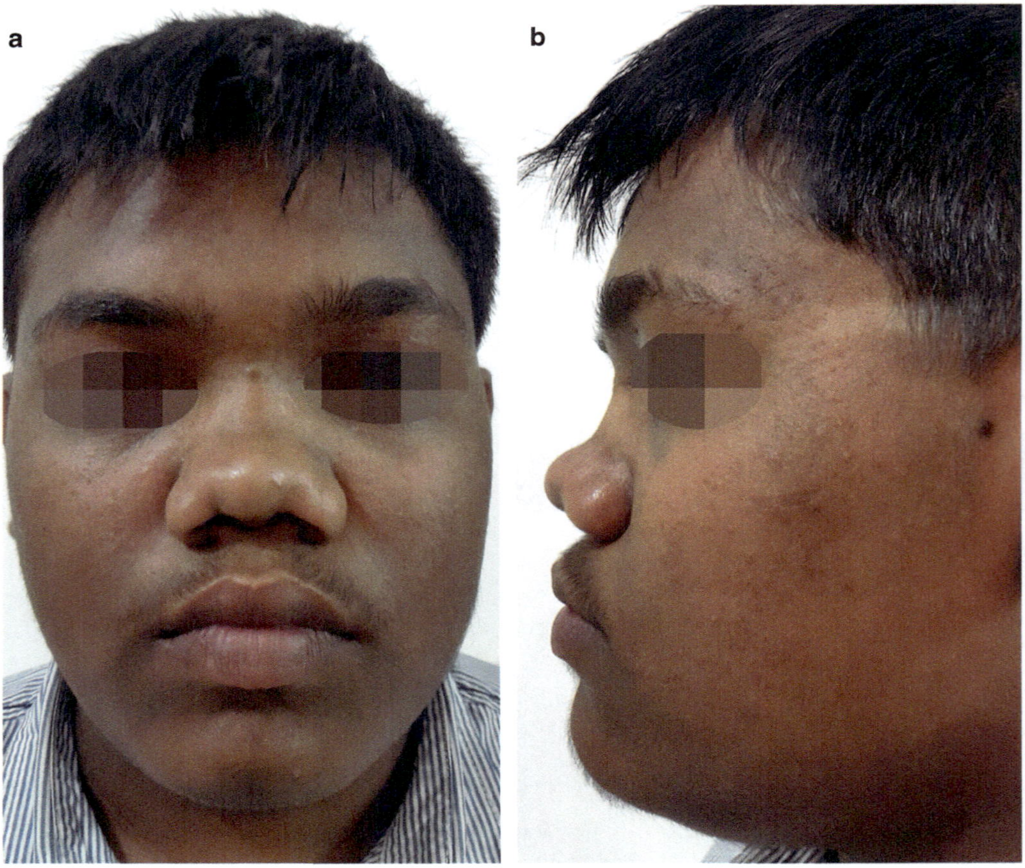

Fig. 2.7 South

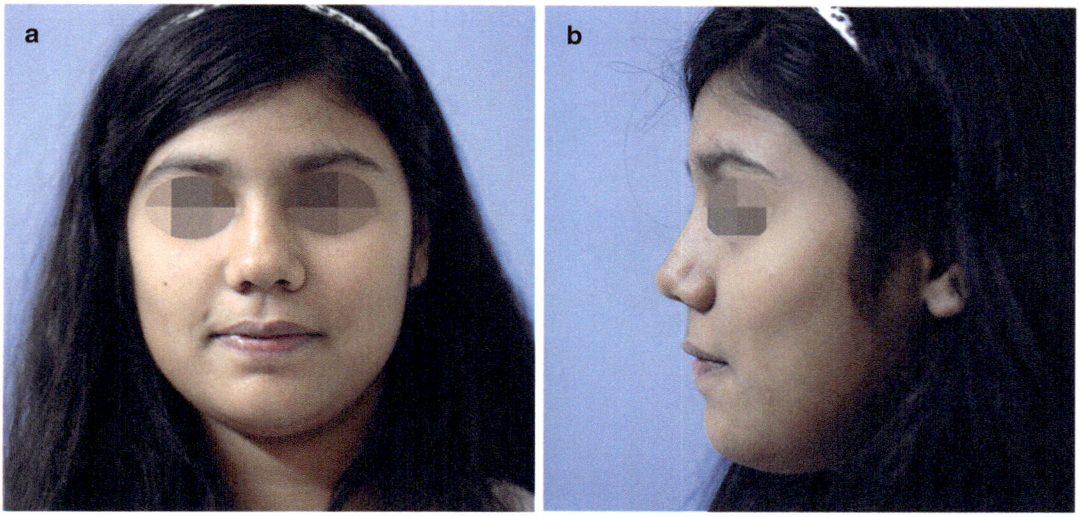

Fig. 2.8 North-East

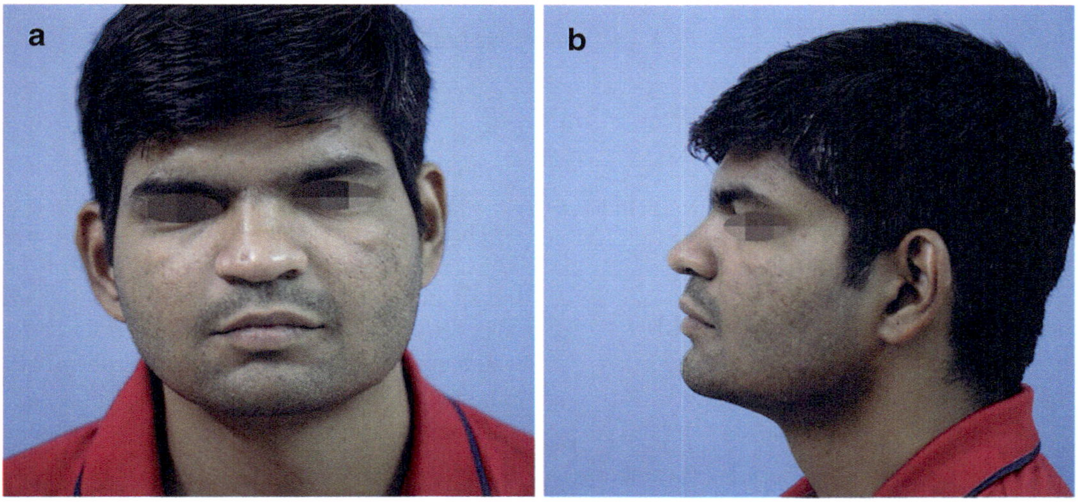

Fig. 2.9 West

3. *Nasal Width* (Fig. 2.10)

The ideal width of the nasal bony vault depends on several factors such as facial width, nasal length, tip sharpness and skin thickness. The Indian feature of a broad face width frequently is due to a wide nasal bony vault. However, it is usually acceptable when the width is two-thirds of the alar base width or two-thirds of the intercanthal distance. Wide nasal bones are not rare among Indian patients belonging to Southern, Western, North-East and Central India. However, it is very uncommon in Northern group of patients. Correction of wide nasal bones is commonly done by using medial and lateral osteotomies to move the nasal bone inwards.

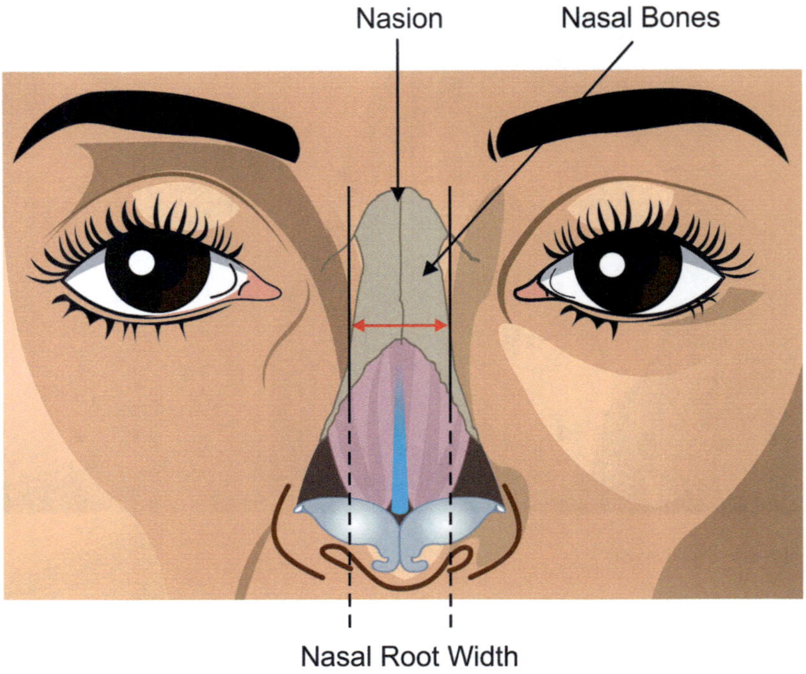

Fig. 2.10 Nasal width

2.4 Nasal Index

The nasal index is the ratio of nasal width to nasal height.

2.4.1 Nasal Index (Doddi et al.)

$$\frac{\text{Width of nose} \times 100}{\text{Height of nose}}$$

It varies greatly among different anthropological groups and in different climate zones. In dry climates, noses often tend to be narrower, whereas in humid climates, noses often are smaller and wider.

A higher index is suggestive of a broad nose, whereas a lower index value is indicative of a narrow nose:

- Nasal index <70—leptorrhine nose—commonly seen in Caucasians
- Nasal index 70–85—mesorrhine nose—commonly seen in Asians
- Nasal index >85—platyrrhine nose—commonly seen in Africans

The mean nasal index of Indian population is 72.81 ± 7.29, thus suggesting that most of the Indian populations have a mesorrhine (asian) nose. North Indians have a leptorrhine nose which equates well with the fact that they have long, narrow noses.

How do all these really influence the operative planning?

- Complete understanding of the patient's concerns and realistic expectations of nasal surgery.
- The goal of maintaining ethnic identity congruent with the patient's facial features.
- Recognising the limitations imposed by ethnic anatomical features and the slightly increased risk of certain complications.
- Morphing the outcome produced by a software can be helpful in grounding patients' expectations.

3 Evaluation of Rhinoplasty Patients

Main

The nose is the most prominent organ of the body which has an important aesthetic and functional significance. When a patient with an intention of changing the shape of the nose visits your OPD, a thorough pre-operative evaluation of the patient is essential.

Physical and psychological changes can either be a positive or negative impact on the patient post-surgery. Patient selection is the most challenging task for the surgeon. Evaluation of physical deformity and psychological framework of the patient, patient's expectation and limitation of our surgical skills are always taken into consideration.

This chapter is a brief overview of some of the important criteria of patient's selection. For a more detailed information on any of these topics, the reader may refer to other sources.

This chapter is broadly discussed under the first and second visits of the patient.

3.1 During Patient's First Visit

3.1.1 Patient's Approach to Surgery

Patient's perception of the defect must be understood. His/her motivation for surgery is an important factor that must be paid attention to. For example, not getting good bridal/groom offers, to impress people in their life, can be an underlying motivation. This will help the surgeon to be cautious of a patient having unrealistic expectations, which can sometimes indicate an underlying psychiatric disturbance. Discussion with their family and friends can help to resolve/understand the patient's perspective better. Clarity must be maintained regarding the patient's expectations of the post-operative results from that of a surgeon. This is very important in revision cases, and adequate time must be spent with the patients and their family members to explain the expected outcomes and possible complications.

3.1.2 Surgeon's Approach to Surgery

It is important that patient's expectation is the same as the projected outcome by the surgeon. Minimal deformities may pose a problem.

After more than nearly few thousand rhinoplasties, with a few failures, the most important aspect before proceeding to the next stage of assessment, I strongly feel, is to know your own limitations and to contemplate one's capability to take up the surgery or if it has to be referred to your teachers. There will be many more opportunities in the future and so, kindly don't hesitate to take guidance of senior experienced rhinoplasty surgeons rather than trying to be too brave in the initial stages of one's career. Performing rhinoplasties is a lifelong learning curve. So when the patient is in the OPD, surgeon must think if they really want to take the patient up for surgery.

V. Ghaisas, *Indian Ethnic Rhinoplasty*, https://doi.org/10.1007/978-981-16-2478-0_3

3.1.3 Examination

3.1.3.1 General Examination

- A person's height is an important factor:

For example, small nose with an upturn tip may not suit tall people.

- Both conchae have to be felt and checked for the availability of cartilage if need be.
- For rib graft harvesting—A lean person will be easier to harvest from.

3.1.3.2 Examination of the Nose

- *Evaluation of the skin*

Most important in Indian patients—

The skin and soft tissue cover of the nose contribute to the overall shape of the nose. Hence, skin pinch test (SPT) is done to assess the thickness of the skin. This is discussed in detail in Chaps. 6 and 9.

- *Osseo-cartilaginous assessment*—whether wide or narrow and if it is a deviated, saddle, hump or irregular deformity.
- Cold spatula test for misting and Cottle's and modified Cottle's test for internal nasal valve obstruction.
- Tip recoil to check if weak or strong.
- Bernoulli's phenomenon for external valve collapse on forceful inspiration and expiration (Figs. 3.1 and 3.2).
- Alar pathology if pinched or flared.
- Columella if retracted, deviated or broadened.
- Vestibule if stenosed or broad.
- Anterior rhinoscopic examination is done with headlight, Thudicum's nasal speculum and nasal endoscope to assess the size of the turbinate—presence/absence of hypertrophy—which may require treatment. If there is presence of allergic rhinitis, *the patient must be informed that rhinoplasty surgery is not going to relieve allergic symptoms.*

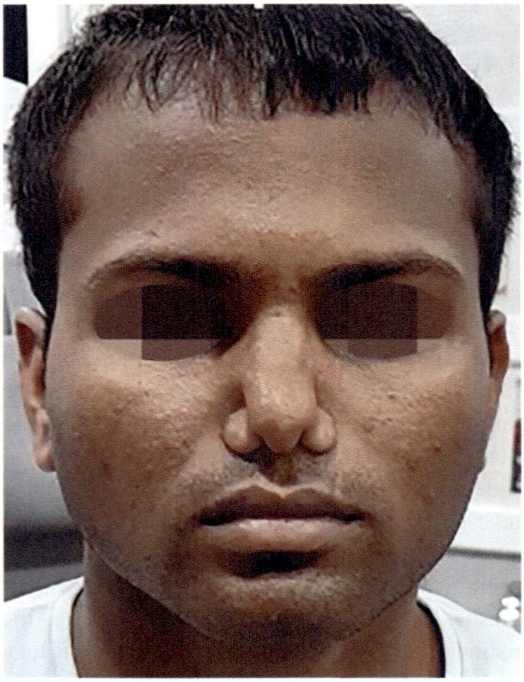

Fig. 3.1 ENV during inspiration

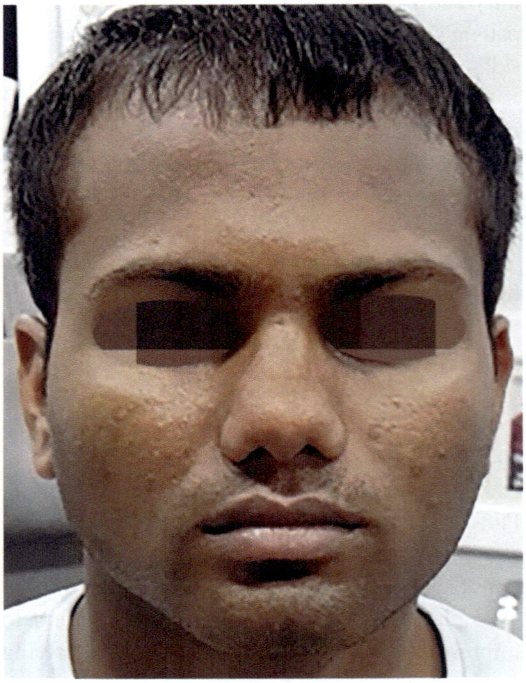

Fig. 3.2 ENV during expiration

3.1.4 Diagnostic Nasal Endoscopy

To rule out any functional aspects, which needs to be tackled simultaneously.

If not done in the OPD, it must be done under anaesthesia, when the patient is taken up for surgery. Also, the adult adenoids if present or not can be ruled out.

3.2 Evaluation During Second Detailed Visit of the Patient

3.2.1 Patients' Expectations

It is mandatory to understand what is patient's perception about their nose and face. Knowing their idea of a *beautiful nose* will help us form a decision. It helps if you ask them to pen down their three needs in their coming visit and check if the expectations are realistic

(three things what patients want to change most commonly,

e.g. flaring of the nose, a broad tip and a low dorsum to narrow nose, sharp tip and higher dorsum, respectively) (Fig. 3.3).

3.2.2 Psychological Assessment

- The following features, if seen during the first visit, should serve as a warning sign, and we have to be cautious while dealing with such patients:
  - **Patient walking alone into the OPD**, without any relatives or friends. This is an important signal as a normal Indian patient generally does not take such a leap to undergo surgery all by themselves. However, patients accompanied by strong-headed attendees also to be dealt carefully with, as satisfying them is a harder task than the patient themselves.
  - Unmarried men.
  - Unrealistic expectations.
  - Minimal deformities.

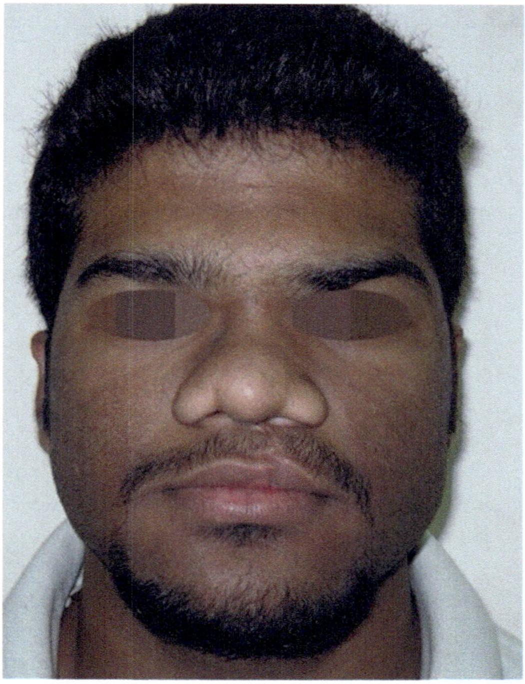

Fig. 3.3 Alar flaring with broad and bulky tip

3.2.2.1 Body Dysmorphic Syndrome

This has been reported in 5% of the patients seeking rhinoplasty. It is usually seen in younger males, who are anxious and excessively worried about their nose. They expect miraculous changes after rhinoplasty. They are always known to blame their nose for their unfortunate difficulties/failures in life. Usually, such patients have a poorer prognosis after rhinoplasty. However, it may be difficult to diagnose this condition and is further compounded by the patient's unwillingness to have a psychiatry referral.

Another point of concern is when a patient begins to praise the doctor unusually. This can be tackled by referring the patient initially to a counsellor. And there should be no hesitation to refer to a counsellor rather than a psychiatrist since psychiatric consultation is still a taboo in India.

In a study by Herrur et al., similar negative predictors of patient satisfaction have been mentioned.

3.2.2.2 Questionnaire

Body Dysmorphic Disorder Questionnaire (BDDQ)

Name____________________________________ Date____________________

This questionnaire asks about concerns with physical appearance. Please read each question carefully and circle the answer that is true for you. Also write in answers where indicated.

1) Are you worried about how you look? Yes No
   - If yes: Do you think about your appearance problems a lot and wish you could think about them less? Yes No
   - If yes: Please list the body areas you don't like:____________________________________

     ____

     ____

Examples of disliked body areas include your skin (e.g. acne, scars, wrinkles, paleness, redness); hair; the shape or size of your nose, mouth, jaw, lips, stomach, hips, etc.; or defects of your hands, genitals, breasts or any other body part.

NOTE: If you answered 'No' to either of the above questions, you are finished with this questionnaire. Otherwise please continue.

2) Is your main concern with how you look that you aren't thin enough or that you might get too fat? Yes No
3) How has this problem with how you look affected your life?
   - Has it often upset you a lot? Yes No
   - Has it often gotten in the way of doing things with friends, dating, your relationships with people or your social activities? Yes No
   - If yes: Describe how:____

     ____
   - Has it caused you any problems with school, work or other activities? Yes No
   - If yes: What are they?____

     ____
   - Are there things you avoid because of how you look? Yes No
   - If yes: What are they?____

     ____
4) On an average day, how much time do you usually spend thinking about how you look? (Add up all the time you spend in total in a day, and then circle one.)

   ______________________ ______________________ ______________________

   (a) Less than 1 hour a day (b) 1–3 hours a day (c) More than 3 hours a day

3.2.3 Background and Ethnicity of the Patient

A rhinoplasty surgeon, especially in specialised rhinoplasty centres and tertiary referral/care centres, many times consults patients from different regions of our country. Patient's background is kept in mind as his/her expectations may differ accordingly. It is often observed that, in metropolitan and larger cities, for higher education, work and career opportunities, internal migration, from different parts of the country, occurs. This thought is always kept in mind. The limitations imposed by ethnic anatomical features should be carefully reviewed and explained to the patient. The goal is to maintain ethnic identity, congruent with the patient's facial features.

3.2.4 Functional Assessment

- A thorough evaluation of the nasal obstruction is done. Unilateral or bilateral and to nasal obstruction caused by the deviated nasal septum per se or by the enlarged turbinates is imperative.
- External nasal valve (ENV) is tested by asking the patient to walk while we observe the ENV at deep inspiration and expiration.
- Associated functional nasal symptoms like polyps, chronic sinusitis, recurrent infections and headache are noted.
- Detailed analysis of the face is done.

3.2.5 Analysis of Facial Aesthetics

The face is divided into three equal horizontal planes (Fig. 3.4). The width of the face is divided into equal fifths. The balance of the midface depends on the equal widths of the key components as shown in Fig. 3.4.

3.2.6 Analysis of the Nose

The mobile part of the external nose consists of the skin and cartilage.

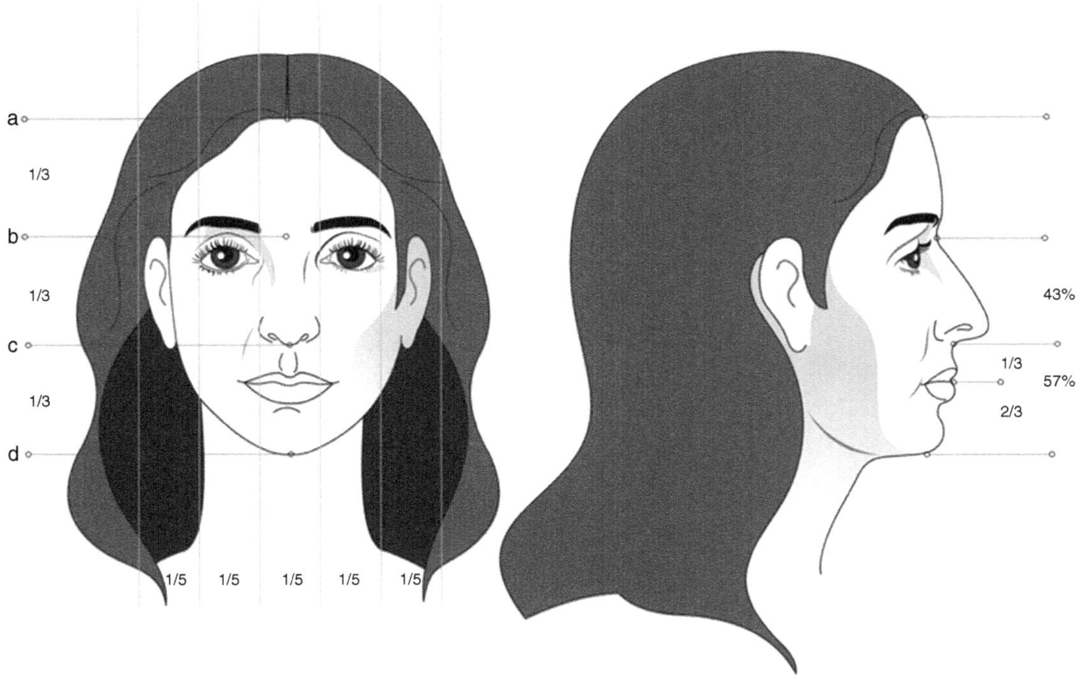

Fig. 3.4 Divisions of the face

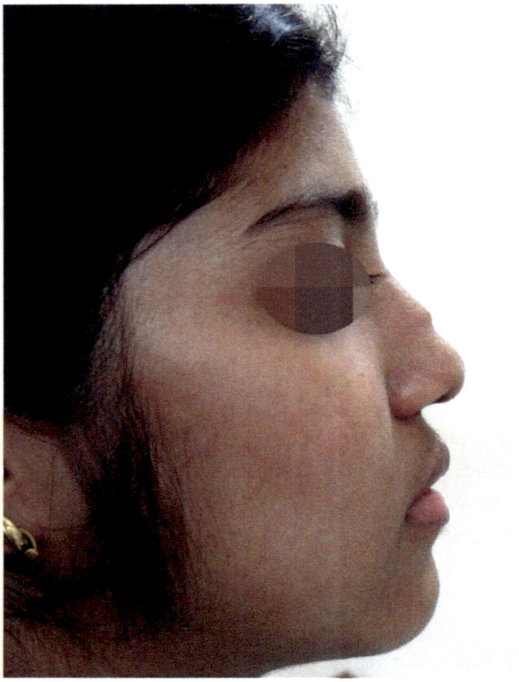

Fig. 3.5 Thin skin

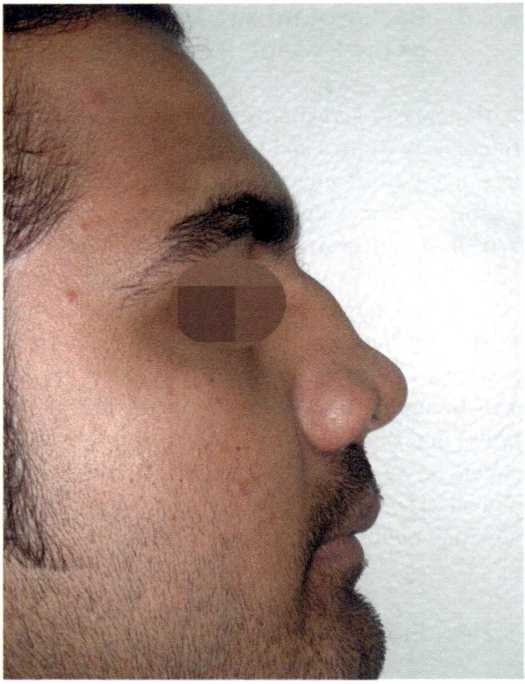

Fig. 3.6 Thick skin

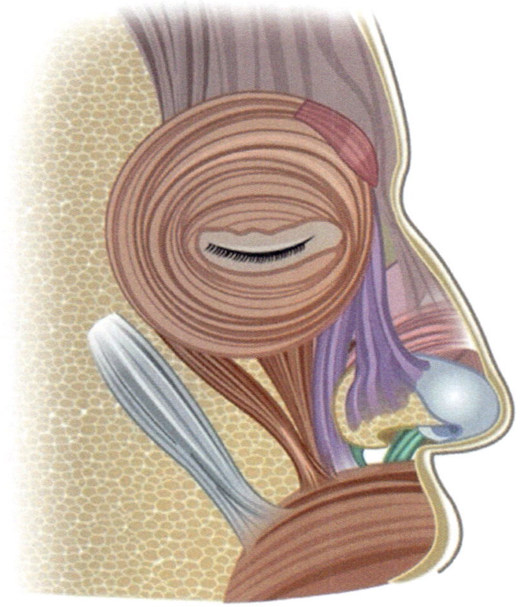

Fig. 3.7 (Ref from Scott & Brown 7th edition)—green-coloured muscle—depressor septi nasi also known as depressor septi, important in rhinoplasty surgery

- *Skin* (Figs. 3.5 and 3.6)

In Indians, a geographic/regional difference has been noted in the skin of the nasal dorsum. This has an important implication in the results of rhinoplasty.

Special importance is given for the type of skin in tertiary care and specialised centres since patients come for rhinoplasty from different areas of the country.

A quick analysis of the skin to know the texture, hydration, evenness, if free from disease and tolerance to sun/oil is important. A thorough examination to understand the skin thickness and the fibro-fatty tissue underneath is done by skin pinch test. Skin texture, quality and the nature of the subcutaneous fibro-fatty show variance across our country. Patients from northern region have thin skin and from the south have thick skin.

- *Muscles* (Fig. 3.7)

The muscles of facial expression take origin from the underlying bone. Many of them are

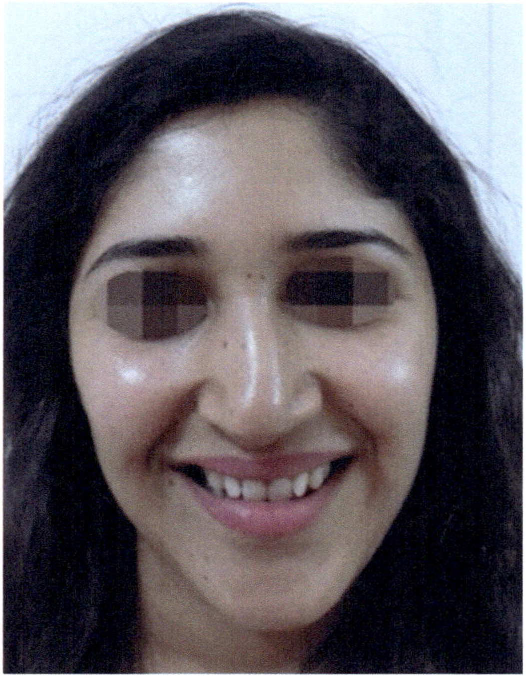

Fig. 3.8 Depressor septi muscle

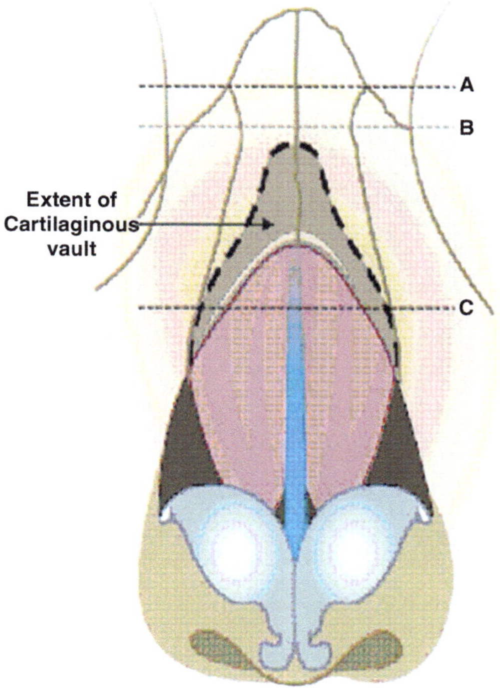

Fig. 3.9 Osseo-cartilaginous framework of the nose—The cartilaginous framework is formed by septal cartilage, two upper nasal cartilages and two lower alar cartilages. The bony nasal framework is formed by the nasal bones, ascending process of maxilla and nasal process of frontal bones. The skin is adherent to the cartilages, but mobile over the bones

named according to their actions, and actions of others may be inferred from their positions.

Depressor septi is an important muscle in rhinoplasty (Fig. 3.8)

An active depressor septi muscle can accentuate a drooping nasal tip while one smiles or speaks and shortens the upper lip on animation. The release and transposition can improve the tip-upper lip relationship in dynamic function.

- *Osseo-cartilaginous vault* (Fig. 3.9)

3.2.6.1 Pre-operative Clinical Correlation

1. *Bony pyramid* (Figs. 3.10 and 3.11)
    - Symmetry—if present or not.
    - Shape in relation to the entire nose.
    - Size of the bony pyramid noted in relation to cartilaginous part.
- Nasofrontal angle is calculated.
- Normal is around 130 degrees.

2. *Cartilaginous framework* (Figs. 3.12 and 3.13)

To look for any of the following deformities and document in detail:

- Saddle deformity
- Hump deformity
- Deviation
- Irregularities on the dorsum

3. *Nasal tip* (Figs. 3.14 and 3.15)

The tip of the nose is the apex of the nose. This part of the nasal anatomy needs a lot of attention, during pre-operative evaluation of the

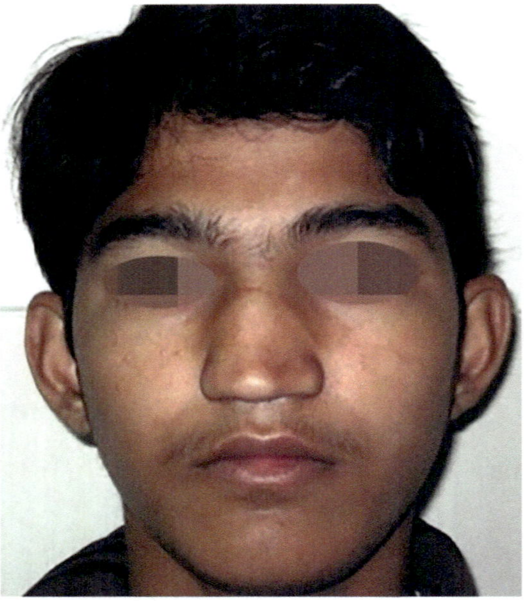

Fig. 3.10 Wide bony dorsum with nasal bones asymmetrical

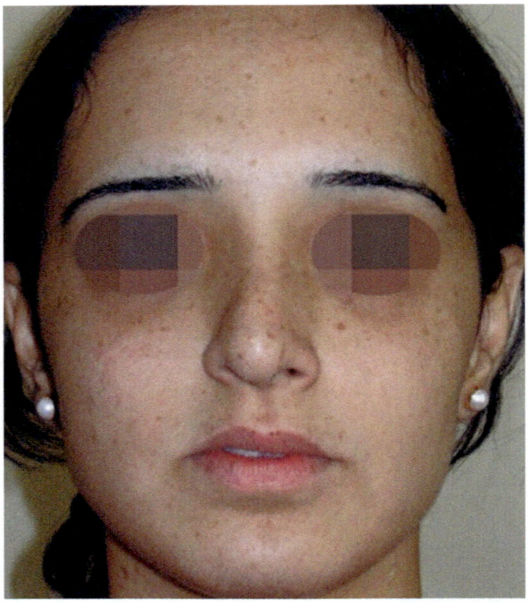

Fig. 3.11 Narrow bony dorsum

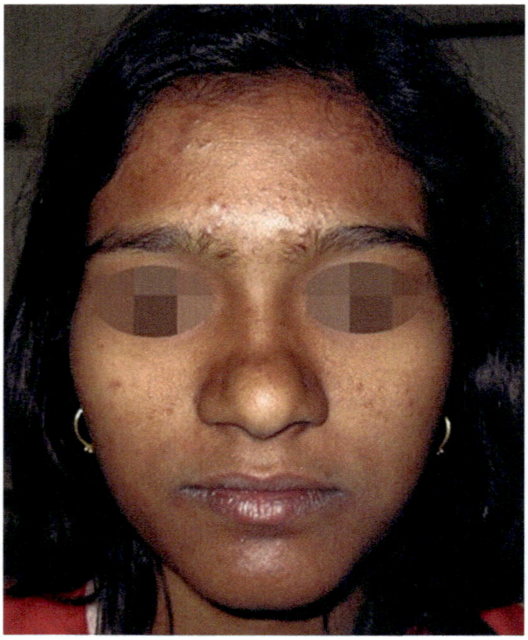

Fig. 3.12 Saddle deformity with narrow dorsum

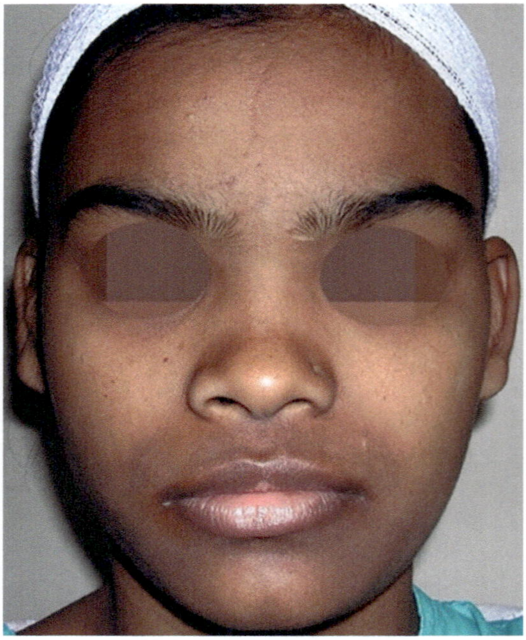

Fig. 3.13 Saddle deformity with wide dorsum

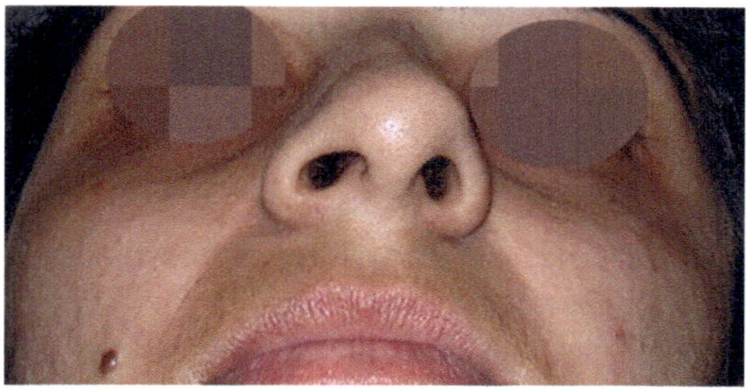

Fig. 3.14 Bulbous tip with deviation to the left

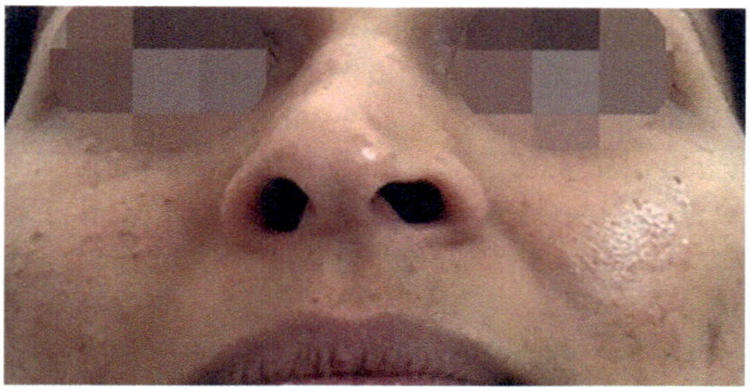

Fig. 3.15 Left alar collapse

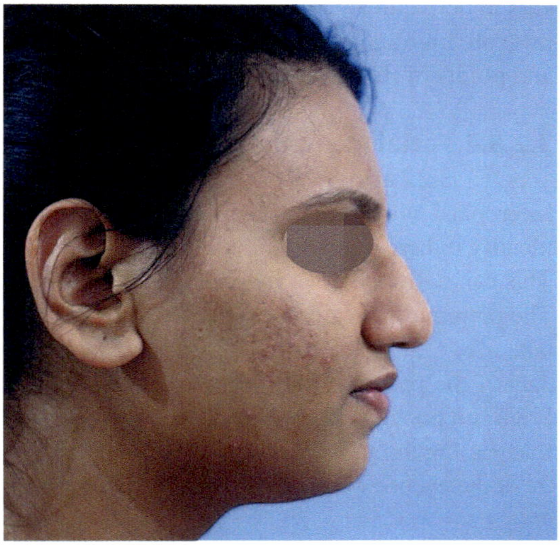

Fig. 3.16 Lateral view for pre-operative measurements

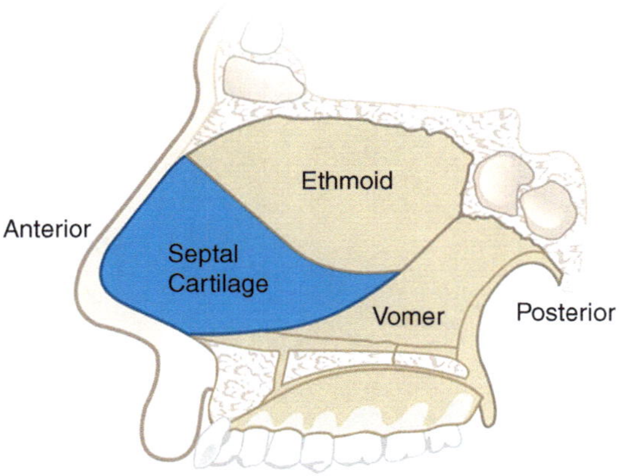

Fig. 3.17 Medial wall of nasal cavity—nasal septum

patient of rhinoplasty. (Details of the tip will be discussed in the Chap. 9.)

4. *Pre-operative facial measurements* (Fig. 3.16)

- Nasofrontal angle:

Indian patients prefer to have deep nasofrontal angle.

- Dorsum—if smooth or irregular.
- Projection—overprojected or underprojected.
- Rotation—uprotated or downrotated tip.
- Nasolabial angle.
- Columellar show—is the gap between the columella and the nostril edge. This is seen in alar insufficiency or if the septum is protruding outwards.

Angles in Indian noses:

- Nasofacial angle is 30–40 degrees.
- Nasolabial is 90–95 in M and 100–110 in F.
- Nasofrontal is 130 degrees.

5. *Nasal septum* (Fig. 3.17)

This is formed by the bony and cartilaginous framework with a small caudal membranous part forming columella.

Deviation—type of deviation and caudal location to be noted.

Ant. nasal spine palpation and if it is in the centre or dislocated is checked.

Probing of the septum to know the available cartilage is sufficient—can be correlated with CT scan of PNS asked.

3.2.6.2 Internal Nasal Valve (Fig. 3.18)

It's a triangular area with a cross-sectional area of 50–70 mm^2. It is formed by the lower margin of triangular cartilage, head of inferior turbinate, septum. It is defined as the narrowest portion of the human airway. This accounts for almost two-thirds of the total nasal airway resistance, and hence collapse or stenosis of this area is thought to be one of the common causes of nasal obstruction.

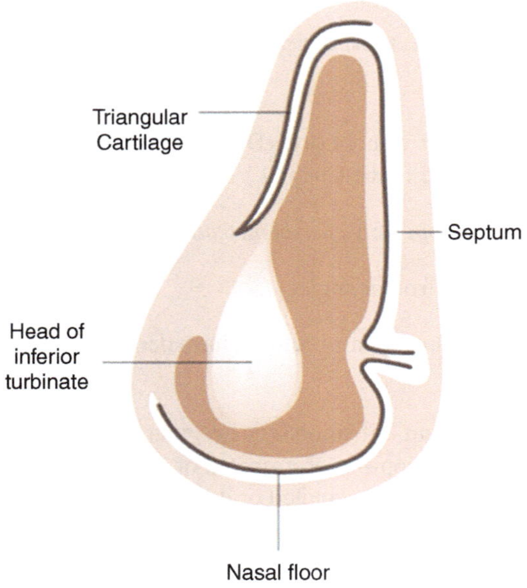

Fig. 3.18 Internal nasal valve

3.2.6.3 Analysis of Artistic or Aesthetic Beauty of the Face

Dorsal lines and tip-defining points (Figs. 3.19 and 3.20)

With simple classic quarter-lighting arrangement, in the front view the diverging lines from radix to tip which depicts the smooth even dorsum underneath and the tip-defining points on the nose are highlighted which are the aesthetic lines and points of the nose.

3.2.6.4 Facial Asymmetry (Figs. 3.21, 3.22 and 3.23)

In crooked nose rhinoplasty, it is very crucial to identify if there is any significant facial asymmetry. This can easily be done by photographic analysis. The prerequisite is a proper front view photograph taken from a minimum of 5 ft distance with both ears of the patient equally seen on the sides, in a Frankfurt horizontal plane. Then, a straight vertical line passing through the midpoint between the centre of the eyebrows is drawn vertically downwards,

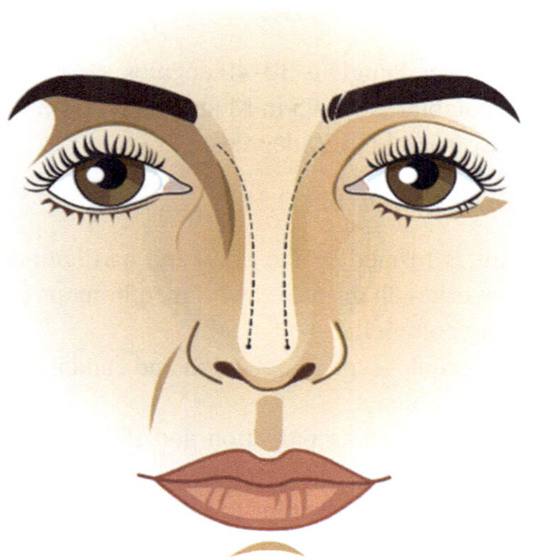

Fig. 3.19 Dorsal aesthetic lines and tip-defining points

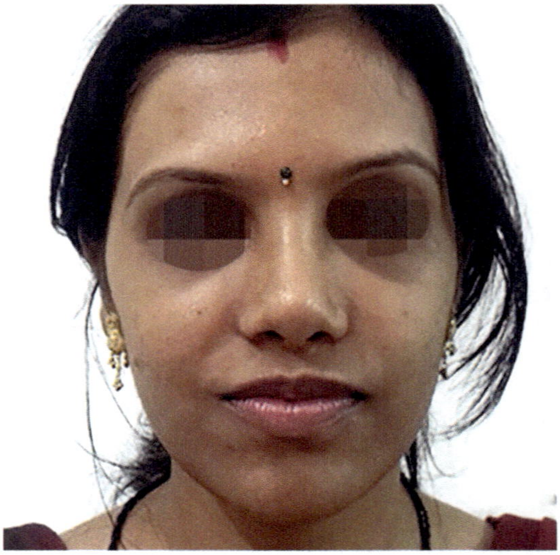

Fig. 3.20 Corresponding picture showing dorsal aesthetic lines and tip-defining points

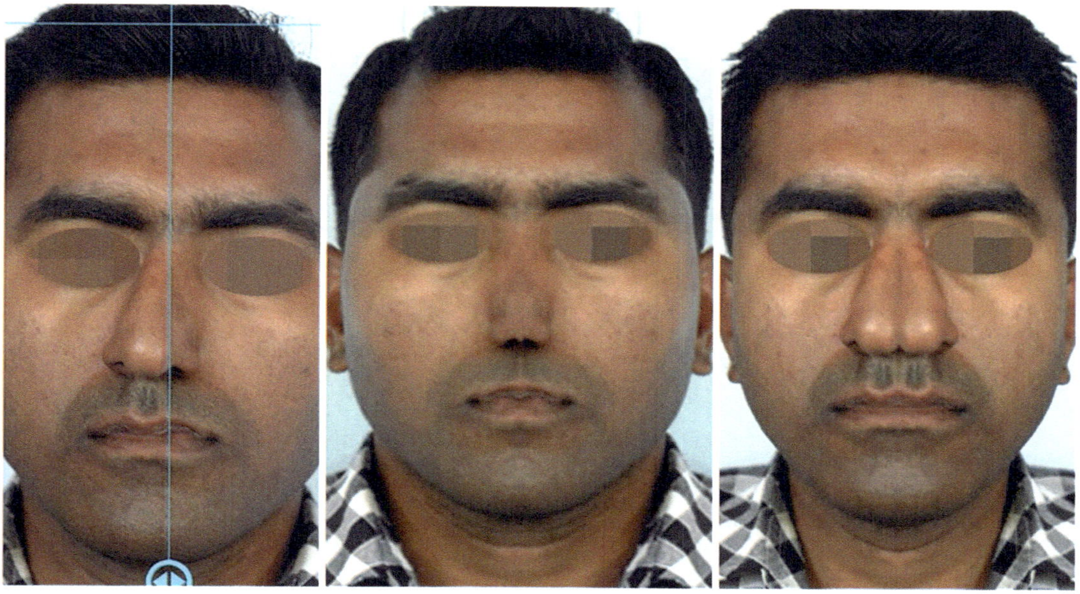

Figs. 3.21–3.23 (left: Fig. 3.21): Vertical line drawn through the centre of the forehead doesn't pass through the centre of the philtrum; (middle: Fig. 3.22): Duplicating the left side of the face; (right: Fig. 3.23): Duplicating the right side of the face

and the surgeon should note if it passes through the centre of the philtrum. If it does, then the face is symmetrical, and if doesn't, then there is a definite facial asymmetry. Asymmetry, if any, should be brought to notice of patient, and guarded prognosis should be given in such cases of facial asymmetry. In cases of facial asymmetry, the nose should be aligned straight from the root of the nose to camouflage the deformity maximally.

3.2.6.5 Photography

Photographic documentation is of vital importance, not only for records but also as an aid to a surgeon's learning process. Digital library is maintained for photographs of the patients.

Camera

My choice is a Canon camera with macro lens.

In a mobile phone camera, clarity is not satisfactory according to my opinion.

Camera with HDR in mobile camera is not equally good but acceptable.

And selfie mode should be avoided since it causes camera fisheye effect.

Patient's photographs are taken in five views. These are frontal, lateral, basal, oblique and eagle's view. The nose in dynamic state has to be noted and documented with photographs if present, that is, the patient's nose is examined while smiling.

- Frontal view (Figs. 3.24 and 3.25)—both ears to be equally visualised
- Lateral view (Figs. 3.26 and 3.27)—opposite eyelashes not to be seen
- Basal view (Figs. 3.28 and 3.29)—nasal tip is in between both the medial canthi
- Oblique view (Figs. 3.30 and 3.31)—45-degree view
- Bird's view—from above (Fig. 3.32)

3.2.6.6 Medical Photography (Figs. 3.33, 3.34, 3.35, 3.36 and 3.37)

3.2.6.7 Rhinomanometry (Fig. 3.38)

Four-phase rhinomanometry helps to evaluate and deduce the underlying nasal disorder such as turbinate hypertrophy, deviated nasal septum and more. Active rhinomanometry is done at our centre, and the nasal obstruction is documented through a graph plotted against airflow and pressure. (This will be explained in detail in Chap. 5.)

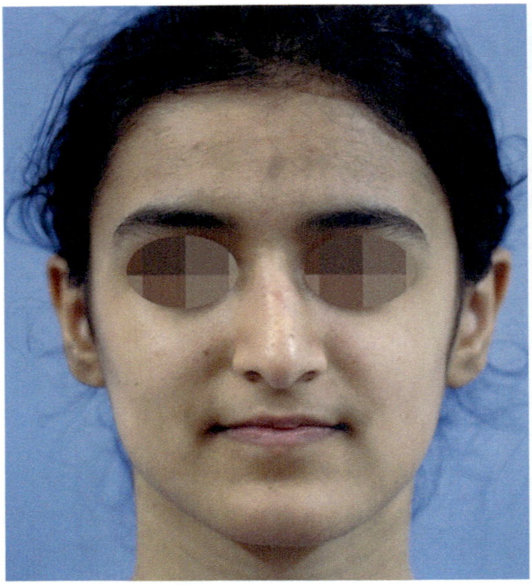

Fig. 3.24 Frontal view

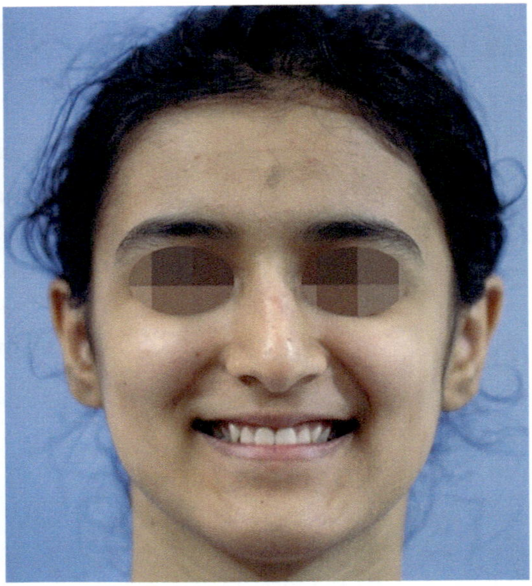

Fig. 3.25 Frontal view with a smile

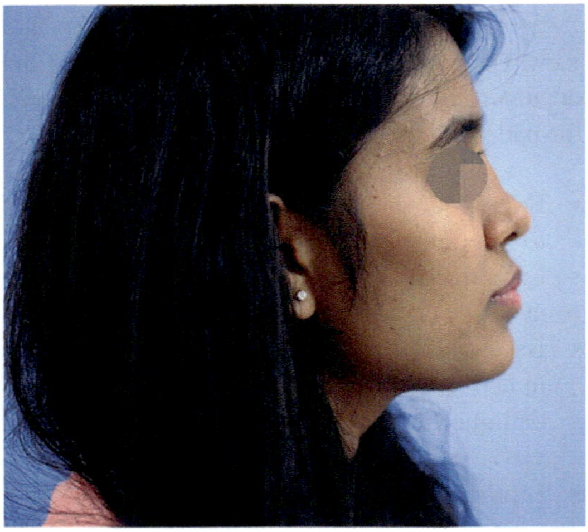

Fig. 3.26 Right lateral view

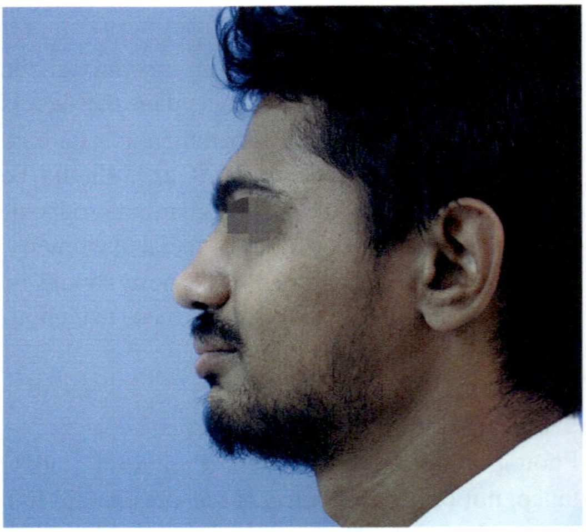

Fig. 3.27 Left lateral view

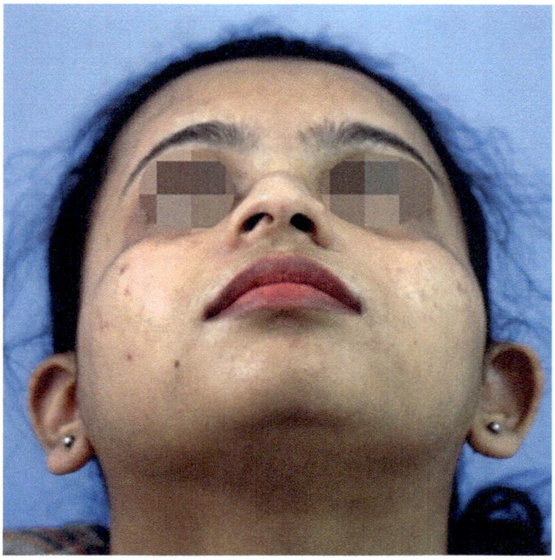

Fig. 3.28 Basal view

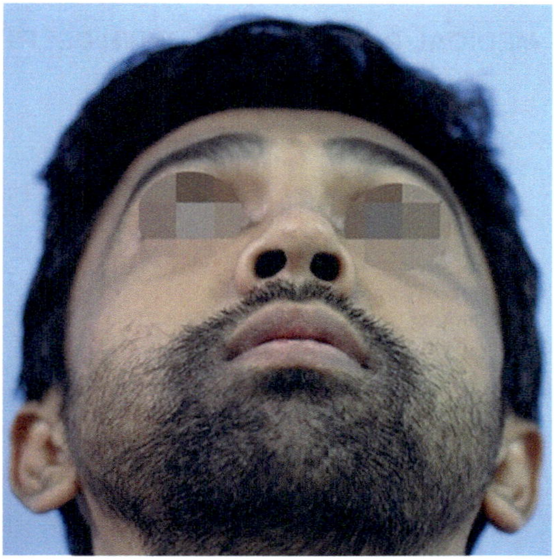

Fig. 3.29 Basal view

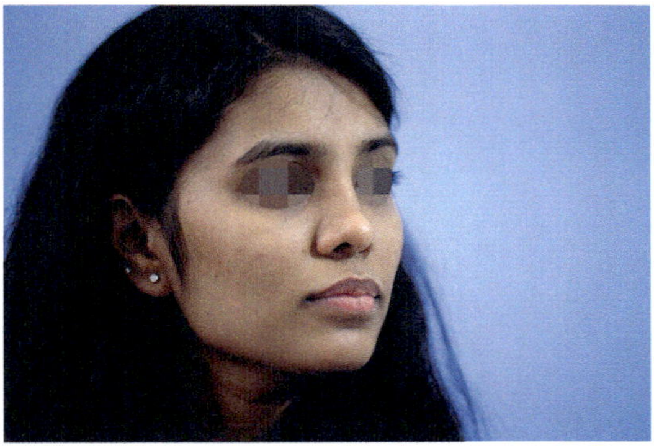

Fig. 3.30 Oblique view

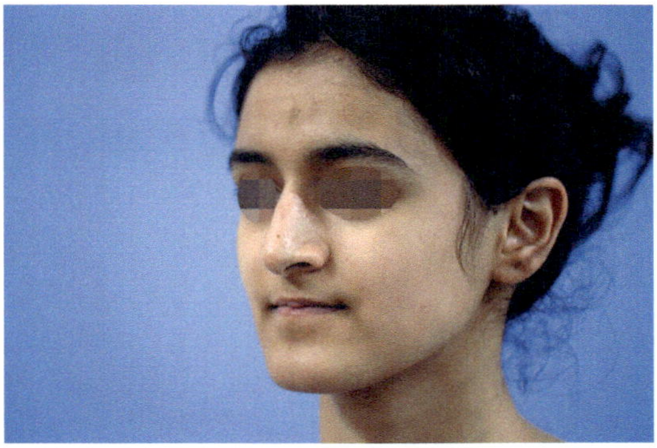

Fig. 3.31 Oblique view

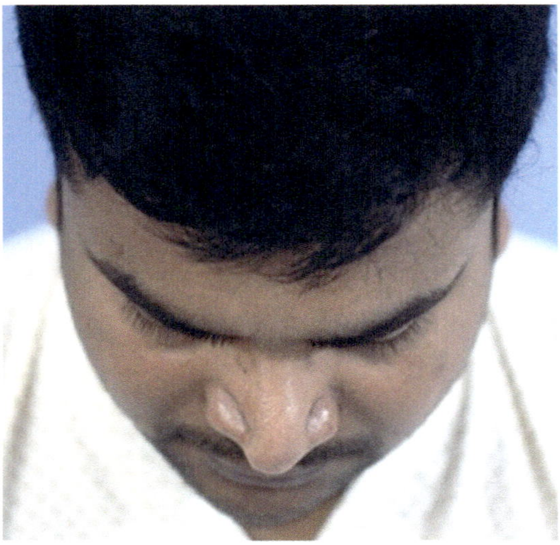

Fig. 3.32 Bird's view

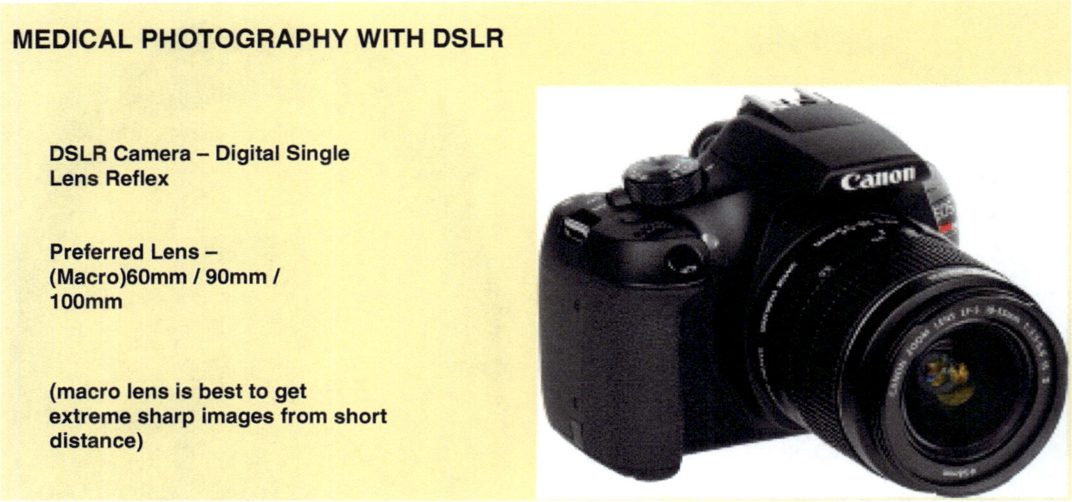

Fig. 3.33 DSLR

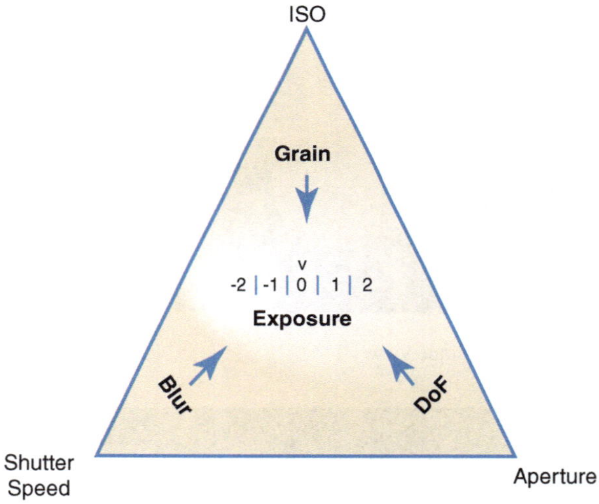

Fig. 3.34 Details of camera settings

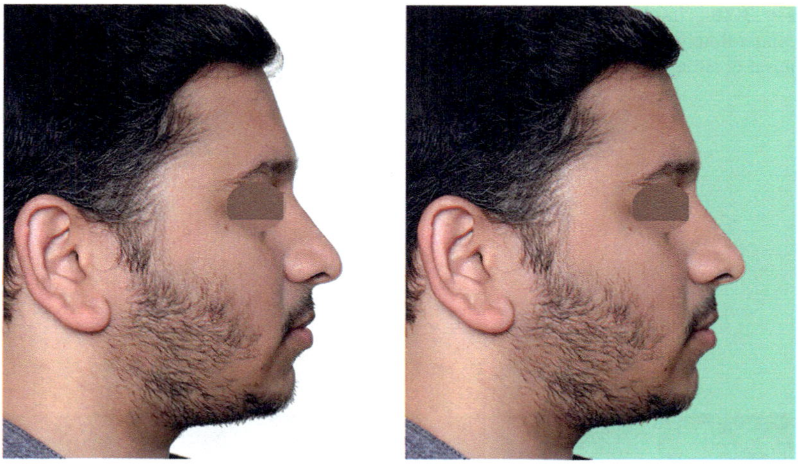

Fig. 3.35 Precautions to be taken during photography

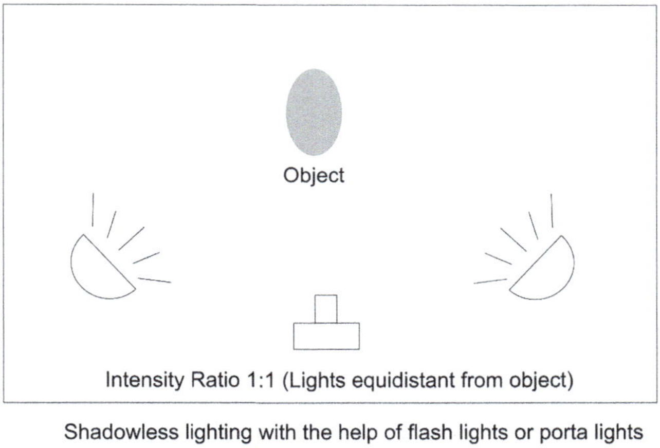

Fig. 3.36 Lighting setup

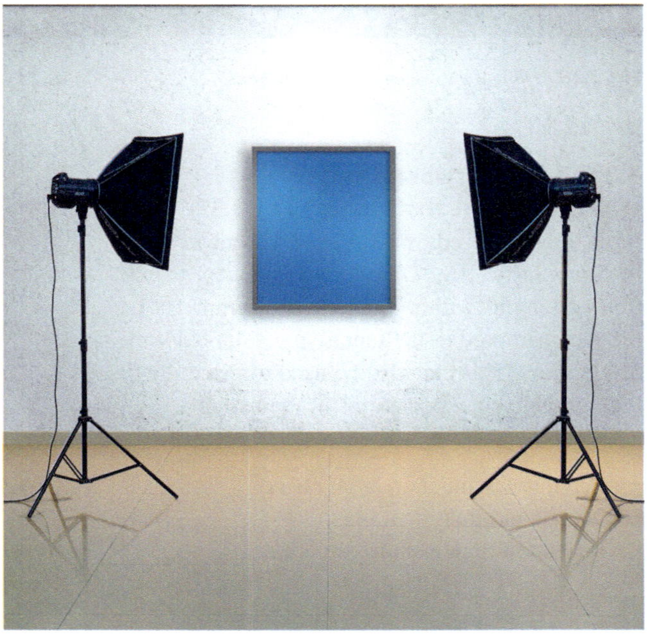

Fig. 3.37 Photography: background and lighting setup

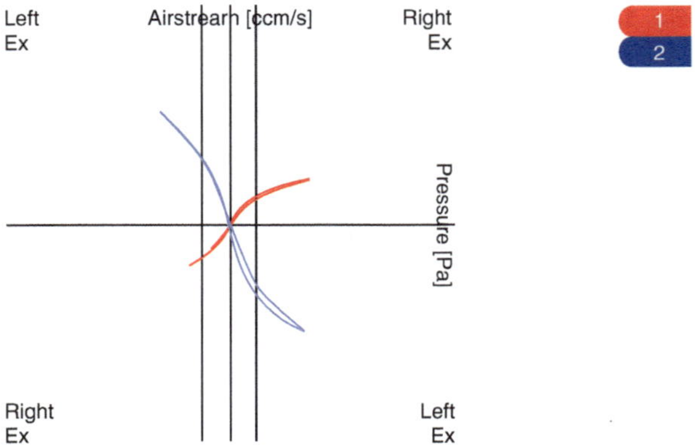

Fig. 3.38 Graph of rhinomanometry—bilateral non-sloping curves indicating no nasal obstruction

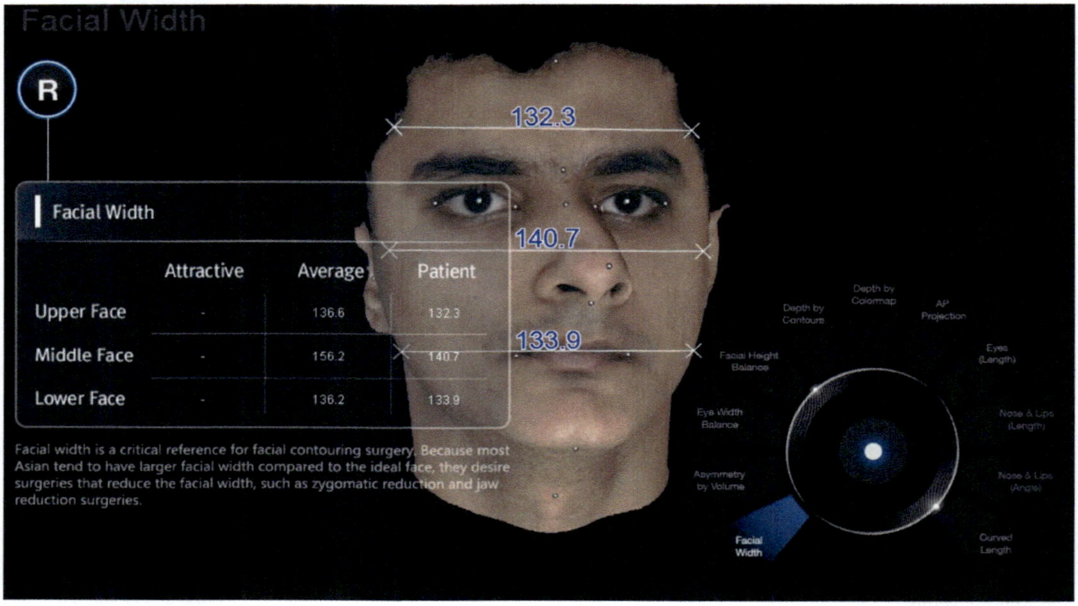

Fig. 3.39 3D software scanning and analysis

3.2.6.8 3D Software Analysis and Reconstruction (Fig. 3.39)

It is a double-edged weapon and is recent advance in rhinoplasty. By 3D software analysis, valuation of length, width, angles and asymmetry of the face can predict the tentative results but with disclaimers. This can also be used to grind down high unrealistic expectations of the patients.

3D facial imaging system is for:

- Facial assessment and diagnosis
- Design and treatment planning
- Treatment review and evaluation

Plan of action is further discussed and the need for grafts from different sites is explained. Discussing pre- and post-operative photographs of other patients related to their deformity improves the rapport and their confidence.

Routine pre-operative haematological tests and CT scan of paranasal sinus are advised. The patients are asked to review with the reports along with their family.

It is important to meet the family as they can talk about psychological aspects of the patient and how concerned is the patient about his deformity.

CT PNS
Two important views are coronal and axial. It is also helpful to rule out sinusitis and to check for the status of the adenoids.

It is helpful to confirm the position of ANS.

In sagittal view, the skin thickness can be measured.

Also in 3D configuration, nasal bones can be studied.

In a 0.5 mm thickness cut, the cartilage can also be studied in detail.

CT of the Thorax
CT of the thorax is done in young females of 18–20 years of age group if rib graft is considered. This helps in ruling out calcification of the rib as it may pose a difficulty in graft harvesting.

Also, it helps if patient has a history of smoking, to rule out lung pathology and of course to rule out our pandemic disease COVID-19.

Chest X-ray
For preanaesthetic check-up

DETAILED CONSENT

GHAISAS ENT HOSPITAL
Govind 1248-B Deccan Gymkhana,
Pune 411004
PMC/LCBP/0506/01279

Name of patient: .... Age: ...... Sex: ......
Reg No.:..................Address:
....

Diagnosis: Crooked nose deformity/saddle nose deformity/hump nose/.................

Operation title: Septorhinoplasty primary/revision

I, ...the undersigned give consent for my own operation.

The following procedure will be performed:
Surgery of the nose (rhinoplasty) is an operation frequently performed by surgeons. This surgical procedure can produce changes in the appearance, structure and function of the nose. Rhinoplasty can reduce or increase the size of the nose, change the shape of the tip, narrow the width of the nostrils or change the angle between the nose and the upper lip. This operation can help correct birth defects and nasal injuries and help relieve breathing problems.

There is not a universal type of rhinoplasty surgery that will meet the needs of every patient. Rhinoplasty surgery is customised for each patient, depending on his or her needs. Incisions may be made within the nose or concealed in inconspicuous locations of the nose in the open rhinoplasty procedure. Internal nasal surgery to improve nasal breathing can be performed at the time of the rhinoplasty.

Grafts used during the surgery to augment (increase) or reshape the nose shall be taken from the patient's own body so as to avoid the possibility of rejection of graft material.

Conchal cartilage (ear bowl cartilage) removal as graft material rarely can give rise to mild to moderate deformity of the ear shape/bleeding and swelling at the site of removal. Incision taken is inconspicuous and placed behind the ear. This in no way interferes with the hearing capacity neither has any bearing on the function of the ear.

Rib cartilage harvesting is done for revision or severely deformed or as per the preference in individual case. Harvesting is done from the chest wall which leaves an obvious scar and can have considerable post-operative pain/relieved by medication. It rarely can cause injury to underlying structures which may need additional hospitalisation.

The best candidates for this type of surgery are individuals who are looking for improvement, not perfection, in the appearance of their nose. In addition to realistic expectations, good health and psychological stability are important qualities for a patient considering rhinoplasty surgery. Rhinoplasty can be performed in conjunction with other surgeries.

The expected outcome and likelihood of success is:
Good/fair/poor……..

Risks of the procedure: There are risks and complications with this procedure. They include but are not limited to the following.
General risks:

- Bleeding could occur and may require a return to the operating room. (Is the patient on blood-thinning drugs such as warfarin, aspirin, clopidogrel or dipyridamole?)
- Infection can occur, requiring antibiotics and further treatment.
- Small areas of the lung can collapse, increasing the risk of chest infection. This may need antibiotics and physiotherapy.
- Increased risk in obese people of wound infection, chest infection, heart and lung complications and deep vein thrombosis (DVT).
- Cardiac arrest and death as a result of this procedure.

Specific risks:

- With any type of activity, there is inherent risk. An individual's choice to undergo a surgical procedure is based on the comparison of the risk to potential benefit. Although the majority of patients do not experience these complications, you should discuss each of them with your surgeon to make sure you understand the risks, potential complications and consequences of rhinoplasty.

Bleeding—It is possible, though unusual, that you may have problem with bleeding during or after surgery. Should post-operative bleeding occur, it may require emergency treatment to stop the bleeding, or require a blood transfusion. Do not take any aspirin or anti-inflammatory medications for 10 days before surgery, as this contributes to a greater risk of bleeding. Hypertension (high blood pressure) that is not under good medical control may cause bleeding during or after surgery. Accumulations of blood under the skin may delay healing and cause scarring

Infection—Infection is quite unusual after surgery. Should an infection occur, additional treatment including oral or intravenous antibiotics might be necessary.

Scarring—Although good wound healing after a surgical procedure is expected, abnormal scars may occur both within the skin and the deeper tissues. Scars may be unattractive and of different color than the surrounding skin. There is the possibility of visible marks from sutures. Additional treatments including surgery may be needed to treat scarring.

Damage to deeper structures—Deeper structures such as nerves, tear ducts, blood vessels and muscles may be damaged during the course of surgery. The potential for this to occur varies with the type of rhinoplasty procedure performed. Injury to deeper structures may be temporary or permanent.

Unsatisfactory result—There is the possibility of an unsatisfactory result from the rhinoplasty surgery. The surgery may result in unacceptable visible or tactile deformities, loss of function or structural malposition after rhinoplasty surgery. You may be disappointed that the results of rhinoplasty surgery do not meet your expectations. **Additional surgery may be necessary should the result of rhinoplasty resolve after rhinoplasty.**

Numbness—There is the potential for permanent numbness within the nasal skin after rhinoplasty. The occurrence of this is not predictable. Diminished sensation (or loss of skin sensation) in the nasal area may not totally resolve rhinoplasty.

Asymmetry—The human face is normally asymmetrical. There can be a variation from one side to the other in the results obtained from a rhinoplasty procedure.

Chronic pain—Chronic pain may occur very infrequently after rhinoplasty.

Skin disorders/skin cancer—Rhinoplasty is a surgical procedure to reshape both internal and external structures of the nose. Skin disorders and skin cancer may occur independently of a rhinoplasty.

Allergic reactions—In rare cases, local allergies to tape, suture material or topical preparations have been reported. Systemic reactions, which are more serious, may occur to drugs used during surgery and prescription medicines. Allergic reactions may require additional treatment.

Delayed healing—Wound disruption or delayed wound healing is possible. Some areas of the face may not heal normally and may take a long time to heal. Areas of the skin may die. This may require frequent dressing changes or further surgery to remove the non-healed tissue.

Long-term effects—Subsequent alterations in nasal appearance may occur as the result of aging, sun exposure or other circumstances not related to rhinoplasty surgery. Future surgery or other treatments may be necessary to maintain the results of a rhinoplasty operation.

Nasal septal perforation—There is the possibility that surgery will cause hole in the nasal septum to develop. This occurrence is rare. However, if it occurs, additional surgical treatment may be necessary to repair the hole in the nasal septum. In some cases, it may be impossible to correct this complication.

Nasal airway alteration—Changes may occur after a rhinoplasty or septoplasty operation that may interfere with normal passage of air through the nose.

HEALTH INSURANCE

Most insurance companies exclude coverage for cosmetic surgical operations or any complications that might occur from cosmetic surgery. If the procedure corrects a breathing problem or marked deformity after a nasal fracture, a portion may be covered. Please carefully review your health insurance subscriber information pamphlet.

ADDITIONAL SURGERY NECESSARY

There are many variable conditions in addition to risk and potential surgical complications that may influence the long-term result of rhinoplasty surgery, even though risks and complications occur.

Infrequently, the risks cited are the ones that are particularly associated with rhinoplasty surgery. Other complications and risks can occur but are even more uncommon. Should complications occur, additional surgery or other treatments may be necessary. **The practice of medicine and surgery is not an exact science. Although good results are expected, there is no guarantee or warranty expressed or implied on the results that may be obtained. Infrequently, it is necessary to perform additional surgery to improve your result.**

Statistically worldwide 10% patients need additional surgery planned or unplanned.

FINANCIAL RESPONSIBILITIES

The cost of surgery involves several charges for the services provided. The total includes fees charged by your doctor, the cost of surgical supplies, laboratory test, anaesthesia and outpatient hospital charges, depending on where the surgery is performed. Depending on whether the cost of surgery is covered by an insurance plan, you will be responsible for necessary co-payments, deductibles and charges no covered. Additional costs may occur should complications develop from the surgery. Secondary surgery or hospital day surgery charges involved with revisionary surgery would also be your responsibility.

<u>Alternatives to this procedure</u>: Alternative forms of management consist of not undergoing the rhinoplasty surgery. Certain internal nasal airway disorder may not require surgery on the exterior of the nose. Risks and potential complications are associated with alternative forms of treatment that involve surgery such as septoplasty to correct nasal airway disorders.

Smoking, second-hand smoke exposure and nicotine products (patch, gum, nasal spray): Patients who are currently smoking and use tobacco products or nicotine products (patch, gum or nasal spray) are at a greater risk for significant surgical complications of skin dying, delayed healing and additional scarring. Individuals exposed to second-hand smoke are also at potential risk for similar complications attributable to nicotine exposure. Additionally, smokers may have a significant negative effect on anaesthesia and recovery from anaesthesia, with coughing and possibly increased bleeding. Individuals who are not exposed to tobacco smoke or nicotine-containing products have a significantly lower risk of this type of complication. Please indicate your current status regarding these items below:

____________ I am a non-smoker and do not use nicotine products. I understand the risk of second-hand smoke exposure causing surgical complications.

____________ I am a smoker or use tobacco/nicotine products. I understand the risk of surgical complications due to smoking or use of nicotine products.

It is important to refrain from smoking at least 6 weeks before surgery and until your physician states it is safe to return, if desired.

Female patient information: It is important to inform your plastic surgeon if you use birth control pills and oestrogen replacement, or if you believe you may be pregnant. Many medications including antibiotics may neutralise the preventive effect of birth control pills, allowing for conception and pregnancy.

Intimate relations after surgery: Surgery involves coagulating of blood vessels, and increased activity of any kind may open these vessels leading to a bleed, or haematoma. Increased activity that increased your pulse or heart rate may cause additional bruising, swelling and the need for return to surgery and control of bleeding. It is wise to refrain from sexual activity until your physician states it is safe.

Medications: There are many adverse reactions that occur as the result of taking over the counter, herbal and/or prescription medications. Be sure to check with your physician about any drug interactions that may exist with medications that you are already taking. If you have an adverse reaction, stop the drugs immediately and call your plastic surgeon for further instructions. If the reaction is severe, go immediately to the nearest emergency room. When taking the prescribed pain medications after surgery, realise that they can affect your thought process. Do not drive, do not operate complex equipment, do not make any important decisions, and do not drink any alcohol while taking these medications. Be sure to take your prescribed medication only as directed.

PATIENT COMPLIANCE

Follow all physician instructions carefully; this is essential for the success of your outcome. It is important that the surgical incisions are not subjected to excessive force, swelling, abrasion or motion during the time of healing. Personal and vocational activity needs to be restricted. Protective dressings and drains should not be removed unless instructed by your plastic surgeon. Successful post-operative function depends on both surgery and subsequent care. Physical activity that increases your pulse or heart rate may cause bruising, swelling, fluid accumulation around implants and the need for the return to surgery. It is important that you participate in follow-up care, return for aftercare and promote your recovery after surgery.

DISCLAIMER

Informed-consent documents are used to communicate information about the proposed surgical treatment of a disease or condition along with disclosure of risks and alternative forms of treatment(s). This document is based on a thorough evaluation of scientific literature and relevant clinic practice to describe a range of generally acceptable risks and alternative forms of management of a particular disease or condition. The informed-consent process attempts to define principles of risk disclosure that should generally meet the needs of most patients in most circumstances.

However, informed-consent documents should not be considered all-inclusive in defining other methods of care and risks encountered. Your plastic surgeon may provide you with additional or different information that is based on all the facts in your particular case and the state of medical knowledge.

Informed-consent documents are not intended to define or serve as the standard of medical care. Standards of medical care are determined on the basis of all of the facts involved in an individual case and are subject to change as scientific knowledge and technology advance and as practice patterns evolve. This informed-consent document reflects the state of knowledge current at the time of publication.

It is important that you have read the above information carefully and have all of your questions answered before signing the consent on the next page.

<u>I acknowledge that the Dr. has explained:</u>

- My medical condition and the proposed procedure, including additional treatment if the doctor finds something unexpected. I understand the risks, including the risks that are specific to me.
- The anaesthetic required for this procedure. I understand the risks, including the risks that are specific to me.
- My prognosis and risks of not having the procedure.
- The procedure may include a blood transfusion.
- I have been explained that excessive bleeding, infection, cardiac arrest, pulmonary embolism and complications like this can arise suddenly and unexpectedly while undergoing operative procedure or anaesthesia.
- During surgery suspected body tissues could be removed for histopathological examination.
- I give consent for any change in anaesthesia or operative procedure at the time of surgery.
- I have been made aware that after the above operation and anaesthesia, some complication may arise, and I believe that to avoid

such complications, if any appropriate care is needed, it shall be taken by surgeon and anaesthetist or any other doctor suggested by them.

- That there is no ICU in this hospital but this hospitalhasatie-upwith…………………….. hospital which has ICU backup and patient will be shifted there in case of any complication so that appropriate care can be taken of.
- I have been explained that after surgery I might need to take some medications for a particular period of time as per my medical condition and as per prescribed by doctors. After surgery I will have to regularly follow up with my doctor as per his orders.
- I was able to ask questions and raise concerns with the doctor about my condition, the proposed procedure and its risks and my treatment options. My questions and concerns have been discussed and answered to my satisfaction.
- I understand I have the right to change my mind at any time, including after I have signed this form but, preferably following a discussion with my doctor.
- I understand that images or video footage may be recorded as a part of and during my procedure. I consent to the photographing or televising of the operation(s) or procedure(s) to be performed, including appropriate portions of my body, for medical, scientific or educational purposes.
- Provided my identity is not revealed by the pictures for medical, scientific and educational purpose only.
- Website or social media with no identity revealed (eye closed).
- Everywhere without eye closure.

(Please tick your option)
Photographs will be used

- For purposes of advancing medical education, I consent to the admittance of observers to the operating room.
- I accept that medicine is not an exact science and understand that no guarantees can be given to the results and understand these limitations.
- I have read the above writing/the above writing has been read out to me and is explained to me in the ……...language by……………………….(interpreter) which I understand.
- I have understood the aforesaid and I am giving my consent willingly with sound mental state without any coercion, undue influence, fraud, misrepresentation or mistake of facts.
- I request Dr. ………………………to perform upon me the above-mentioned procedure.
- The competent courts in Pune will have jurisdiction in relation to any claim/dispute arising from or relating to the procedure(s) mentioned herein.

Declaration by doctor: I declare that I have explained the nature and consequences of the procedure to be performed, and discussed the risks that particularly concern the patient.

I have given the patient an opportunity to ask questions and I have answered these.

- **DoctorPatient/Guardian**
- Sign…………………………………... Sign/lt thumb imp................................
- Name………………... Name………………………………………………………
- Address……………….. Address……………………………………………
- Date…………………….. Date…………………….Age…..
- Time……… Time…………..
- **Witness** 1 **Witness 2**
- Sign……………………
Sign………………………………...
- Name……….. ……………………
Name…………………………………………..
- Relation with patient….. ……… Relation with patient………………………………
- Address…….. ……………. Address……
- Date…………….Age……….
Date…………………..Age………
- Time……. Time…………

POST-RHINOPLASTY INSTRUCTIONS

1. Keep the head higher than the level of the heart for 48 hours—head end elevation.
2. Change the gauze under the nose if and when it is soiled.
3. Take pain medications as needed.
4. Take antibiotics two times daily for 10 days.
5. Keep the head out of water when bathing or shower.
6. Call the hospital and take necessary advice from any attending ENT surgeon regarding any problems faced by you.

Basic Rhinoplasty Surgery

4

Main

The variable anatomy of the nose and many techniques available make rhinoplasty difficult. This chapter is about basic surgery and, sticking to this, helps us to tackle most of the rhinoplasty cases.

4.1 Operative Planning

After careful analysis of the nose and face, as discussed in the pre-operative evaluation, an operative plan, expected deformity after opening and stepwise surgical plan have to be noted. This plan and expected deformities should be rewritten after the end of the surgery. As you gain experience, pre-operative deformity predictions and operative planning will start matching with the actual results and findings.

Operative steps followed at our centre:

- General anaesthesia induction.
- Local infiltration.
- Application of pressure with an ice-cold gauze piece after wearing operative light-mounted loupes (Fig. 4.1). While applying pressure, evaluation of the deformity and revision of planning are kept in mind.
- Scrubbing and painting with Betadine scrub.
- Draping.
- Cutting vibrissae with aseptic precautions.

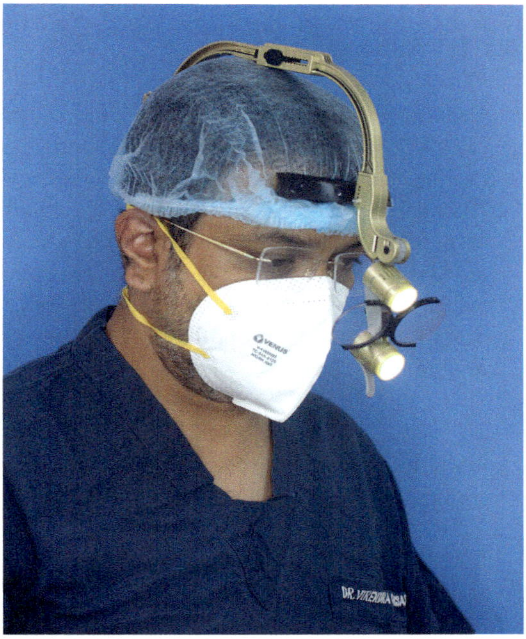

Fig. 4.1 Operative light mounted with loupes

- Incision.
- Parallel graft harvesting by other colleague if costal cartilage harvesting is planned.
- Exposure.
- Reassessment of deformities and operative plan.

V. Ghaisas, *Indian Ethnic Rhinoplasty*, https://doi.org/10.1007/978-981-16-2478-0_4

- Assessing lower alar deformity.
- Septoplasty.
- Treatment of upper 1/3—osteotomy correction of convexity and drilling nasal bones.
- Mid 1/3—segmental hump resection and spreader grafts/flaps.
- Lower 1/3—tip plasty.
- Treatment of the dorsum.
- Closure.
- Alaplasty.
- Doyle splint placement.
- Taping and POP cast application.
- Extubation.

4.1.1 Anaesthesia

- General—total intravenous anaesthesia (**TIVA**) with less or no inhalational support is the best form of anaesthesia for rhinoplasty. Hypotensive anaesthesia is essential, which helps in a good intraoperative field and reduces the tissue oedema subsequently with decreased post-operative recovery period. A combination of sevoflurane, propofol and dexmedetomidine is preferred.

- Local infiltration with 0.2% ropivacaine with adrenaline is preferred.

  Infiltration has the following benefits:

I. Vasoconstriction and good surgical field
II. Good dissection plane in the vestibular skin
III. Eases the dorsal skin and septal flap elevation
IV. Long-acting anaesthesia
V. Enhanced post-operative analgesia

In general, rhinoplasty patients have lesser pain threshold. In case a patient complains that the post-operative pain is unbearable, this would reflect on the future visit of patients in consulting us which is usually their close relatives and friends. This is counteracted by local infiltration.

Infraorbital and supratrochlear block is given. Followed by that a good alar base, columellar, marginal area and on the dorsum (external nasal nerve—terminal branch of anterior ethmoidal nerve), infiltration is given (Figs. 4.2, 4.3, 4.4, 4.5 and 4.6).

After the infiltration, while applying pressure with cold gauze piece, deformity is reassessed. Then after, a good scrubbing of the nose and face is done. And by anticipating the need for a graft, a thorough painting of the graft site area is done.

Draping of the face meticulously yet firmly is mandatory. Vibrissae are trimmed carefully using a 15 No. blade.

Sites of local anaesthesia infiltration are shown in Figs. 4.2, 4.3, 4.4, 4.5 and 4.6.

4.1.2 **Incision** (Figs. 4.7, 4.8, 4.9 and 4.10)

Alar rim is pulled upwards with the help of alar retractor, and at the same time, the middle finger of the left hand is used to press down the lower alar cartilage to make the caudal border prominent to take a proper marginal incision with a 15 No. blade (Fig. 4.7). Columellar side incision is placed 3 mm behind the border during which injury to the soft triangle is avoided.

Starting at the Infracartilaginous incision, using blunt scissors, dissection is done on both sides abutting to the cartilage but not injuring the cartilages. Skin envelope is dissected in the supraperichondrial plane till the dorsum. At this stage, columellar incision is done by 11 No. sharp blade at the narrowest portion of the columella in an inverted V-shaped manner. And thus the bonnet of the nose is opened.

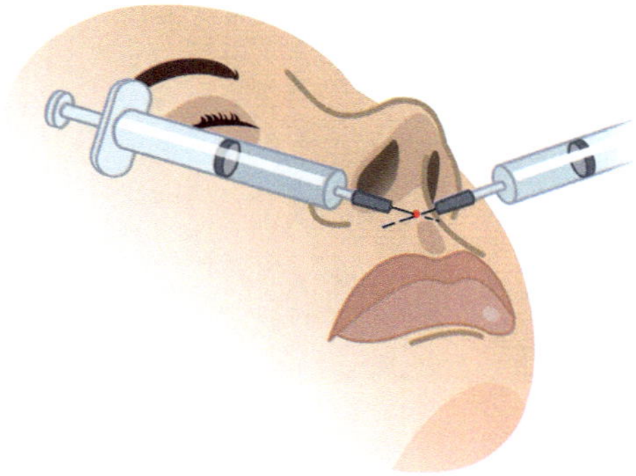

Fig. 4.2 Alar base

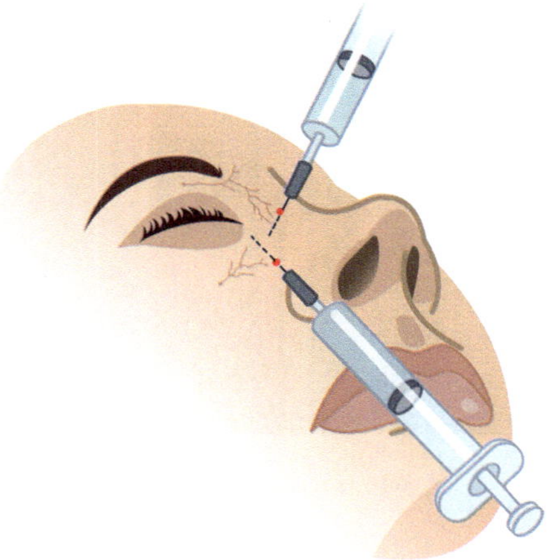

Fig. 4.3 On the dorsum to block external nasal nerve and lateral osteotomy site

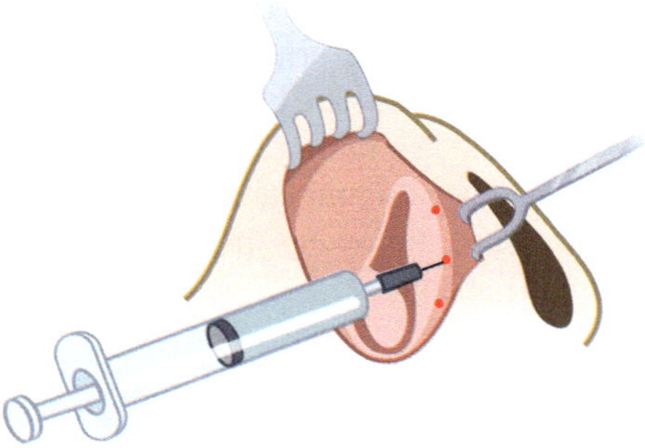

Fig. 4.4 Columella

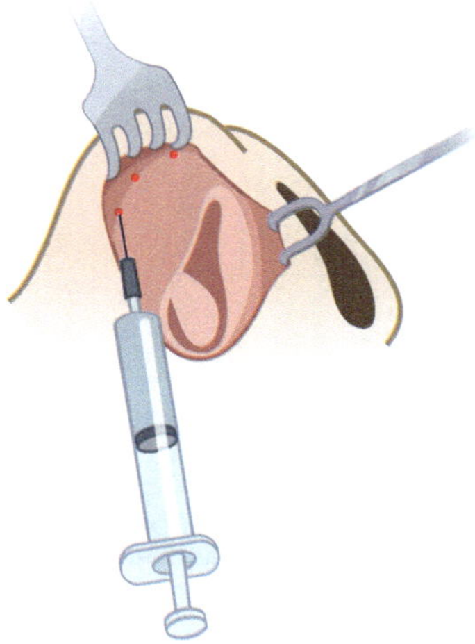

Fig. 4.5 Alar margin

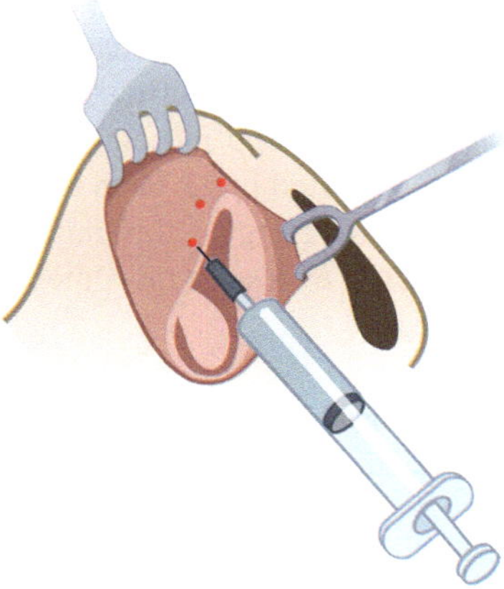

Fig. 4.6 The scroll area

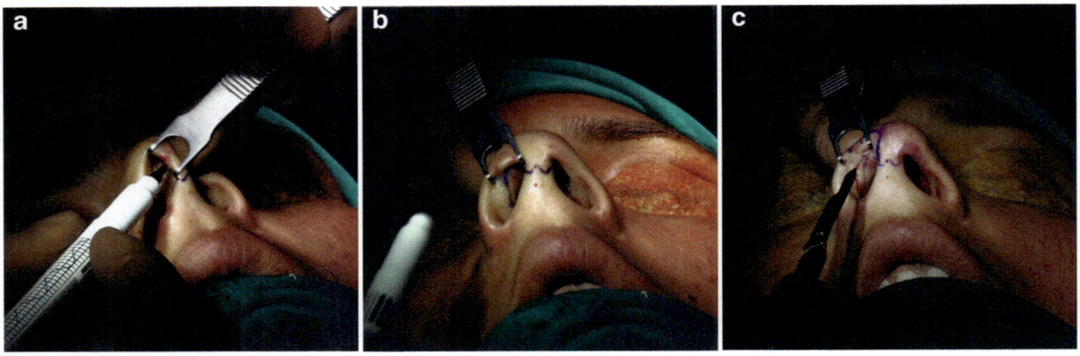

Fig. 4.7 (**a**, **b**, **c**) Infracartilagenous incision

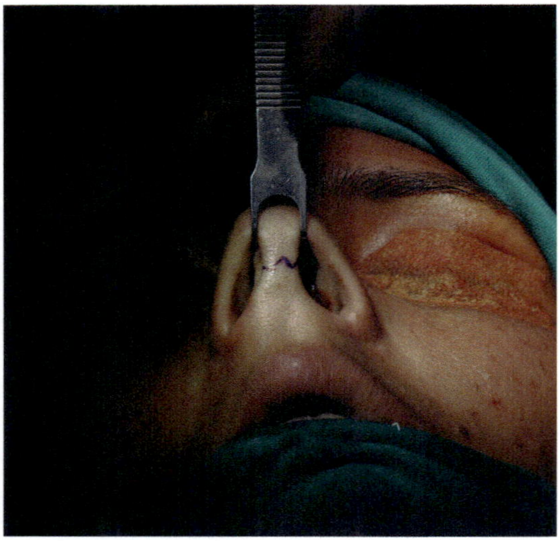

Fig. 4.8 Columellar incision

4.1.3 **Dissection** (Figs. 4.11, 4.12, 4.13 and 4.14)

Following skin flap elevation, dissection is continued with blunt scissors up to the level of nasofrontal angle with minimal lateral dissection. However, if large unequal nasal bones are expected or when loose tension-free skin is desired in severe saddle noses, lateral dissection is done till nasofacial groove or medial canthal level.

Horizontal or vertical incision is taken on the periosteum of the nasal bones for periosteal elevation and nasal bone exposure by holding the skin flap with Aufricht retractor. This is important so as to ensure direct contact of our graft with nasal bones, and eventually periosteum will grow over the graft. In addition, in the late postoperative period, the graft may be easily felt and there is an increased chance of displacement.

Note that in hump deformities, it is advocated to use rasping over the bare bone rather than with periosteum. And also during hump removal, preserved flapped periosteum can be used for draping the dorsum following hump removal in thin-skinned patients.

4.1.4 **Approach to the Septum** (Figs. 4.15, 4.16, 4.17, 4.18 and 4.19)

With sharp scissors, interdomal ligament is cut, following which the membranous part of the septum is dissected to approach the caudal border of the cartilaginous septum. During which one can encounter depressor septi muscle which most of the time is appreciated in deviated type of noses. The purposeful severing of this muscle will be needed in cases of excessive movement of the tip during smiling.

Note: Hence during pre-operative evaluation, change in the position of the tip if present is noted and documented.

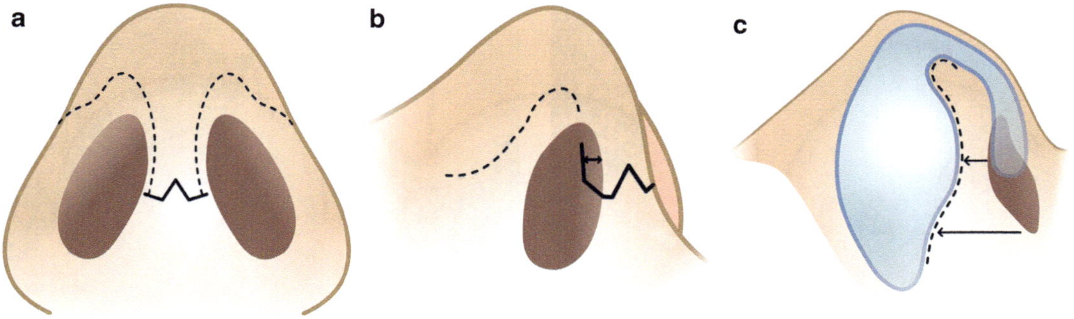

Fig. 4.9 (**a**, **b**, **c**) Incision: Basal view, lateral

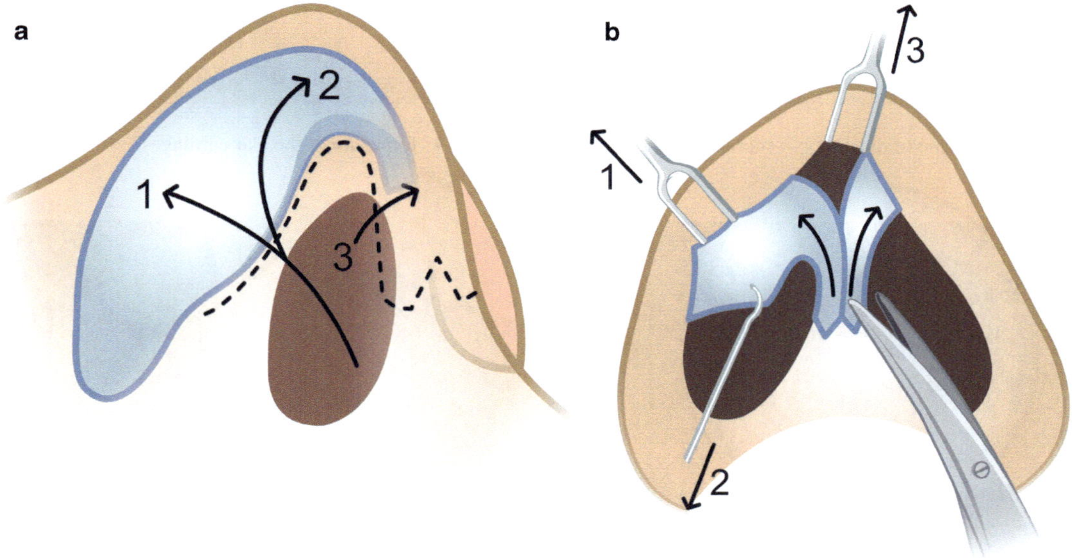

Fig. 4.10 (**a**, **b**) Bidirectional exposure

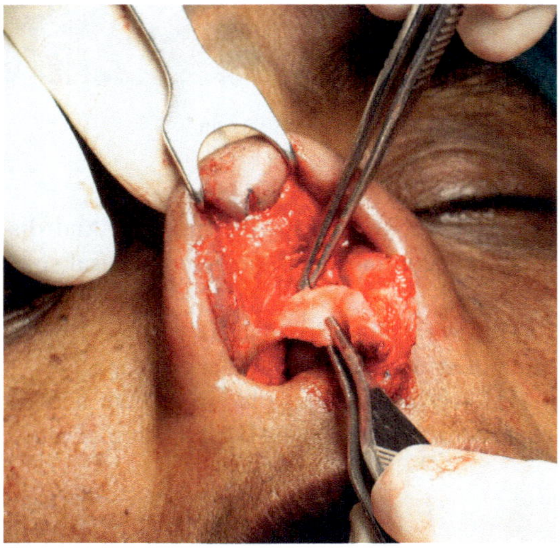

Fig. 4.11 Elevating the skin envelope

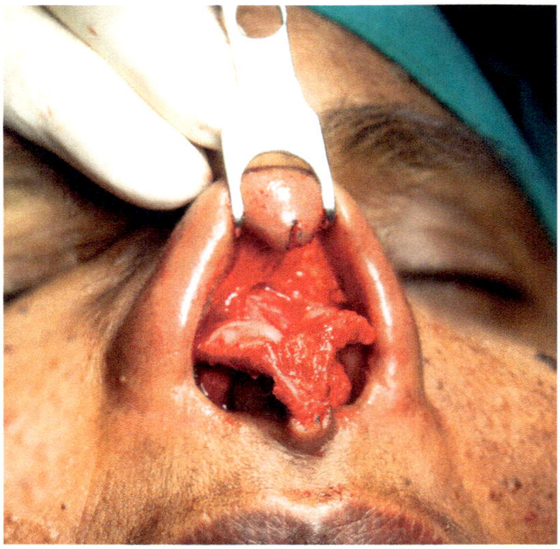

Fig. 4.12 Retraction of skin flaps

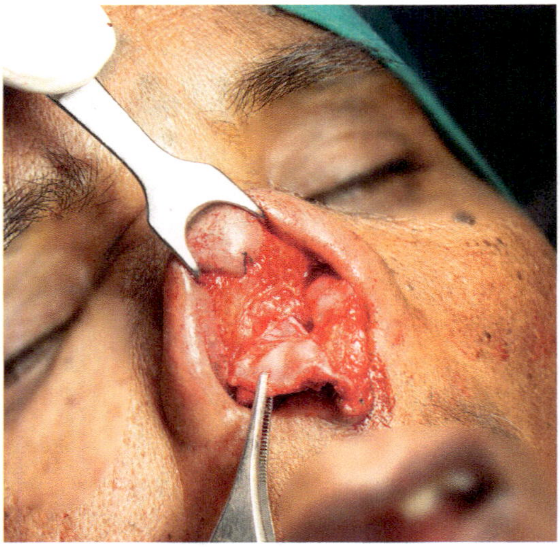

Fig. 4.13 Plane of dissection—supraperichondiral

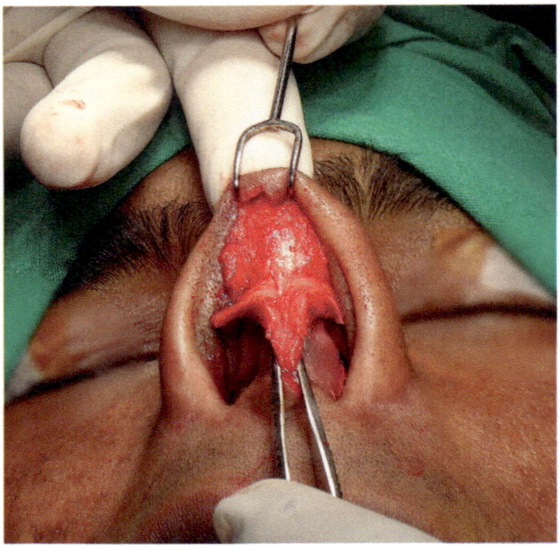

Fig. 4.14 Exposure of the alar cartilages

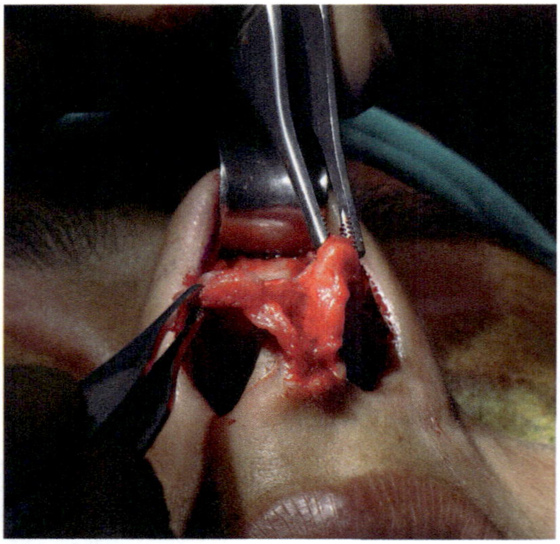

Fig. 4.15 Dissection of membranous septum

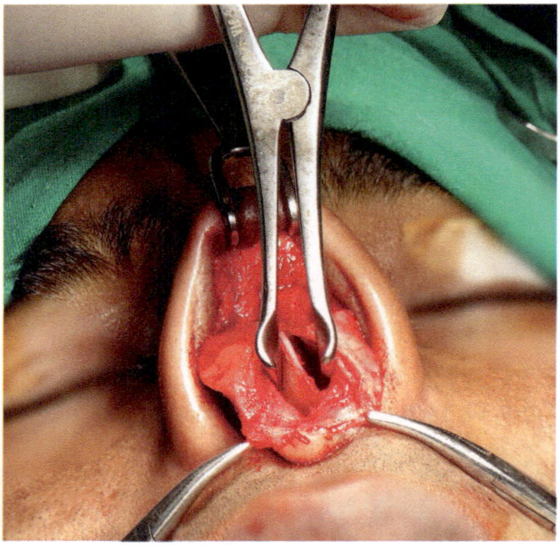

Fig. 4.16 Exposure of nasal septum

Further, anterior septal angle is identified, and with the sharp scissors, septal subperichondrial plane is reached. Dissection of the septum on both sides is done completely. Attachment of the upper lateral cartilage with the septum on either side is cut with 11 number blade or with straight scissors to expose the septum completely without injuring the mucosa. And dissection is continued till the anterior nasal spine is exposed.

Following this, tip analysis is done for creation of symmetrical lower alar cartilage.

If lower alar cartilage is broad, then it needs cephalic trimming leaving behind 8 mm of caudal

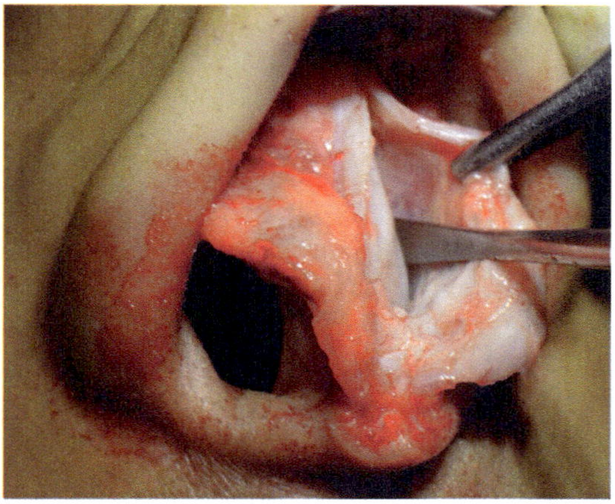

Fig. 4.17 Septal subperichondrial plane dissection

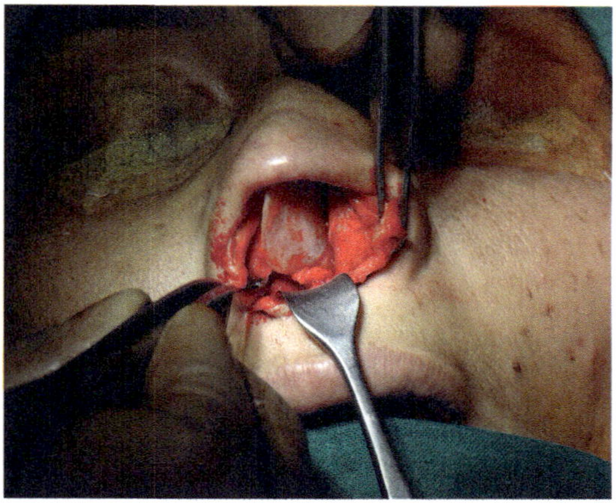

Fig. 4.18 Bilateral septal elevation done

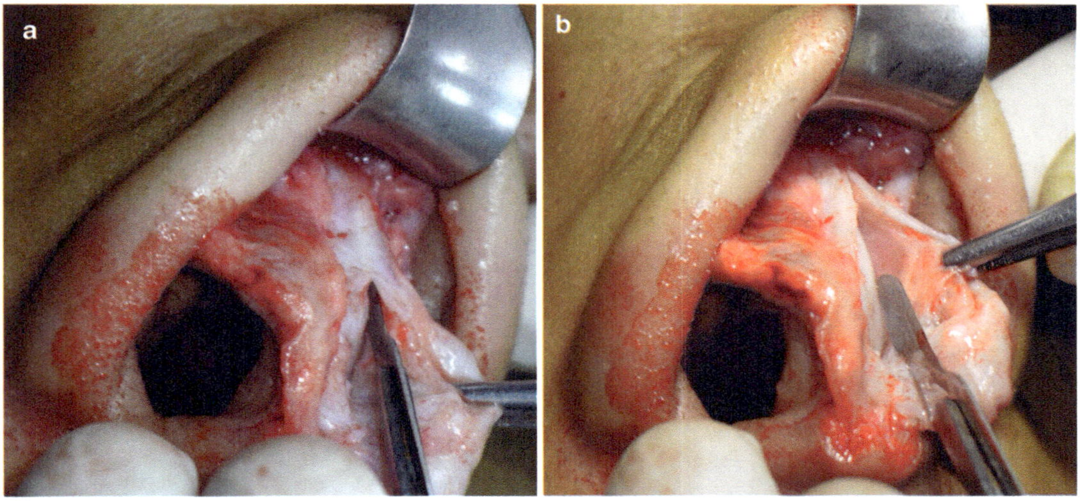

Fig. 4.19 (a, b) Cutting of upper lateral cartilage on either side

border of lateral crura (Fig. 4.20). If cartilage is weak, then it is better to infold it after vestibular skin dissection. Kindly note that this trimming should not be overdone as it can give external valve collapse, pinching and upward rotation of the tip.

For infolding 5-0 PDS suture is used after stabilising the infolded cartilage flaps with 26-gauge-long needles.

Dorsal hump reduction is done prior to septoplasty as it is safe to keep at least 10 mm of the dorsal strip. Dorsal hump is reduced in graduated segmental manner than block resection. Overresection is avoided by systematic step-by-step reduction.

Preferred method for bony hump reduction is rasp, diamond burr or piezoelectric device depending on the availability (Figs. 4.21 and 4.22).

After exposure and assessment, cartilaginous (septal) hump is planned to be removed. Then, if at all excess upper lateral cartilage is present, they can be used as septal flaps.

However, in small humps upper lateral cartilages are shaved and spreader grafts are used (Fig. 4.23a, b).

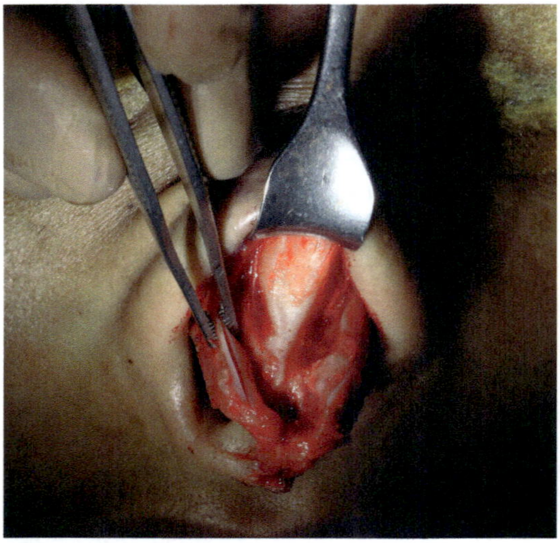

Fig. 4.20 Cephalic trimming

4.1.5 Septoplasty

It is an important procedure because 60% of revision rhinoplasty is due to inadequate septoplasty or secondary to excessive resection.

During rhinoplasty, after retaining the caudal and dorsal 1 cm L-shaped strut, the remaining part of the septum can be taken out which can be used a graft material. Without making a sharp angle at the L strut.

Deviated ethmoid should be cut with double-action scissors, and then forceps is used to remove the bone to avoid injury to the cribriform plate which can be used for splinting later on if need be. Deviated maxillary crest can be removed by gouge and hammer or by drill (Figs. 4.24, 4.25 and 4.26).

Anterior nasal spine is an important structure which is kept in mind. We can drill the deviated part and manipulated to the centre but not be removed in any case. Many a times one has to drill the spine to fix the antero-inferior part of the cartilaginous septum and one has to carefully drill it with sharp and small Lindemann's burr (Fig. 4.27).

During septoplasty, it is very important to elevate the mucoperichondrial flaps without any

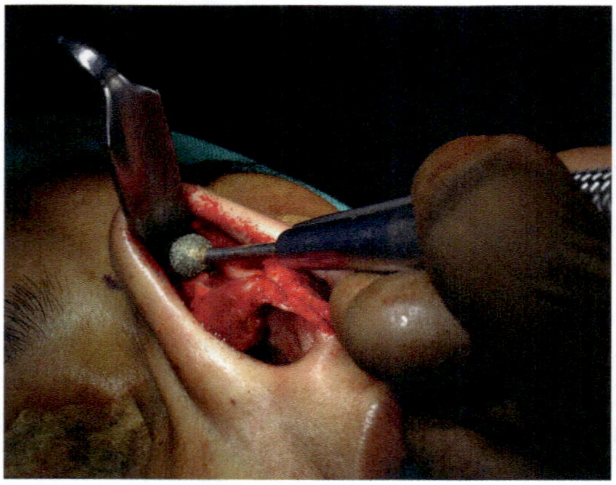

Fig. 4.21 Coarse diamond burr for bony hump reduction

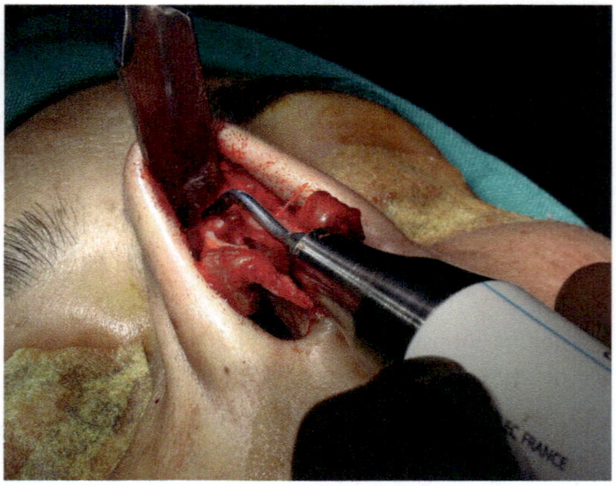

Fig. 4.22 Piezoelectric device for bony hump reduction

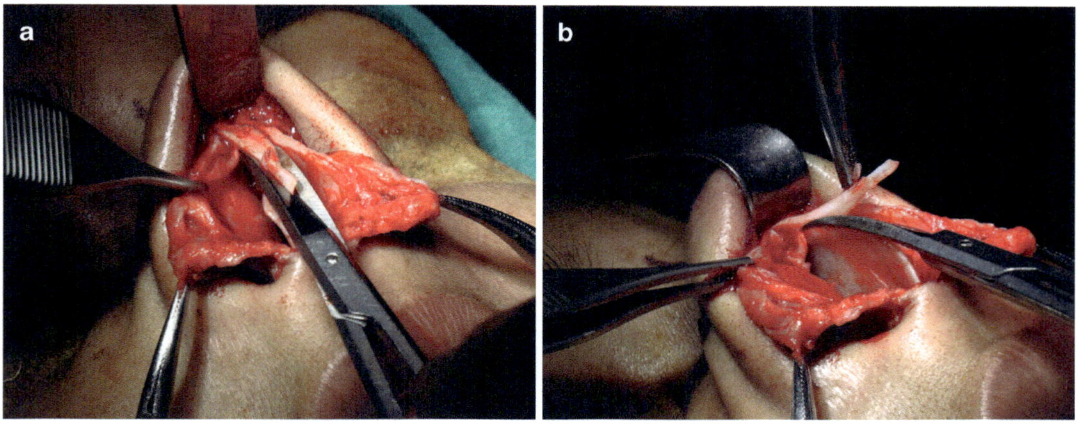

Fig. 4.23 (**a**, **b**) Cutting of shaving the cartilaginous hump

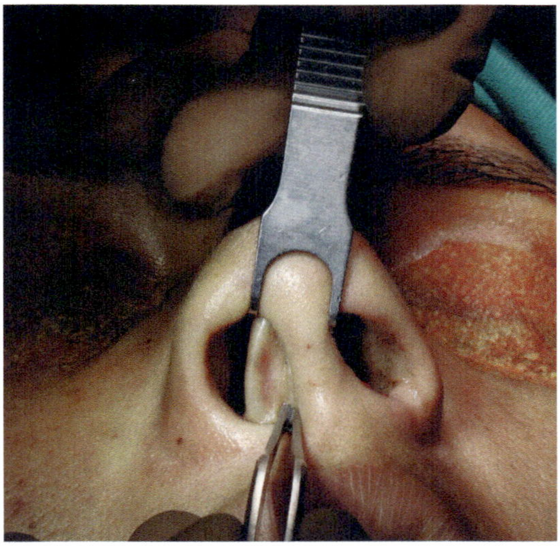

Fig. 4.24 Pre-operative picture of caudal dislocation

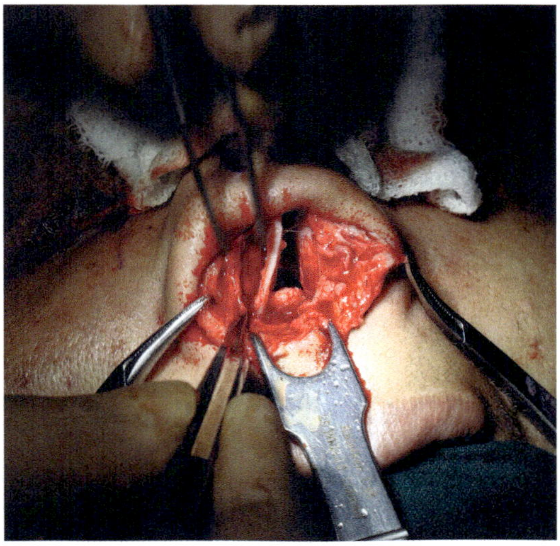

Fig. 4.25 Intraoperative picture showing caudal dislocation with anterior nasal spine at the centre

tear. Care should be taken to avoid two-sided mucosal tear at corresponding areas to prevent or avoid septal perforation.

In central and northern India, noses have characteristic large septal cartilages, and septal cartilage remains as the choice for grafting.

4.1.6 Osteotomy (Figs. 4.28, 4.29, 4.30, 4.31 and 4.32)

Paramedian Osteotomy In this osteotomy we break the attachment of the nasal bones to the nasal septum. This is a straight 5 mm osteotome line

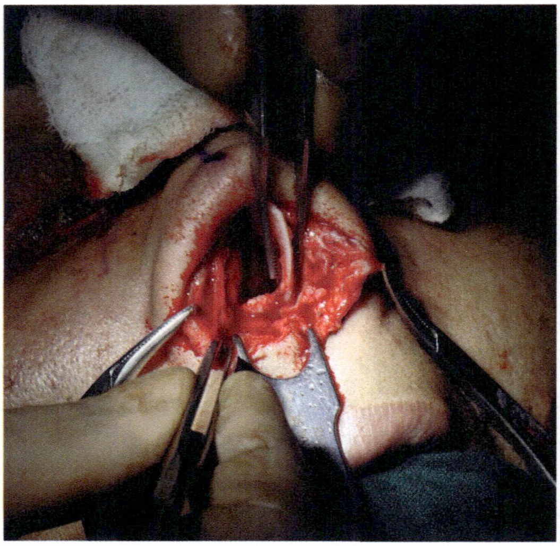

Fig. 4.26 Caudal septum: swing door technique

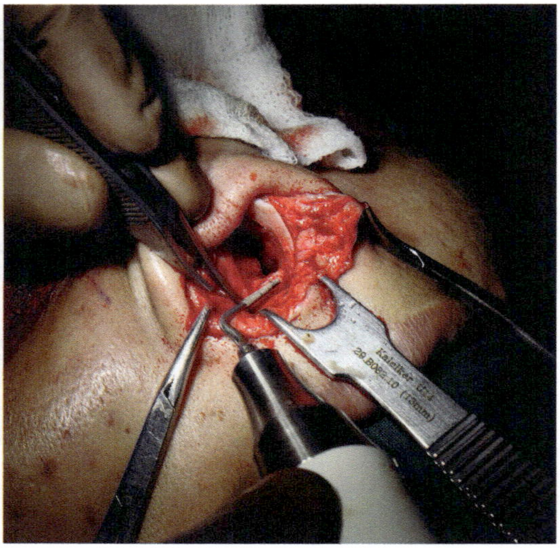

Fig. 4.27 Drilling a hole in ANS (here with piezo, can be done with Lindemann's burr) to fix the caudal septum with 3-0 PDS

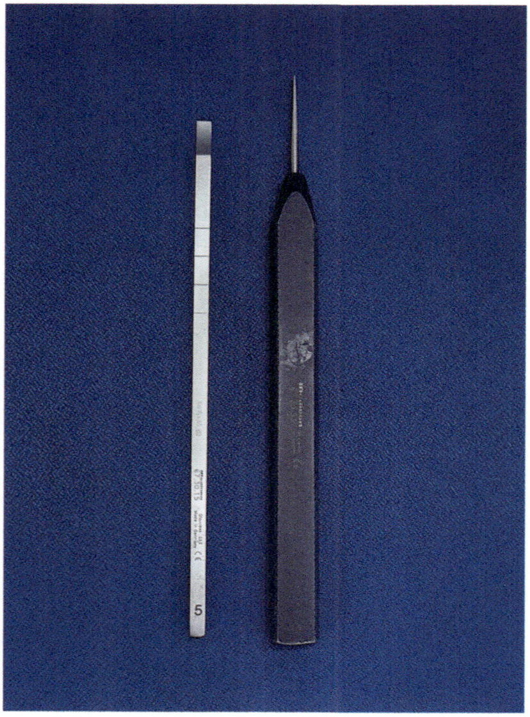

Fig. 4.28 and 29 2 mm osteotome, 5 mm osteotome

starting from 'K' junction to the level of medial canthus of the eye. Upper lateral cartilages extend below the nasal bones around 3–5 mm. Thus, this osteotomy damages the upper lateral cartilages. So one has to avoid using blunt osteotome; instead, a sharp 5 mm osteotome (with the non-bevelled edge facing the septum) or Lindemann's burr is preferred. These days we prefer to do with piezoelectric device as it helps to avoid injury to the underlying cartilage and adjacent soft tissue.

Lateral Osteotomy External lateral osteotomy is done with the help of a 2 mm osteotome. A small nick is made at the midpoint of the line from the medial canthus to the lobule on the nasofacial groove. Through this nick, an osteotome is introduced, and the periosteum over the bone along the osteotomy line is cut pushing the vessels away, thus avoiding injury to the vessels and subsequent bleeding and oedema. Sometimes, angular vein can get injured. Being in the nasofacial groove, precise continuous osteotomy is done to avoid a step deformity (Fig. 4.33). These are low to low osteotomies.

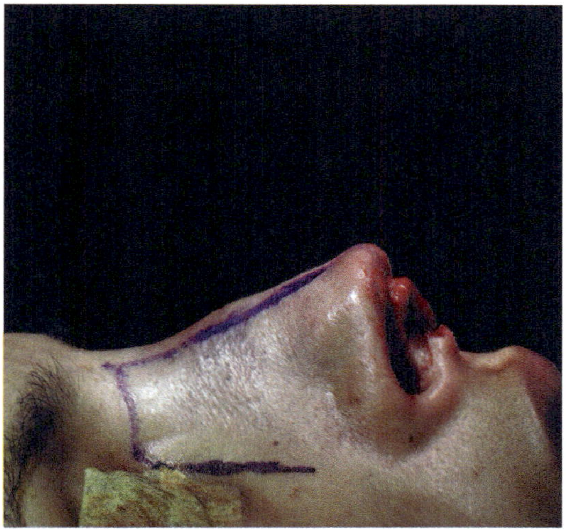

Fig. 4.30 Paramedian osteotomy using piezoelectric device (usually done with a 5 mm osteotome keeping the non-bevelled edge towards the septum)

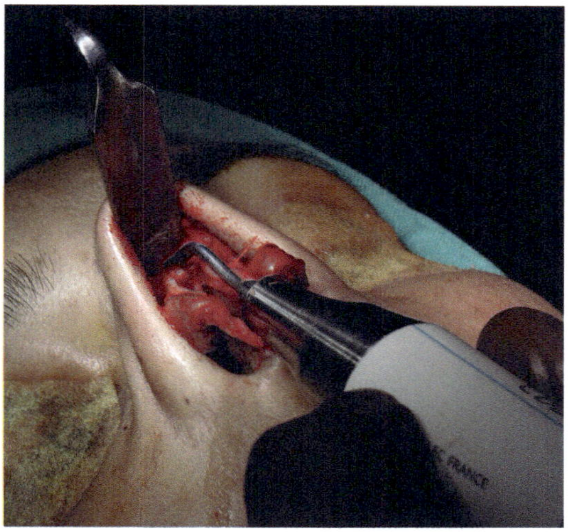

Fig. 4.31 Sharp edge of osteotomy cutting the periosteum along the nasofacial groove

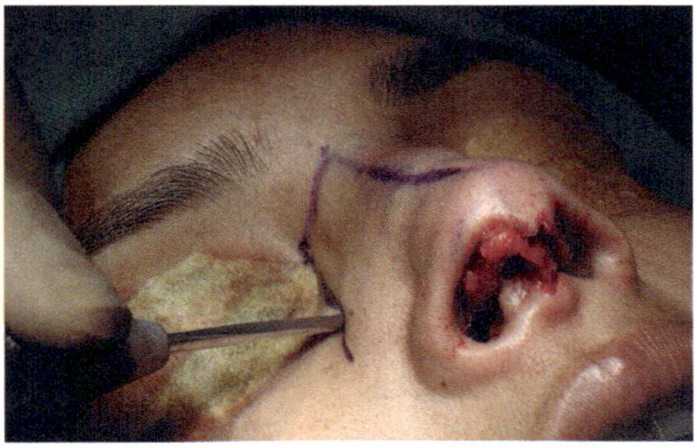

Fig. 4.32 Intranasal lateral osteotomy

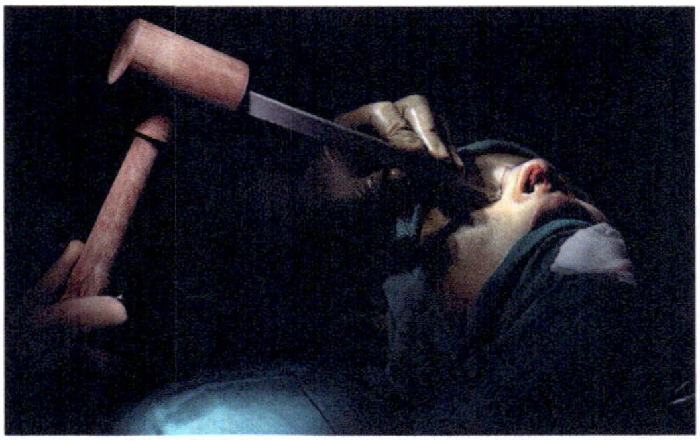

Fig. 4.33 Wooden hammer used for osteotomy

Lateral osteotomy can also be done by intranasal approach (Fig. 4.34) with silver chisel and guard, but we prefer external osteotomy as it is more precise.

Transverse Osteotomy At the midpoint of medial canthus and the dorsum, a nick is made, and again with 2 mm osteotome, osteotomy is done to mobilise the nasal bones.

Rarely if the nasal bones are unequal, then one has to perform intermediate osteotomy. But, I prefer to drill the nasal bones to make it symmetrical with a diamond burr or with piezoelectric device.

We prefer low to low osteotomy (Fig. 4.35), but some prefer low to high osteotomy and avoid separate transverse osteotomy. Some also prefer, high-to-low-to-high osteotomy with preservation

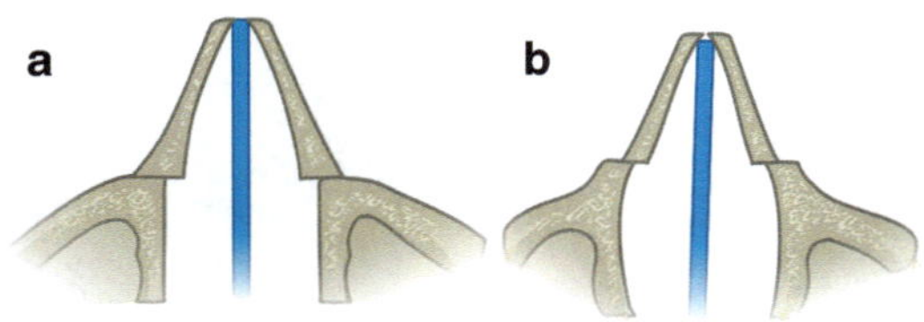

Fig. 4.34 (**a**) Lateral osteotomy done at the correct site. (**b**) Lateral osteotomy done way too medial to the nasofacial groove causing step deformity

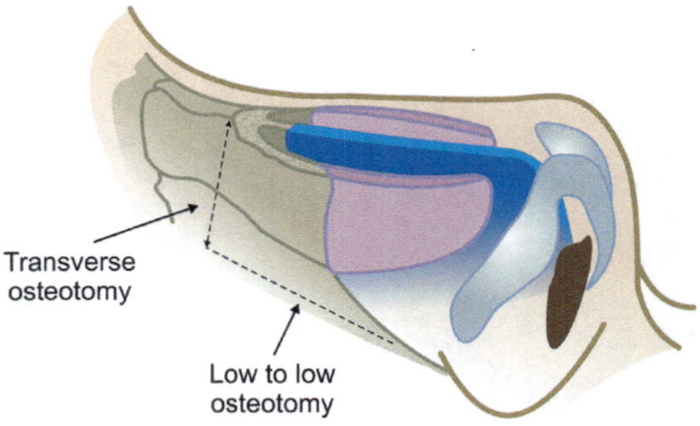

Fig. 4.35 Low to low with transverse osteotomy

of Webster'as trinagle. I think it is only indicated, if the inferior turbinate is located quite high.

4.1.7 Surgery of Middle One-Third of the Nose

Spreader grafts (Figs. 4.36 and 4.37) remain the *mainstay/workhorse* of rhinoplasty in deviated nose to open up the internal nasal valve. In saddle nose, as a part of structural grafting and in hump nose to avoid inverted V deformity, one has to use spreader grafts.

Spreader grafts have three main features:

1. To stabilise the nasal dorsum
2. To give dorsal aesthetic lines
3. To improve the nasal valve area

Length of the spreader graft is measured from just below the nasal bones to a few millimetres till anterior nasal angle. Thickness is generally 1 mm in females and 1.5 mm in males.

Extended spreader grafts are used to lengthen the nose. Spreader flaps (Fig. 4.38) are used in hump noses where upper lateral cartilages are 5 mm more than the height of cartilaginous septum.

You will never regret by applying appropriate size spreader grafts, but one will regret if not used.

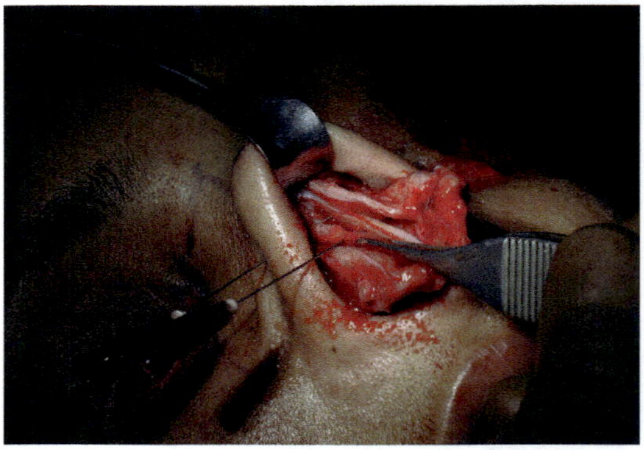

Fig. 4.36 Spreader grafts placed on either side of the septum in between the upper lateral cartilage stabilised with 26-gauge-long needles

4.1.8 Surgery of Lower One-Third of the Nose

Tip Plasty (Few Salient Features Mentioned Here, Detailed Explanation Given in Chap. 9)

The basic tip surgery principle remains to provide stability to the tip either by sutures or by instilling grafts.

Depending on the type of deformity, either a columellar strut or septal extension graft is used in most cases (Figs. 4.39 and 4.40).

Maintenance of lateral crural symmetry is always kept in mind.

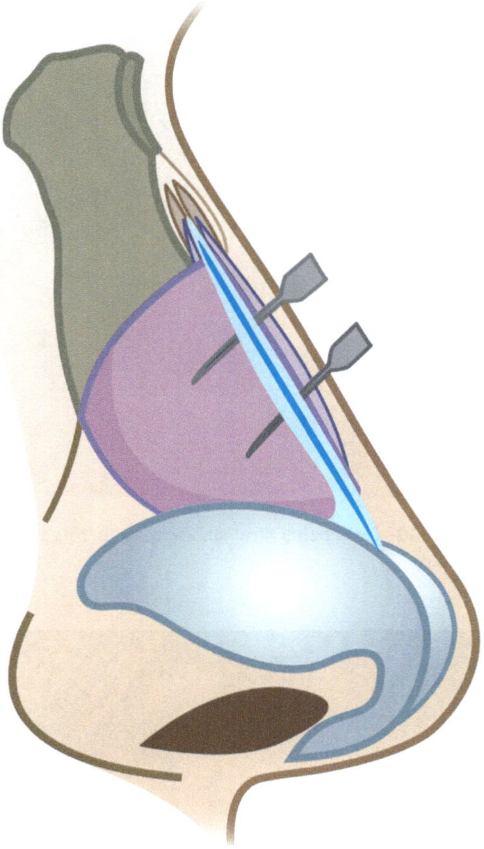

Fig. 4.37 Schematic diagram of spreader grafts fixed on either of the septum

In Indian thick-skinned noses to stabilise the tip, though the domal creation sutures are commonly performed, it is always better to have dorsal onlay grafts.

Ironically, shield grafts have been used in the region of nasal tips since 1895 which has steadily increased in the renewed interest in the procedure.

Rim graft (Fig. 4.41), i.e. alar rim grafting, is a simple and versatile approach to provide additional support to the external nasal valve and for improving the nasal base contour.

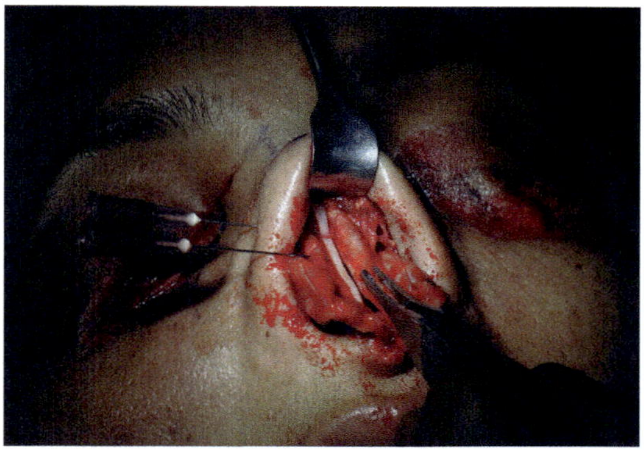

Fig. 4.38 Spreader flaps (held with forceps here) are created if the upper lateral cartilage is more than 5 mm in height of the cartilaginous septum

In Indian noses, all the tips need to be addressed. We tend to counter thicker skin along with weak lateral cartilages in practice, often calling for infolding of the lateral crus, rim grafts and dorsal onlay with shield grafts. If there is less septal tip support, then septal extension graft is used than columellar strut.

In saddle noses, according to height of the nose, augmentation needs to be done.

In deviated noses, osteotomy and tip should be treated, and dorsum should be treated well with fine-diced cartilage.

In hump noses, to recheck if the reduction of hump is adequate, following tip plasty is mandatory.

4.1.9 Closure

Use of 5-0 Vicryl and 5-0 PDS sutures and suturing has to be very precise to avoid scarring in the columellar region. Following closure, free diced cartilage (FDC) filled in a 1 cc syringe is inserted into the nose through the alar margin incision to smoothen the irregularities on the dorsum and tip edges (Fig. 4.42).

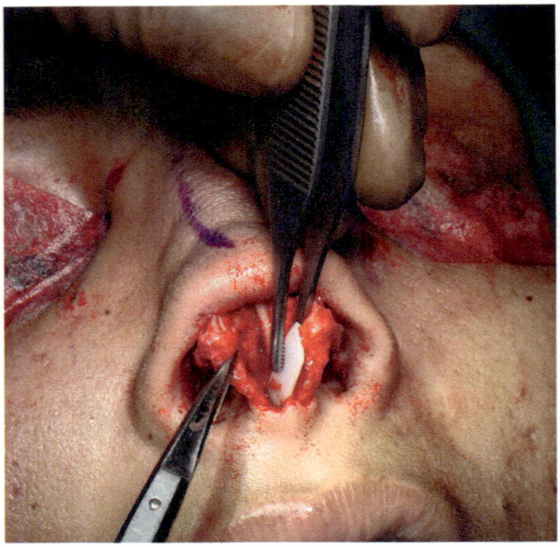

Fig. 4.39 Columellar strut placed in between two medial crura

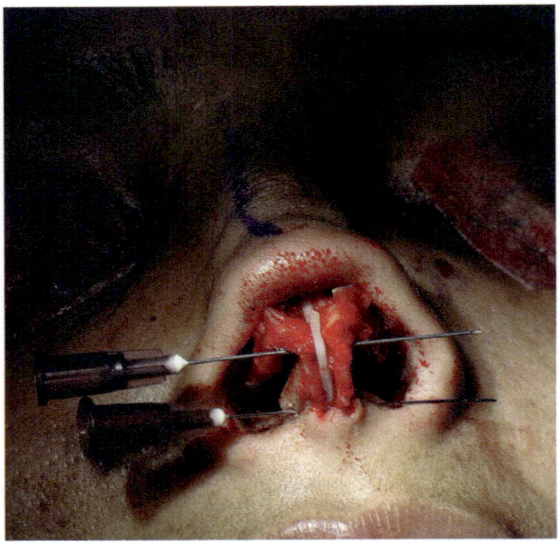

Fig. 4.40 Columellar strut stabilised with 26-gauge-long needles

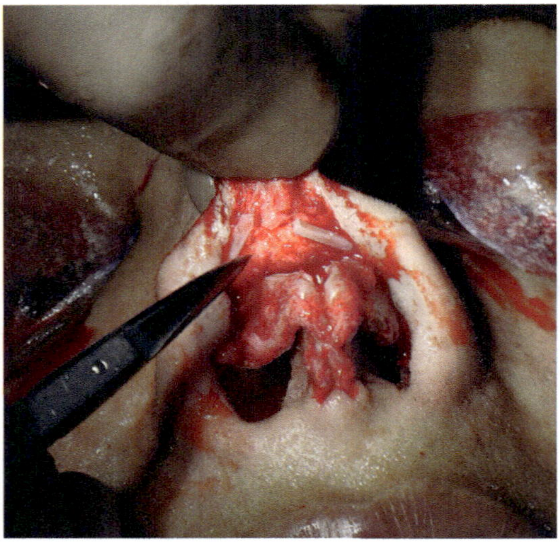

Fig. 4.41 Bilateral rim grafts placed in the pocket created

4.1.10 Alaplasty (Explained in Detail in Chap. 9)

Alaplasty is done either in the same sitting or as a staged procedure.

Commonest alar base reductions are:

1. Nostril sill excision
2. Wedge excision
3. Hockey stick excision

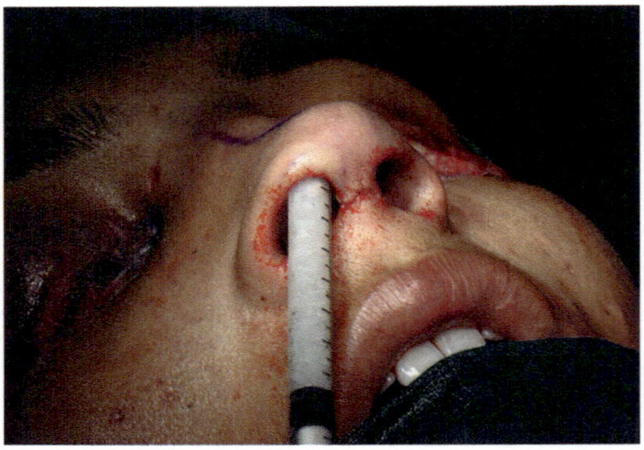

Fig. 4.42 FDC inserted into the nose to smoothen the irregularities

It helps in decreasing the alar show and flare.

It is more commonly required in Indian noses as compared to Caucasian noses.

4.2 Post-Operative Care

Post-operative care is just as important as performing rhinoplasty. To simplify in understanding, it is explained under immediate and late post-op care.

4.2.1 Immediate Post-op Care

(Figs. 4.43, 4.44 and 4.45)

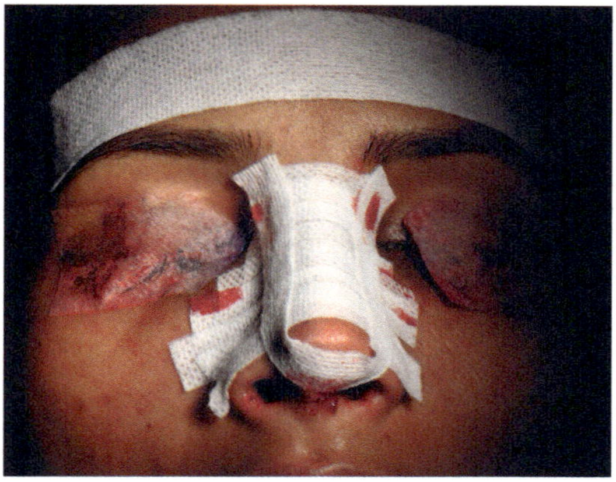

Fig. 4.43 Post-operative taping

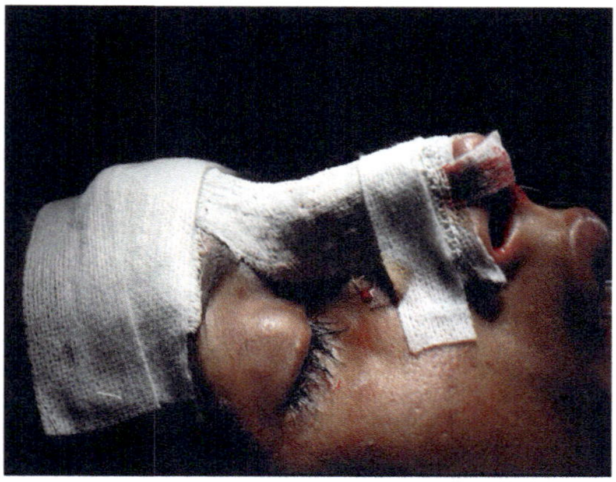

Fig. 4.44 Post-operative plaster of Paris

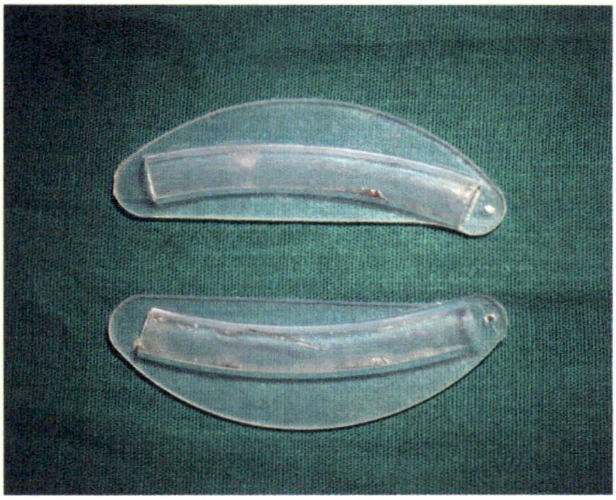

Fig. 4.45 Doyle nasal splints placed in both nasal cavities following surgery and removed after 5 days

This is accounted from the time you finish the surgery to 10 days post-operative.

Dressing has to be done with taping from glabella to tip. This is to be done in a pyramid fashion with each tape covering half of the previous tape:

- Check for postnasal bleeding.
- Head end elevation.

Plaster of Paris is applied over the tape if osteotomies are performed, and it is maintained for 10 days.

And both are kept for 10 days along with the sutures. However, we also use internal nasal splints which will keep the nostrils partially blocked, and this will be removed after 5 days.

Medications

- Antibiotics
- Anti-inflammatory
- Antihistaminics
- Saline nasal spray with decongestant

These are advised for 10 days in a primary case, but saline spray is continued for 1 month:

- Before dressing, ensure patient has had food to avoid vasovagal/hypoglycaemic attack.
- Regular dressing with warm water/saline to remove crusting.
- Keep the incision site clean and moist with ointment.
- Cast removal is done by a gentle rocking motion.
- Taping removal done gently with saline or benzoin by not stretching the skin.

4.2.2 Late Post-op Care

Visits of the Patient

It is on the 5th day, 10th day and after 1 month, 3 months and 1 year following surgery unless otherwise called for. Final post-operative result will be decided after one entire year, and no revision or secondary surgery is considered within 1 year. However, after 3 months one can know as to how their nose will look eventually because the oedema would have settled completely. Post-operative photographs are taken after 3 months and after 1 year.

4.3 Documentation

This is very important where each intraoperative step with pre- and post-operative photographs is kept in one place to revisit and know what was done to the patient on follow-ups. This is of huge advantage in a learning curve to know what better can be done in the subsequent surgeries.

4.4 Note on Piezoelectric Device

It is a true revolution for nasal bones in rhinoplasty. Piezoelectricity is very powerful and therefore can cut highly mineralised bone.

It is used:

1. *To narrow or reduce an open roof following dorsal hump removal*
2. *Straighten deviated nasal bones*
3. *Narrow a broad nasal dorsum*
4. *Reduce dorsal height*
5. *Out-fracture or widen previously narrowed nasal bones*

It decreases the risk of damage to surrounding soft tissues and critical structures as nerves, vessels and mucosa.

When compared to traditional osteotomy, it helps in:

(a) *Reducing bleeding during surgery and in immediate post-operative period*
(b) *Minor oedema*
(c) *Periorbital ecchymosis*
(d) *No visible scarring*

Nasal Septum

5

Main

With more than 2000 rhinoplasties done and a predominant number being secondary/revision surgeries in the last few years, I emphasise enough the need to understand the septum and its pathology and addressing these issues for the successful outcome of rhinoplasty surgery. An understanding of anatomy of the septum, a thorough clinical examination for assessment of the septum pre-operatively and a meticulous planning of tackling the septal deformity if present will help to avoid the risk of complications and need for cumbersome revision procedures. This is of vital importance especially in post-traumatic nasal deformities.

Septum is a midline structure (Fig. 5.1) forming the most important structure for ENT surgeons in rhinoplasty. Since we are trained in detail about septum during our training period, it is not a hard task to tackle septal problems. For plastic surgeons, it is however quite mandatory to learn septoplasty while venturing into the field of rhinoplasty or take an ENT surgeons' assistance for septoplasty. It is interesting to know that the pathology of the septum ranks high among the deformities of the human body. So, understand-

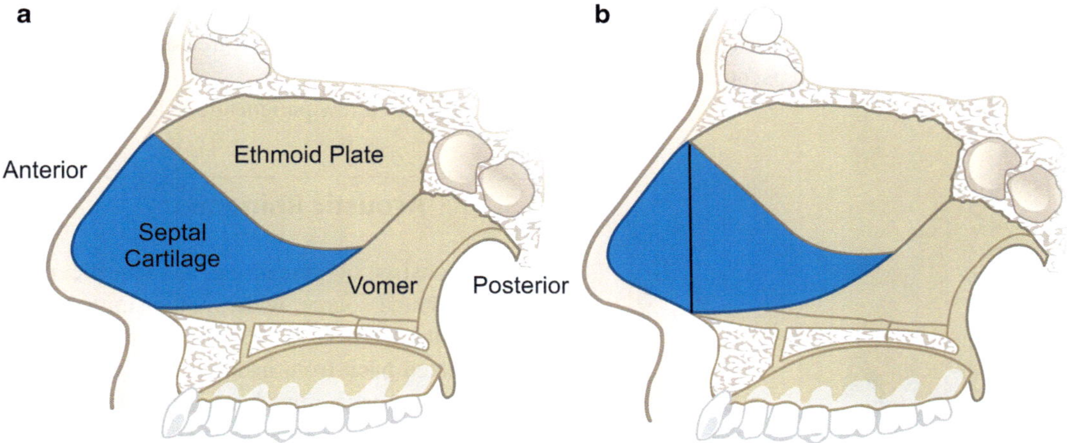

Fig. 5.1 (**a**, **b**) Medial wall of nasal cavity—septum. Vertical black line (Cottle's line) drawn from the frontal process of nasal bone to nasal spine of maxillary crest divides the septum into anterior and posterior segments

V. Ghaisas, *Indian Ethnic Rhinoplasty*, https://doi.org/10.1007/978-981-16-2478-0_5

ing the degree and location of the deformity, which determines the possibility and severity of symptoms, is important.

5.1 Internal Nasal Valve Area (Fig. 5.2)

It is defined as the narrowest portion of the human airway. This forms almost two-thirds of the total nasal airway resistance; hence, collapse or stenosis of this area is thought to be one of the common causes of nasal obstruction. It is a triangular shaped nasal resistor formed by lower margin of ULC, head of inferior turbinate and corresponding aspect of the septum. It has an area of about 50–70 mm^2 forming an angle of about 10–15 degrees.

This area is the one well targeted with rhinoplasty.

Rhinomanometry is important to diagnose nasal obstruction (Figs. 5.3 and 5.4).

It is a functional test of nasal aerodynamics that measures trans-nasal airflow and the pressure gradient allowing nasal resistance to be calculated from these data. It is used for the clinical evaluation of the symptoms of nasal obstruction (Demarrias et al. 2011).

Active rhinomanometry is routinely done for all patients with suspected nasal obstruction at our centre and in all rhinoplasty patients. Here, the pressure-sensing tube is normally taped to

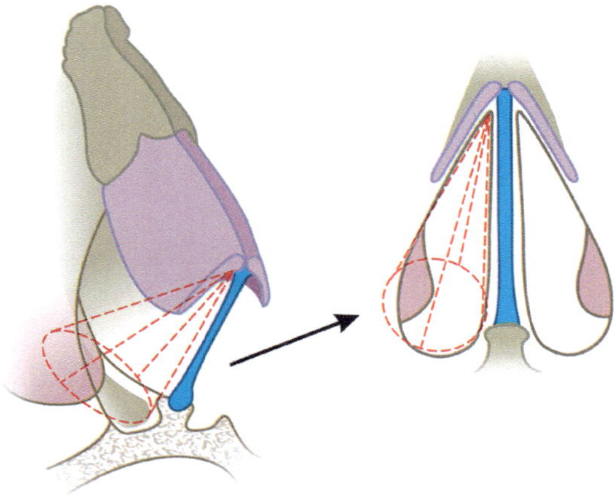

Fig. 5.2 Internal nasal valve area

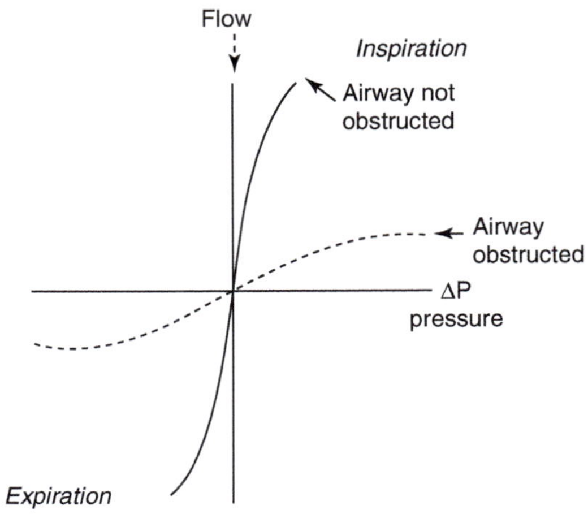

Fig. 5.3 Rhinomanometry graph

one nasal passage. The sealed nasal passage acts as an extension of the pressure-sensing tube to measure pressure in the posterior nares. With this method, nasal airflow is measured from one nostril at a time, and the pressure-sensing tube is moved from one side of the nose to the other. Therefore, the nasal resistance is determined separately for each nasal passage.

Nasal airflow is plotted on a graph against pressure. Normally, it is a sigmoid pressure-flow curve. Patients with genuine nasal obstruction will have high resistance, which is seen as a decreasing slope on the graph. It offers a genuine objective measure of the degree of impairment of nasal airflow.

Graphs of a few patients done at our centre:

5.2 Acoustic Rhinometry

This consists of generating an acoustic pulse from a sound source, which is transmitted along a tube into the nose. The sound from pulse wave is reflected back from inside the nose according to local acoustic impedance. Rhinomanometry and acoustic rhinometry are complementary. Rhinomanometry is a valuable objective test for substantiating nasal obstruction and quantifying nasal resistance. However, acoustic rhinometry is useful for confirming specific sites of airway restriction.

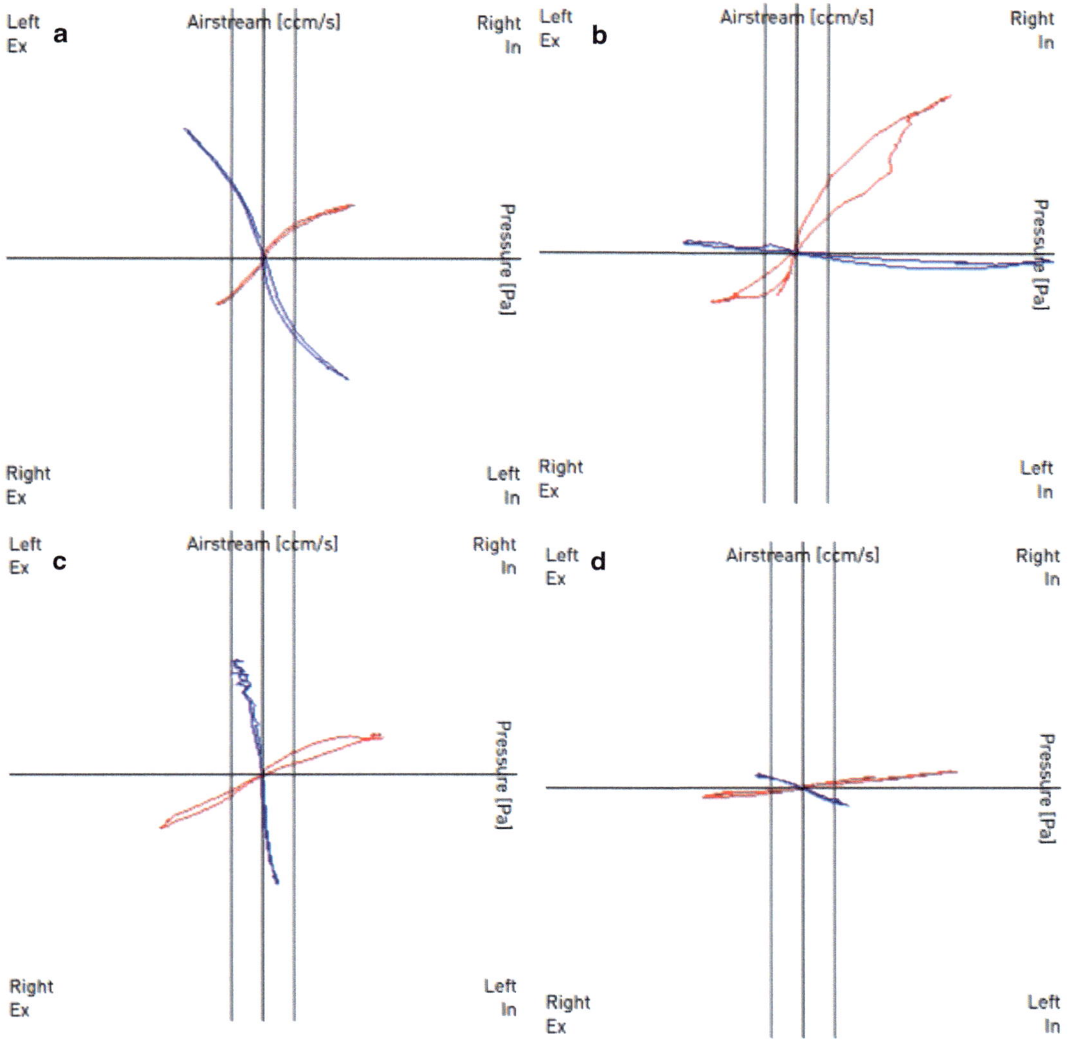

Fig. 5.4 Graph is plotted against pressure produced for airflow (y-axis) and airstream (x-axis). Right—red colour. Left—blue colour

5.3 Etiology of Nasal Septal Deviations

Direct Trauma

- It is frequently associated with damage to other parts of the nose such as fractures of nasal bone, and one should always keep in mind about the effects on the septum during trauma. To simplify further for the beginners, Gray's line is taken into consideration (Fig. 5.5), and any septal fractures anterior to this line tend to be vertically oriented, whereas those posterior to this line are usually horizontally oriented. So, you can keep this in mind while performing septoplasty.

Birth Moulding Theory

- Abnormal intrauterine posture of the foetus may result in compression forces on the nose and upper jaws and cause displacement of the septum during birth (Fig. 5.6a–d).

Differential Growth Between Nasal Septum and Palate

- The nasal septum sometimes is known to grow faster in few people than the palate, and then the nasal septum starts to buckle under pressure.
- Also, it is mostly seen in cases of high-arched palate (paying attention to the presence/absence of high-arched palate is very important for septoplasty and for crest excision); otherwise, an overzealous resection of crest can be done with a resultant palatal perforation.

Congenital malformations, like cleft noses, have very typical septal deviations in the midportion to the cleft side and caudally to the normal side.

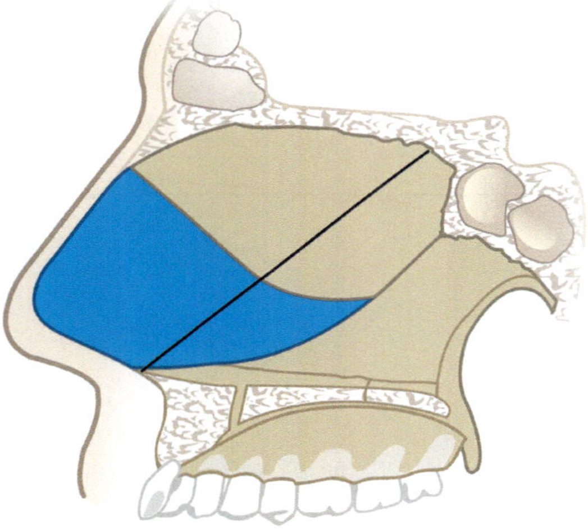

Fig. 5.5 Black line—Gray's line oblique line. (**a**) Septal fractures anterior to this line, vertical; (**b**) septal fractures posterior to this line, horizontal

The diseases of the septum and internal nose septal abscess and granulomatous disease of the nose may cause resorption of the supporting structures leading to collapse of nasal valves and deviation. These cases are characterised by a massive deformation/deformities in all levels of the septum with consequent blockage of one or both nostrils.

5.3.1 Classification of Nasal Septal Deviations

Various classifications of septal deviations are proposed like Baumann classification, Mladina classification, Jang classification and Bahman Guyuron. Yet, there is no universally accepted classification of the septal deviation till now for guiding the surgeon to do proper intervention in treating the problem. However, majority of the currently published classification systems for internal nasal septal deviations can be summarised as C-shaped or reverse C-shaped, S-shaped or reverse S-shaped deviations in the anteroposterior and cephalo-caudal dimensions (Figs. 5.7, 5.8, 5.9, 5.10, 5.11 and 5.12).

So, for the purpose of surgical considerations, classification proposed by Bahman Guyuron is most appropriate, which proposes six classes of septal deviation (Figs. 5.13, 5.14, 5.15, 5.16, 5.17 and 5.18).

1. *Septal tilt* (Fig. 5.13): The most common type of septal deviation is a septal tilt, in which the septum itself has no significant underlying curvature but is tilted to one side because the caudal septum is dislodged to one side of the

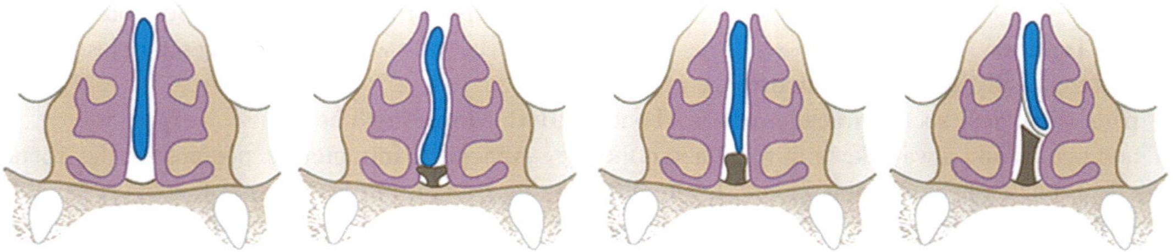

Fig. 5.6 (**a–d**) Septal displacement during birth (**a, c**)—normal (**b, d**)—displaced septum

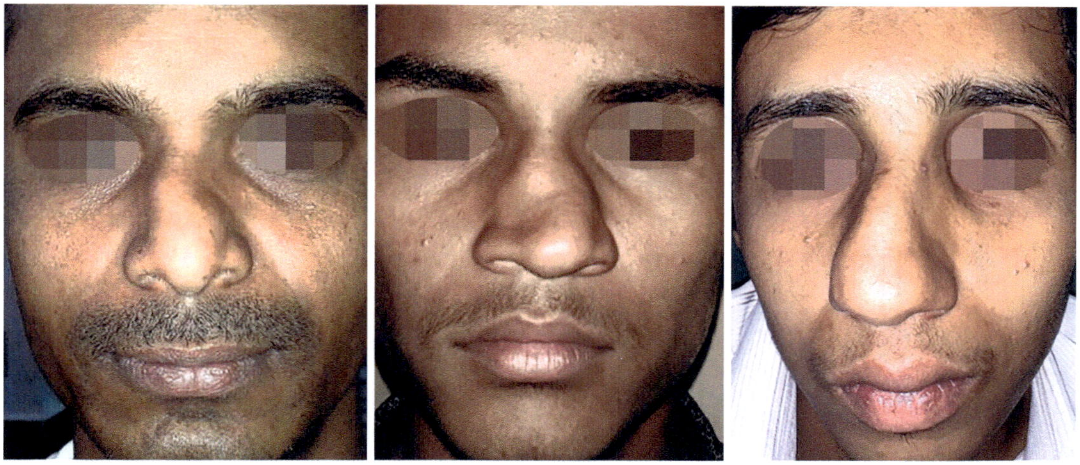

Figs. 5.7–5.9 (left: Fig. 5.7): S-shaped deviation; (middle: Fig. 5.8): Reverse S-shaped deviation; (right: Fig. 5.9): C-shaped deviation

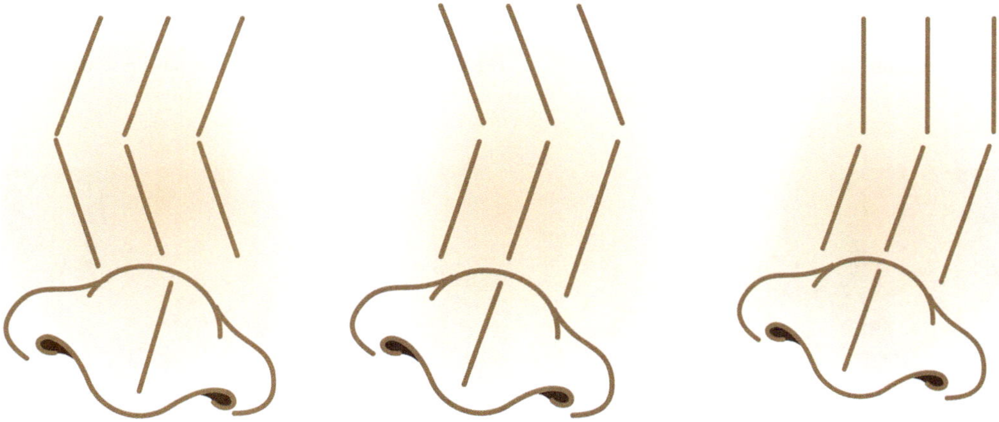

Figs. 5.10–5.12 (left: Fig. 5.10): S-shaped deviation; (middle: Fig. 5.11): Reverse S-shaped deviation; (right: Fig. 5.12): C-shaped deviation

vomer bone. In most cases of septal tilt, the internal dislodgement of the septum is to one side, and the external deviation of the nose is to the opposite side.

2. *C-shaped anteroposterior (caudal) deviation* (Fig. 5.14) is usually associated with deviation of the vomer plate. External reflection of the anteroposterior C deviation is often similar to the septal tilt.
3. *S-shaped anteroposterior (caudal) deviation* (Fig. 5.15) is defined by two opposite curvatures in continuity in the anteroposterior direction. Externally, the anteroposterior deviation will present with a shift of the nose to the left or right. Rarely, the anterior portion of the nose may look totally straight.
4. *C-shaped cephalo-caudal (dorsal) deviation* (Fig. 5.16) is similar to the previous type

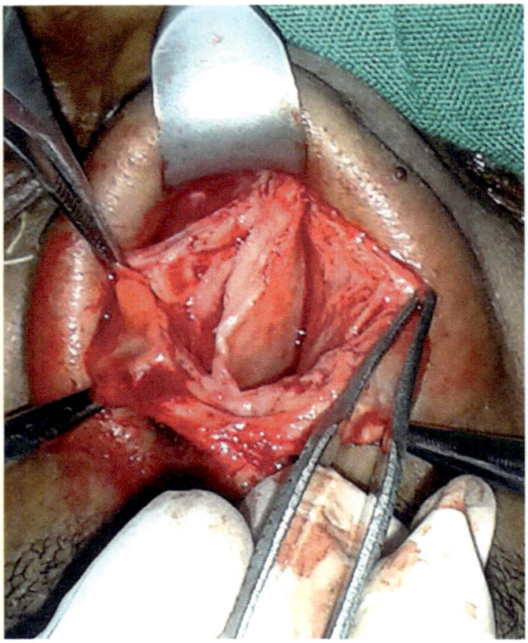

Fig. 5.13 Septal tilt

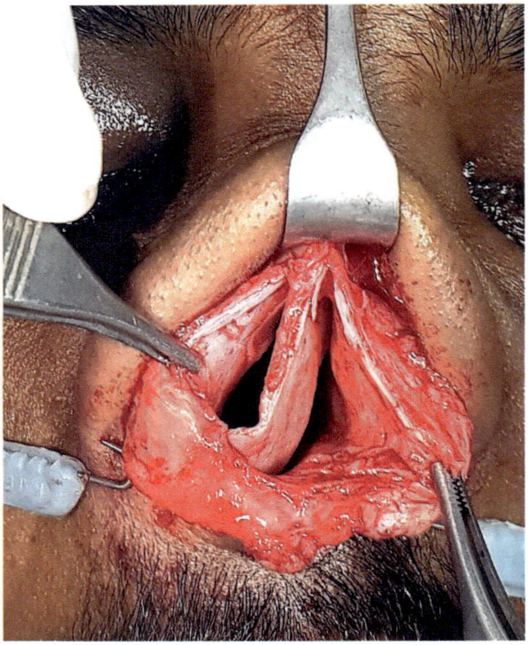

Fig. 5.14 C-shaped caudal (anteroposterior) deviation

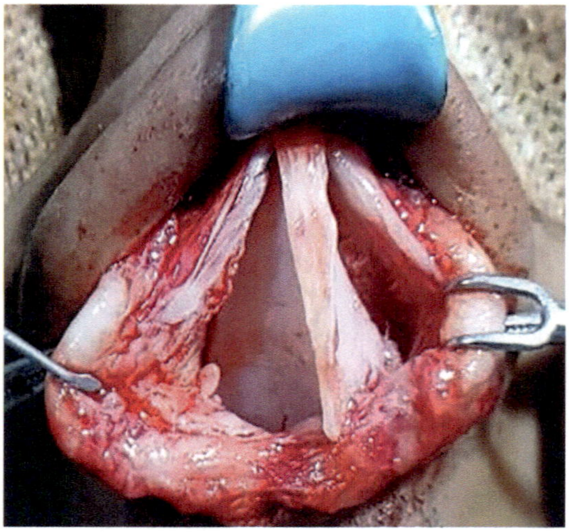

Fig. 5.15 S-shaped caudal (anteroposterior) deviation

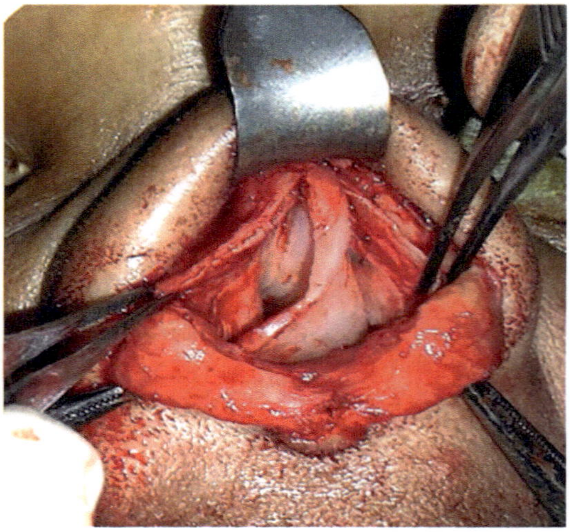

Fig. 5.16 C-shaped dorsal (cephalo-caudal) deviation

except that the curvatures are in cephalo-caudal direction. The external nose follows the pattern of the septal deviation.

5. *S-shaped cephalo-caudal (dorsal) deviation* (Fig. 5.17) is defined by two opposite curvatures in continuity in the cephalo-caudal direction. The external nose follows the pattern of the septal deviation.
6. *Localised deviation or spur* (Fig. 5.18) is the last type of septal deviation. This is a purely functional problem and has no translation to the external shape of the nose.

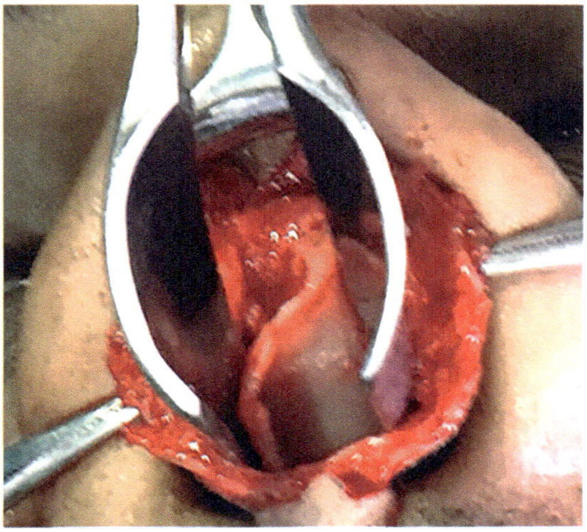

Fig. 5.17 S-shaped dorsal (cephalo-caudal) deviation

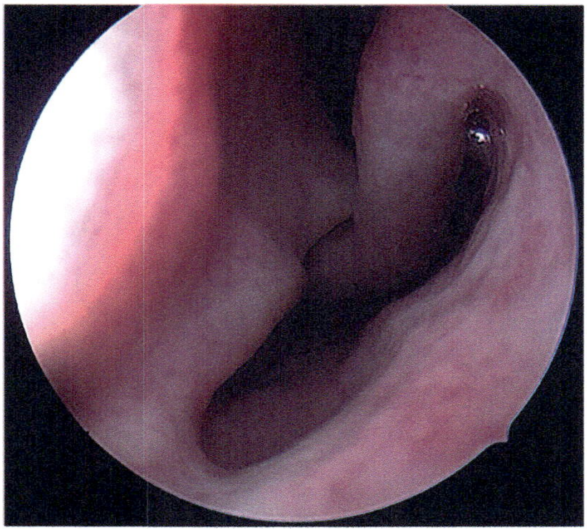

Fig. 5.18 Isolated septal spur

5.3.2 Examination of the Patient

Assessment of the deformity and the internal nasal examination should be done thoroughly.

If associated with rhinitis or sinusitis, it should be treated before surgery.

Associated symptoms with septal deformity which should not be missed are:

- Headache/facial pain
  Nose block leads to sinus infection leading to headache and facial pain.
  Gross deviation may be associated with neurological pain
  because of anterior ethmoidal nerve syndrome (Sluder's neuralgia).
  Epistaxis
  It can occur due to friability of mucosa due to repeated infection.
  It can occur due a stretched vessel over the spur which easily bleeds.
  Air currents are abnormally displaced leading to drying of mucosa and crust formation.
- Anosmia/hyposmia
- Middle ear pathology should be documented prior to the surgery.

5.4 Steps of Septoplasty

1. Approach—Hemitransfixion incision (Fig. 5.19) taken at the caudal aspect of the septum.

However, during rhinoplasty the septum is approached by identifying the anterior septal angle after the membranous septum dissection.

2. Elevation of bilateral mucoperichondrial and mucoperiosteal septal layers (Figs. 5.20 and 5.21). During septoplasty, it is very important to elevate the mucoperichondrial flaps without any tear. There should not be both sided mucosal tear at the same site. If there is any tear, it is better to suture it to prevent septal perforation.
3. Deviated ethmoid is removed with double-action scissors and then by Lucs' forceps to avoid injury to the cribriform plate. Ethmoid plate can be used for splinting later on if needed (Fig. 5.22).
4. Resection of the cartilaginous dorsum leaving behind 1 cm dorso-caudal L strut (Figs. 5.23, 5.24, 5.25 and 5.26).
5. Deviated maxillary crest is removed by gouge and hammer or by drilling.

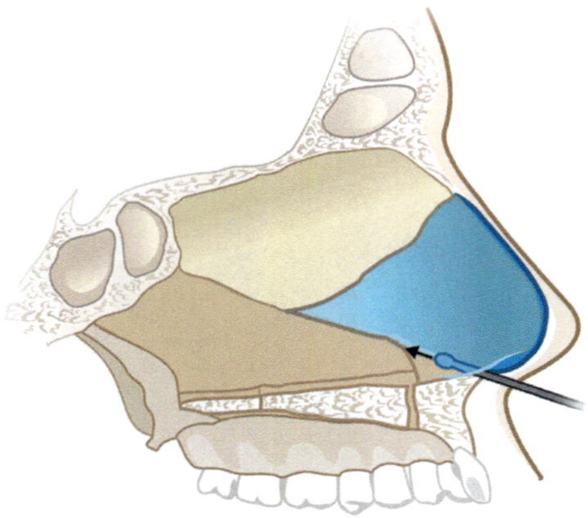

Fig. 5.19 Septal incision

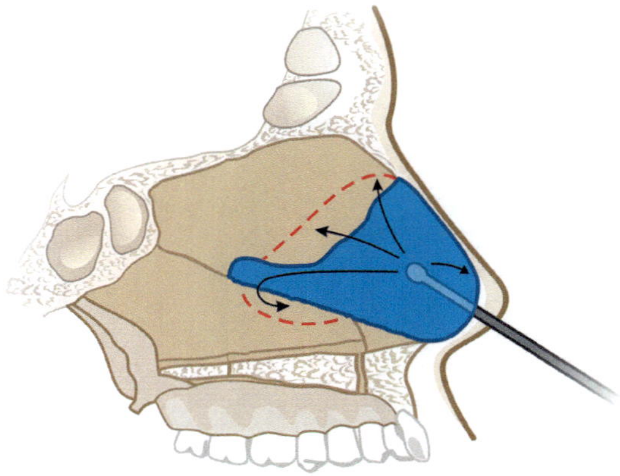

Fig. 5.20 Mucoperichondrial flap elevation

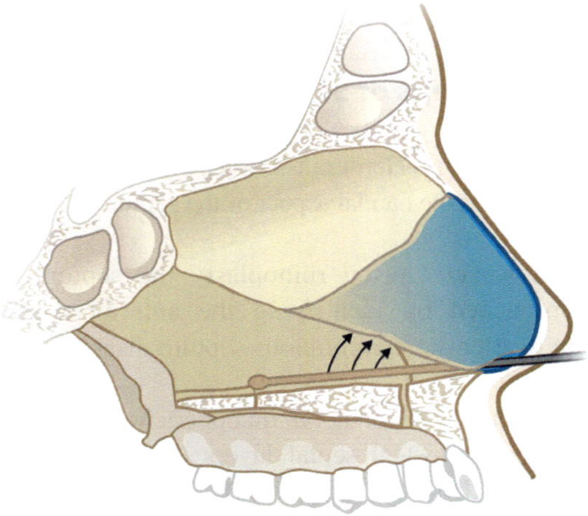

Fig. 5.21 Mucoperiosteal flap elevation

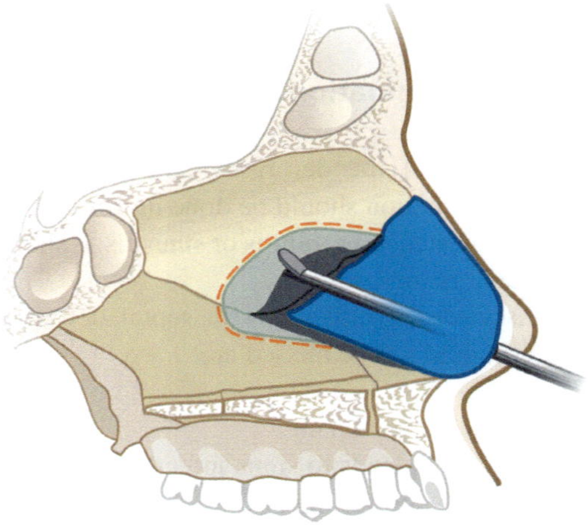

Fig. 5.22 Deviated ethmoid bone removal

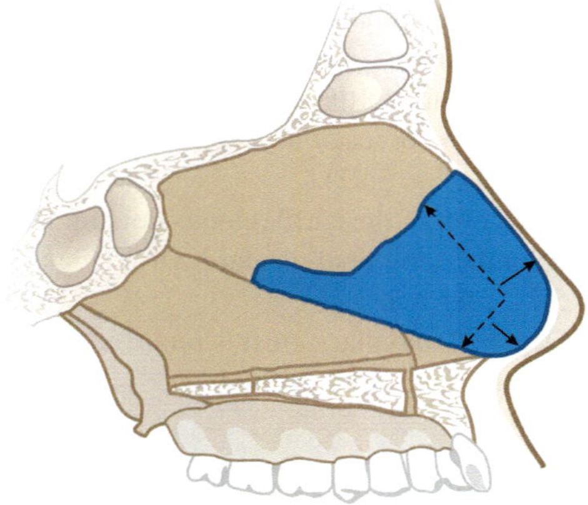

Fig. 5.23 Dorso-caudal L 1 cm strut retained

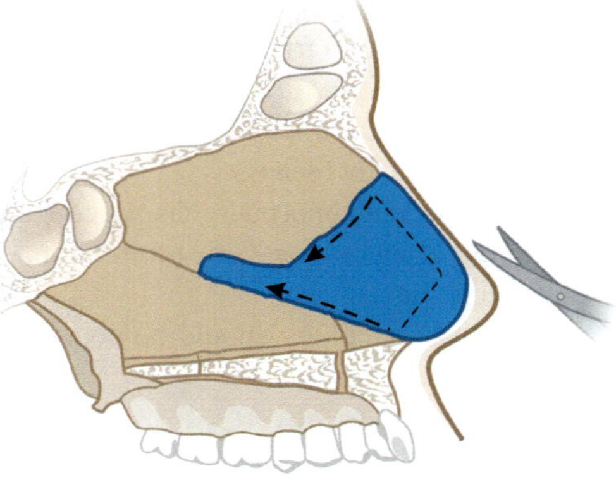

Fig. 5.24 Cartilaginous septum is cut

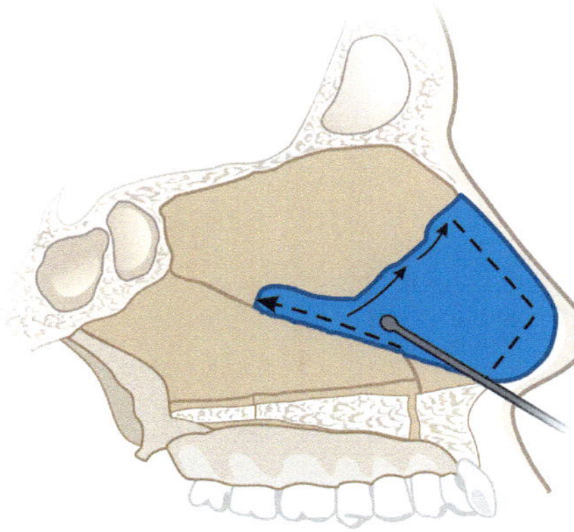

Fig. 5.25 Cartilage separated from posterior and inferior aspect

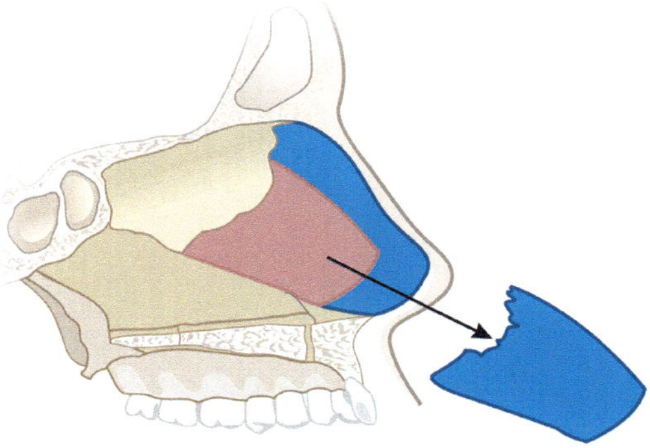

Fig. 5.26 Septal graft harvested

Treating a High Septal Deviation

A high deviation at the internal nasal valve area will cause nasal obstruction and always a challenge to treat via conventional septoplasty. Hence advisable for an open septoplasty and treat further with spreader grafts, ethmoid splint or partial extracorporeal septoplasty (discussed in detail in deviated/crooked nose deformity).

Caudal Dislocation

Anterior nasal spine (ANS) is an important structure usually present in the midline.

Septal attachment from ANS is released to treat caudal dislocation, i.e. a conventional 'swing door technique' is done and sutured to the ANS after drilling it with sharp Lindemann's burr. Partial-thickness scoring is not of much use. However, partial scoring, if done, should be paired with ethmoid splinting. Another method, popularised by Prof. Yong Ju Jang, is that the caudal septal batten graft created from the harvested septal bone was fitted to the desired location, usually on the concave side (but on both sides if concerns about graft tilt were present), and fixed with 5-0 polydioxanone sutures (PDS).

The Indian rhinoplasty surgeon must be mindful of all regional variations, which have an important impact on the surgical outcome. Surgeons outside of India operating on Indian migrants also must keep Indian ethnicity in mind.

5.5 Paediatric Septorhinoplasty

This is a separate entity. Details of which are not discussed here.

However, understanding the development of the septum and the site of ossification centres by the surgeon will help in correction of the nose of the child:

- Two ossification centres appear for the vomer on either side of the cartilage at the anterior end uniting to form a deep bony groove in which the cartilage sits.
- One ossification centre appears for perpendicular plate of ethmoid in the postero-superior aspect, which grows downwards and forwards (Fig. 5.27).

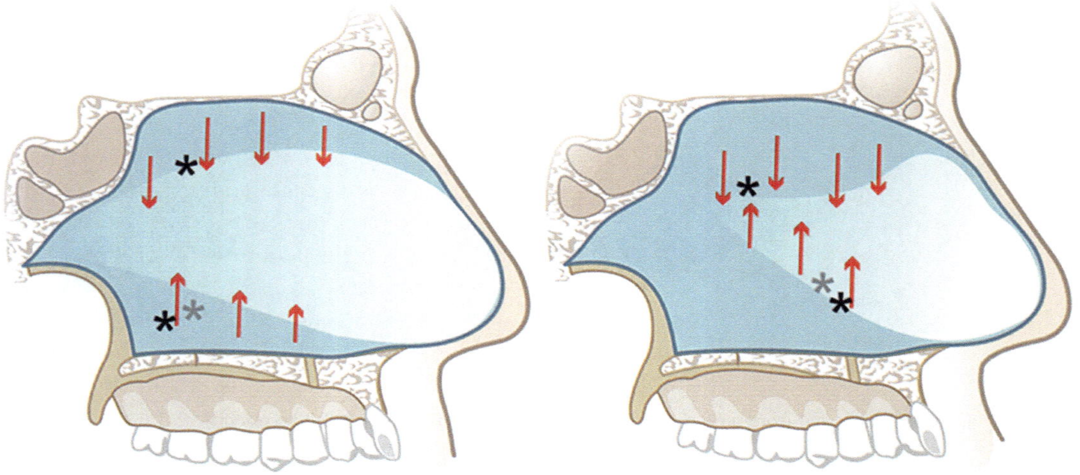

Fig. 5.27 Ossification centres of perpendicular plate of ethmoid and vomer

The primitive septum is entirely made of cartilage. The superior part ossifies to form the perpendicular plate of ethmoid (from the crista galli downwards) and the vomer in the postero-inferior portion, leaving an antero-inferior cartilaginous plate. One should understand the septum and the limitations of septoplasty in paediatric cases, where the growth centres in the bony part must be known and attention must be paid to not damage the developing growing septum.

Saddle Nose Deformity: Augmentation Rhinoplasty

6

Main

Saddle nose deformity, as the name suggests, derives its name from the appearance of the nose on a lateral view, where the dorsal curve resembles the depression in a horse's saddle. It is a pathologic entity, resulting from loss of dorsal height caused by a substantial decrease in the cartilaginous or bony vault. This deformity is very dear to us because this is one of the commonest nasal deformities encountered in the rhinoplasty clinic and perhaps one of the most challenging problems as well.

In our practice, nearly 30% of the patients approaching me for rhinoplasty are the ones requiring augmentation rhinoplasty. The basic principle behind augmentation is like constructing a building which requires a basic strong foundation, proper support system and necessary strengths to cartilage. In the post-op recovery period, one should allow sufficient time for strengthening to occur.

Common causes of saddle noses in our experience:

1. Congenital.
2. Traumatic.
3. Iatrogenic:
   (a) Overzealous septal surgery
   (b) Injudicious resection of dorsum during aesthetic surgery
4. Infection.
   (a) Septal abscess.
5. Additional causes like atrophic rhinitis, granulomatous diseases and malignancy may be associated with a deficient dorsum.

Numerous classifications of saddle nose deformity are proposed. Daniel and Brenner (2006) suggested a classification which considered clinical findings and pathophysiological features for better surgical planning.

6.1 Modified Classification for Indian Patients

As we all know, we have multiple regional variations in India; hence, to have a uniform thought, for simplifying the defect and to have an easier way to treat and surgically manage, we have considered *skin texture* as an additional criterion in the classification.

There are broadly two types of skin (Fig. 6.1):

(a) *Normal or thin skin*—easy to manoeuvre thin skin and the skin is pinchable as it has very less amount of fibro-fatty tissue in supratip area along with strong alar cartilages. Thus, the expected aesthetic results and even subtle changes in the structure are very well drap-

V. Ghaisas, *Indian Ethnic Rhinoplasty*, https://doi.org/10.1007/978-981-16-2478-0_6

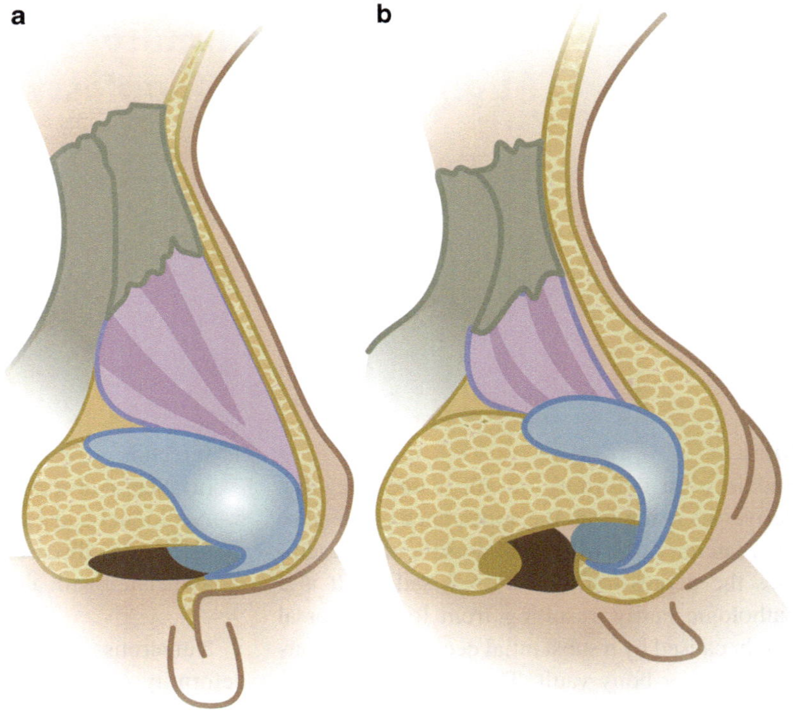

Fig. 6.1 (**a**) Thin skin with less fibro-fatty tissue. (**b**) Thick skin with more fibro-fatty tissue

able. But on the other side, even minor irregularities can be prominently visible.

(b) *Thick skin*—relatively difficult to manoeuvre intraoperatively. It is more forgiving as it generally masks the minor defects. But subtle changes made are difficult to appreciate. Thus, changes made through augmentation are more likely to transmit through a thick skin envelope, and changes made in the form of reduction are less likely to transmit through thick skin.

6.2 Skin Thickness

Skin pinch test is simple yet a very reliable method to test the quality and type of the skin.

Normal or thin skin is easily pinchable which suggests that the fibro-fatty tissue layer also is thin and the skin is pliable, whereas a skin pinch test is difficult in a thick skin which in turn suggests that the fibro-fatty tissue is bulky and tough underneath and will pose surgical problems. It also causes difficulty in adapting to the modified osseo-cartilaginous framework, with the possibility of less satisfactory results for both the surgeon and the patient. The post-operative oedema in thick skin is more noticeable in the supratip area as post-operatively the patient may continue to have some bulbosity or a soft tissue pollybeak deformity. Also, in case of a thick sebaceous skin, removal of subcutaneous tissue, especially in the supratip area, may be undertaken. To control or reduce the resultant dead space, supratip suture can be considered. Secondary defects are commonly encountered in patients with a thick skin. With thin skin, as is seen in the patients from the Himalayan region, extra attention must be paid for the smoothness of the graft. DCF has been my preferred grafting material in such cases.

6.3 Classification

A. *Type 0* (Figs. 6.2, 6.3, 6.4 and 6.5)

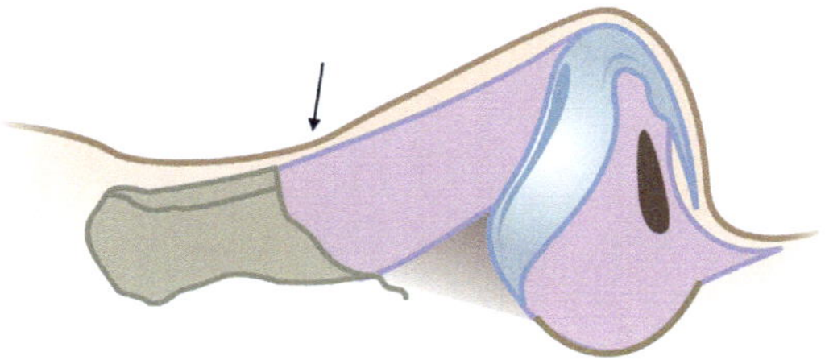

Fig. 6.2 *Type 0* minor deformity seen on the dorsum

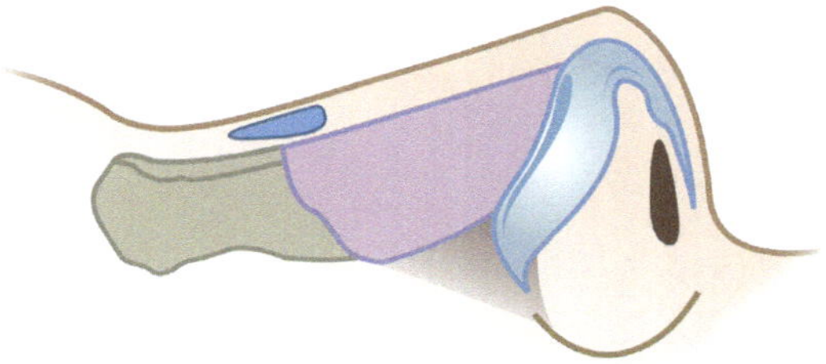

Fig. 6.3 Sketch showing free diced cartilage on the dorsum to mask the pseudo-deformity

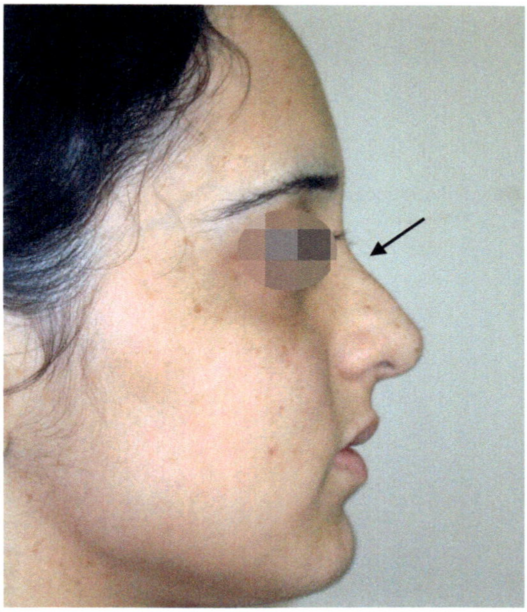

Fig. 6.4 Lateral view pre-op. Arrow showing depression in the bony dorsum

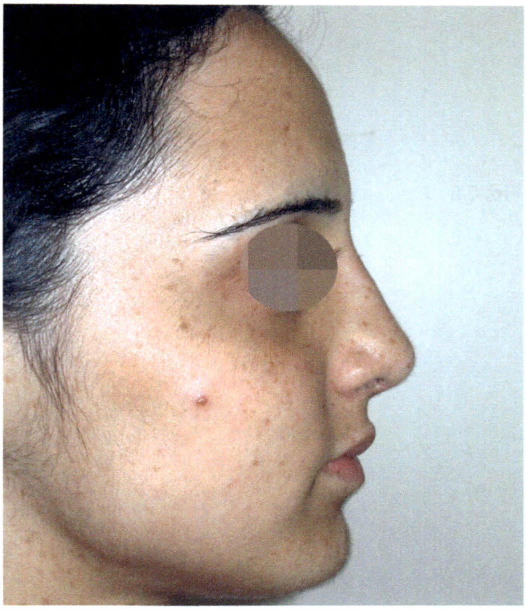

Fig. 6.5 Lateral view post-op. Free diced cartilage has improved the deformity

- Is minor or pseudo-saddle deformity—depression of cartilaginous or bony dorsum. All the other structural integrity is intact. Skin type is mostly thin in these individuals:
  - The correction for these involves minimal augmentation with a fine paste of *free diced* cartilage. It takes care of small irregularities and gives excellent results in thin-skinned patients.

B. *Type 1* (Figs. 6.6, 6.7, 6.8, 6.9 and 6.10)

- Involves greater supratip depression and columellar retraction with minor decrease in septal support. In this type, skin type is thin in most of the individuals:
  - These cases require minor cosmetic concealment by the use of soft tissues like temporalis fascia/rectus fascia or *free diced cartilage* for augmentation of dorsum and columella.
  - Columellar strut or septal extension graft is used to correct the columellar retraction.
  - Minimal supratip depression is dealt by cephalic rotation of alar cartilage.

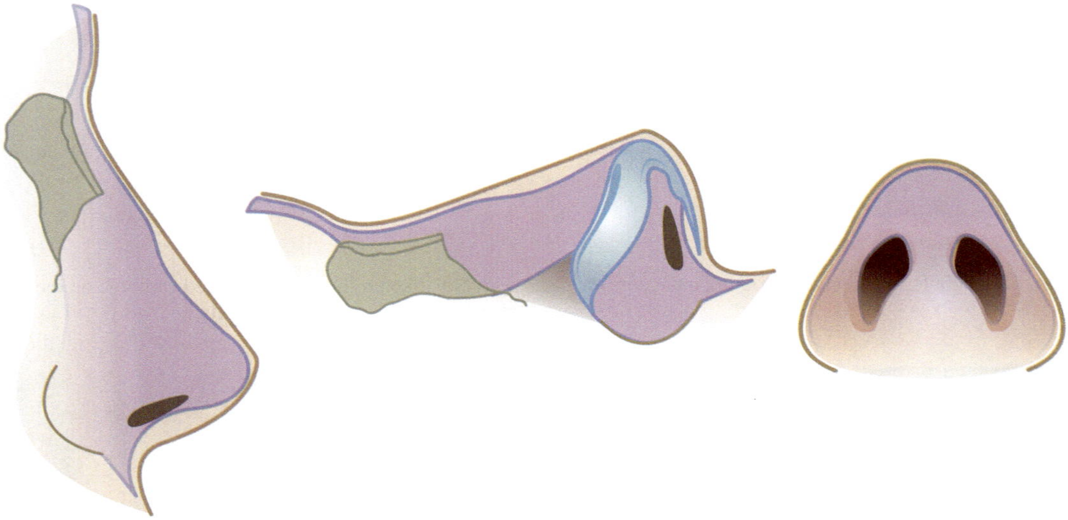

Fig. 6.6 *Type 1 deformity* showing supratip depression with columellar retraction

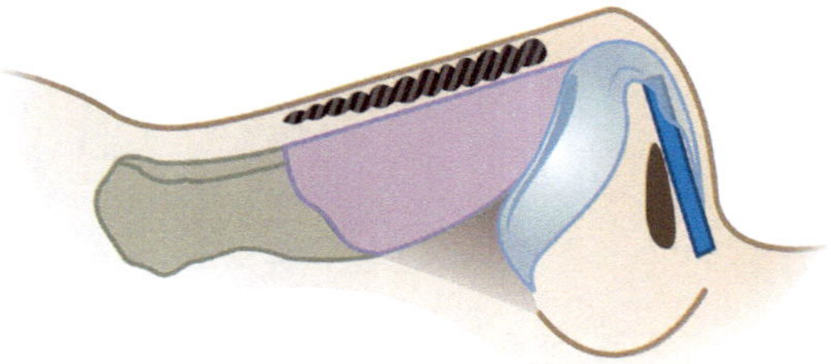

Fig. 6.7 Augmentation by rectus or temporalis facia with or without free diced cartilage

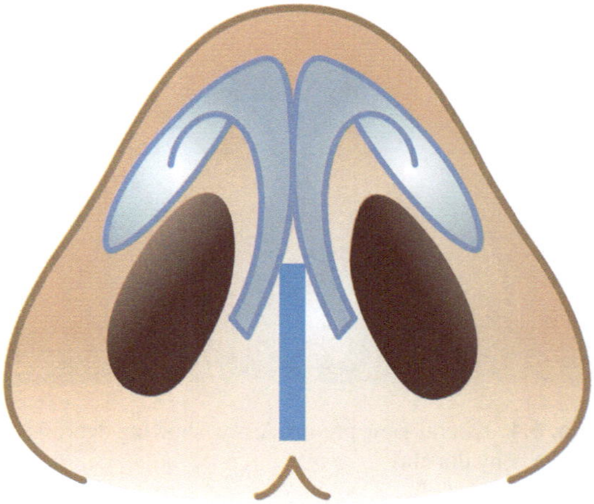

Fig. 6.8 Columellar strut

C. *Type 2* (Figs. 6.11, 6.12, 6.13, 6.14, 6.15, 6.16 and 6.17) deformity has progressive weakening of septal support, collapse of cartilaginous middle vault, columellar retraction and loss of tip support. Nasal obstruction is common, secondary to internal valve collapse. Skin type can be thick or thin in these individuals:

- For this deformity the septal support is established by reconstruction with autologous septal, conchal or costal cartilage. Augmentation is achieved by *DCF* in thin skin and *stacked cartilage with fascia* in thick-skinned individuals. For the valve collapse, extended spreader grafts are used, and columellar retraction is corrected by columellar strut graft or septal extension graft (SEG).

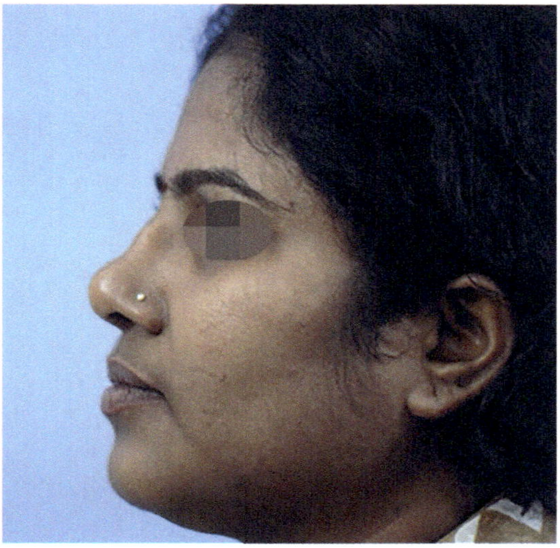

Fig. 6.9 Pre-op lateral view

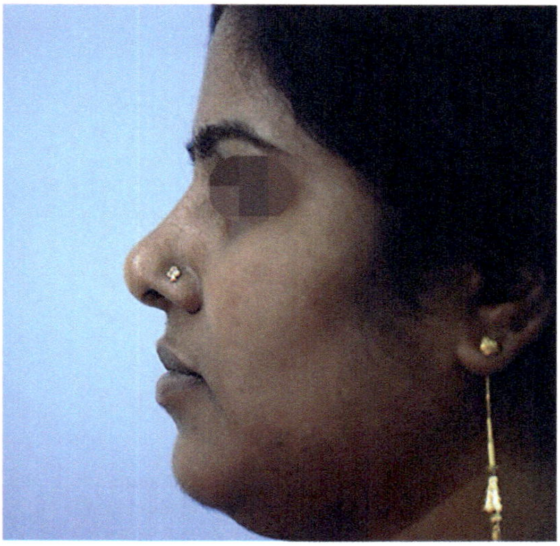

Fig. 6.10 Post-op lateral view

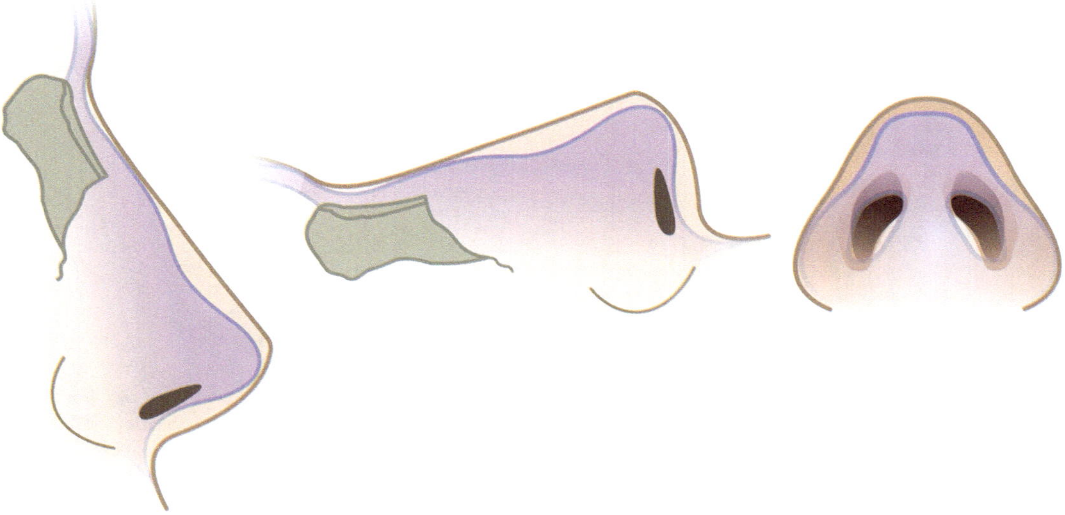

Fig. 6.11 Type 2 deformity showing collapse of cartilaginous vault and columellar retraction

D. *Type 3* (Figs. 6.18, 6.19, 6.20, 6.21, 6.22, 6.23, 6.24, 6.25, 6.26, 6.27, 6.28, 6.29 and 6.30) deformity is indicated by obvious flattening and depression of middle vault. It involves disarticulation of septum or septal perforation, loss of caudal septal support, columellar retrusion, splaying of upper lateral cartilage and upward rotation of the tip. Skin type is mostly thick in these individuals:

- Management is by major composite reconstruction with costal cartilage. Extended spreader grafts are used for lengthening along with septal extension graft (SEG) which is anchored to the anterior nasal spine with establishment of upper lateral cartilage and septal relationship. The tip malpositioning is corrected by suturing techniques and shield and peg tip grafts.

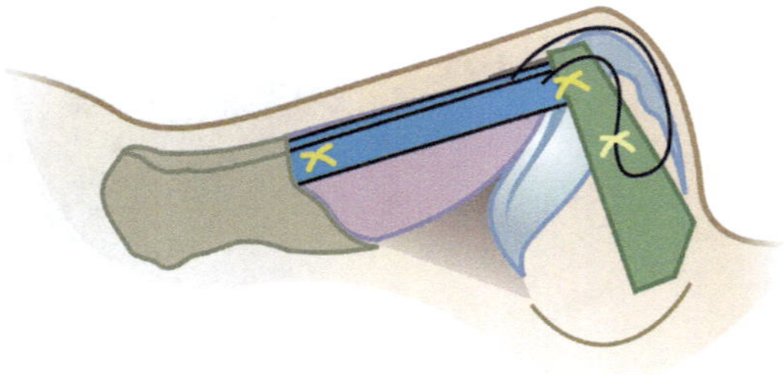

Fig. 6.12 Reconstruction with autologous cartilage. With extended spreader and septal extension graft

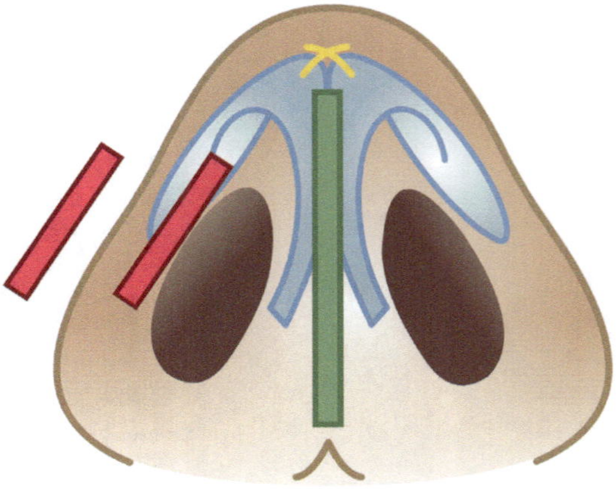

Fig. 6.13 Basal view showing SEG and alar rim grafts

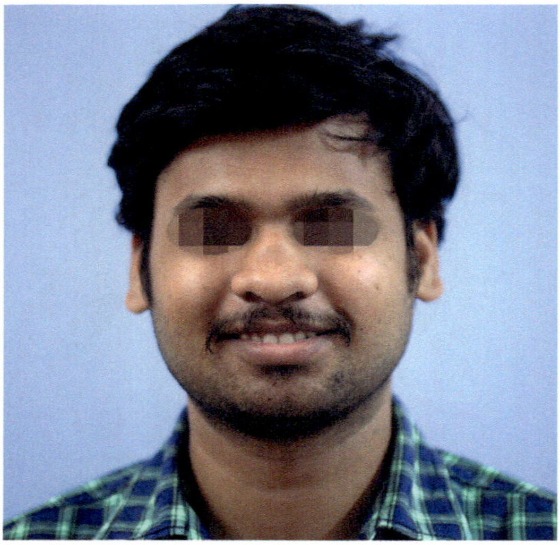

Fig. 6.14 Pre-op frontal view

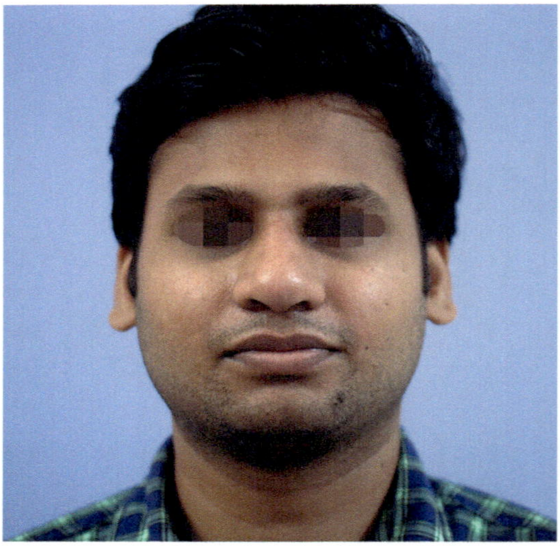

Fig. 6.15 Post-op frontal view

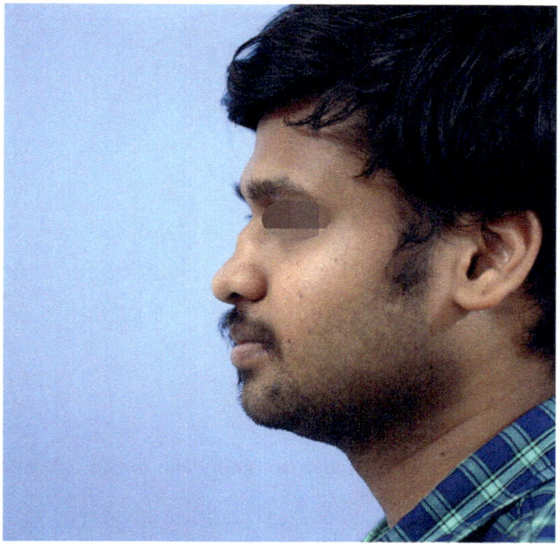

Fig. 6.16 Pre-op lateral view

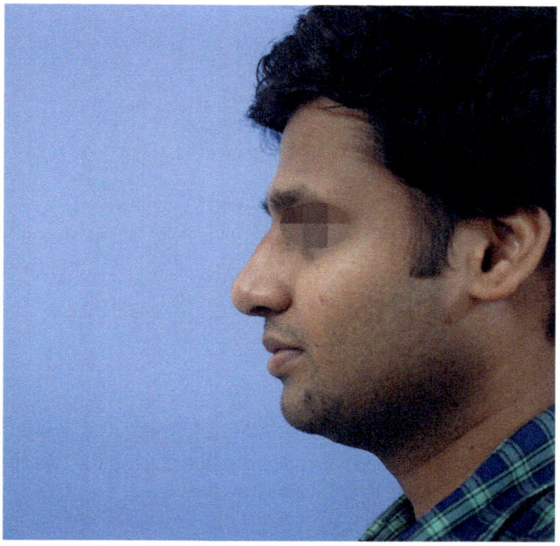

Fig. 6.17 Post-op lateral view

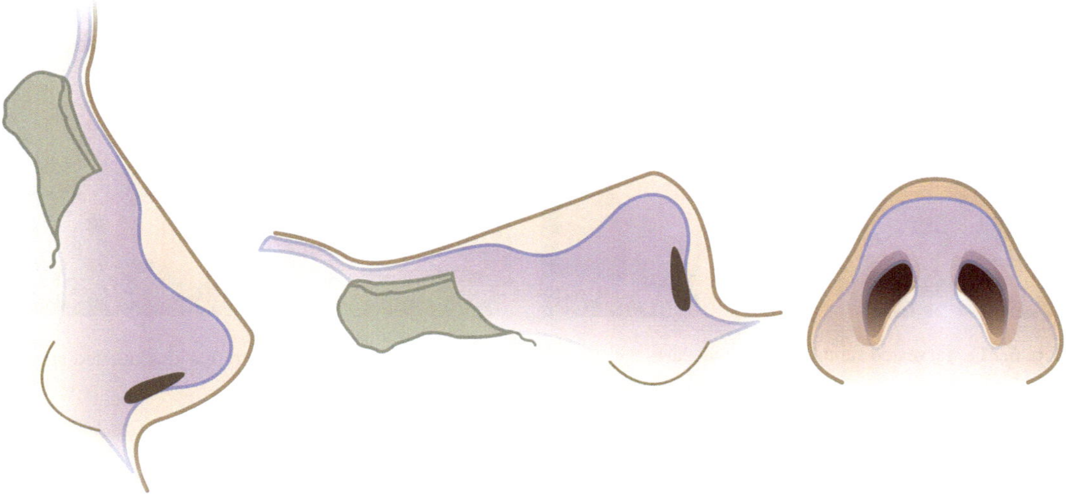

Fig. 6.18 Type 3 deformity with depression of middle vault. Loss of caudal septal support, columellar retrusion and splaying of upper lateral cartilage

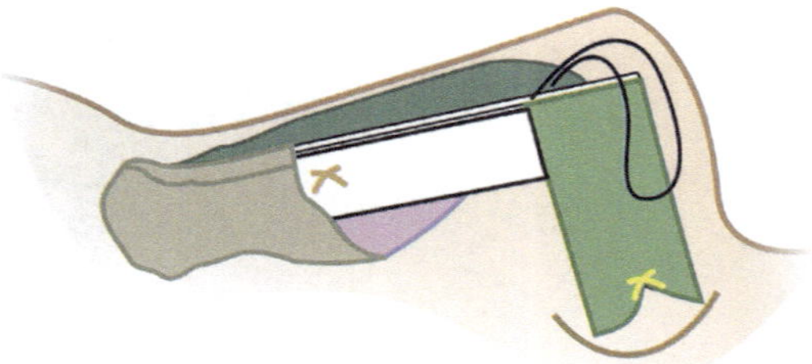

Fig. 6.19 Extended spreader grafts are used for lengthening along with septal extension graft

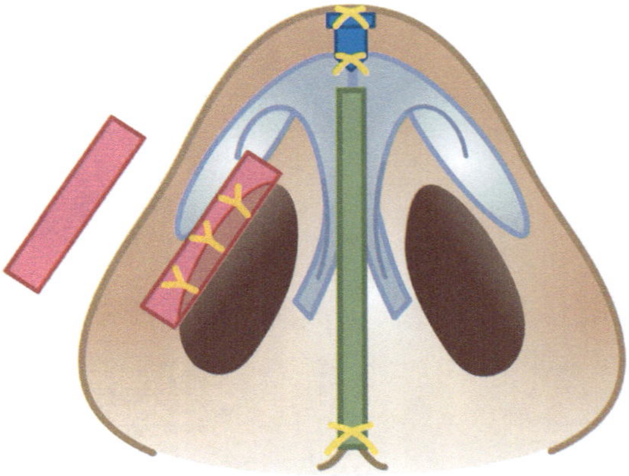

Fig. 6.20 SEG with alar rim grafts and dorsal onlay or peg tip grafts

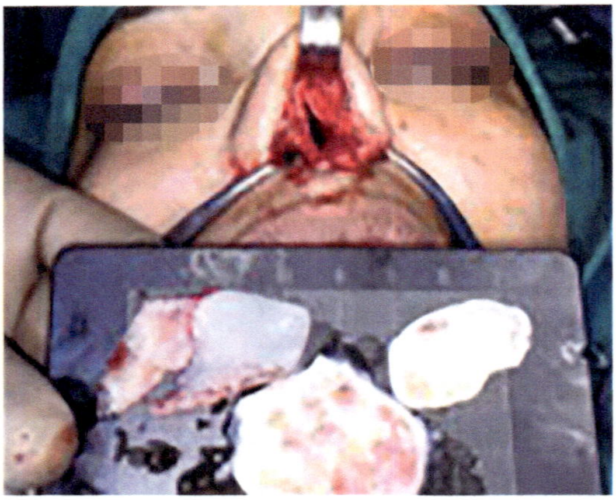

Fig. 6.21 Harvested septal and conchal cartilage

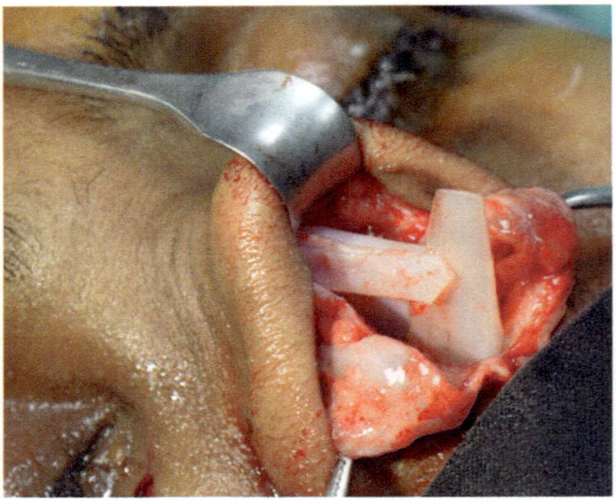

Fig. 6.22 Septal extension graft with extended spreader grafts

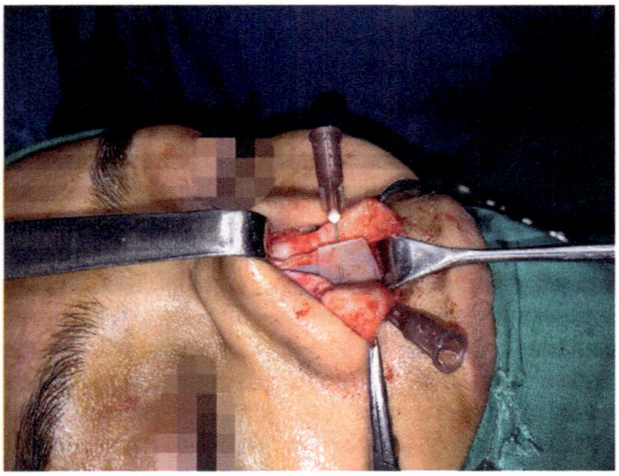

Fig. 6.23 Septal extension graft

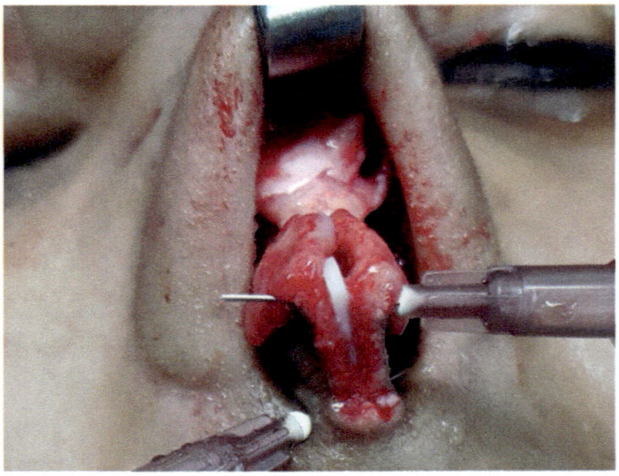

Fig. 6.24 Columellar strut

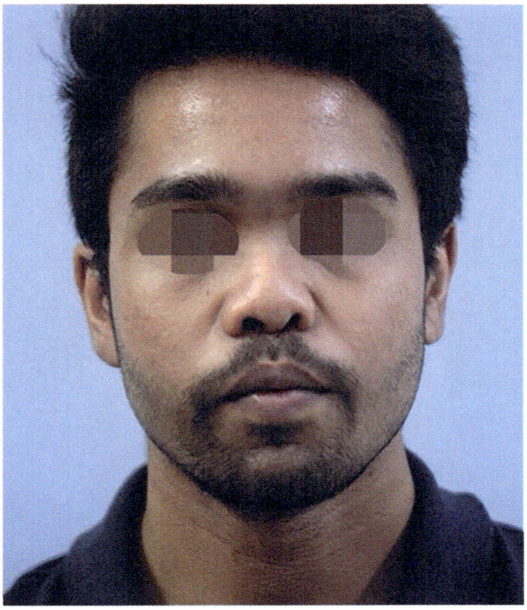

Fig. 6.25 Pre-op frontal view

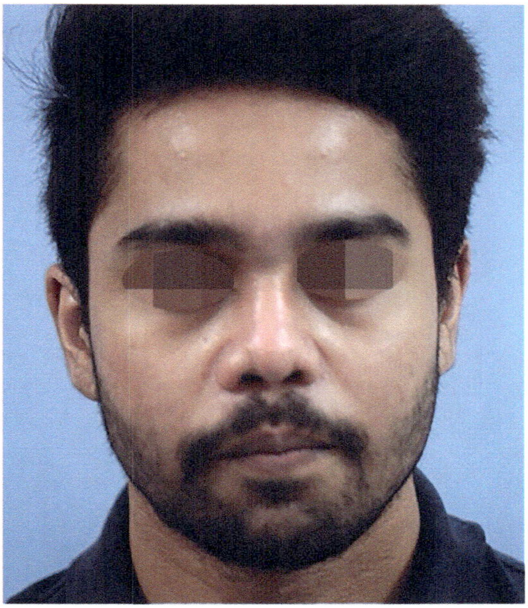

Fig. 6.26 Post-op frontal view

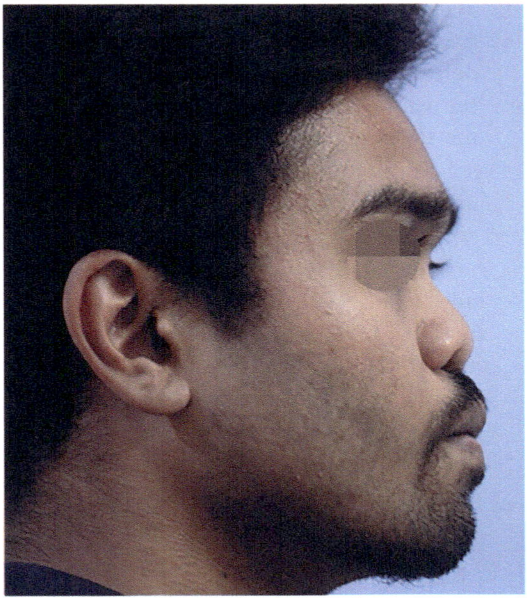

Fig. 6.27 Pre-op lateral view

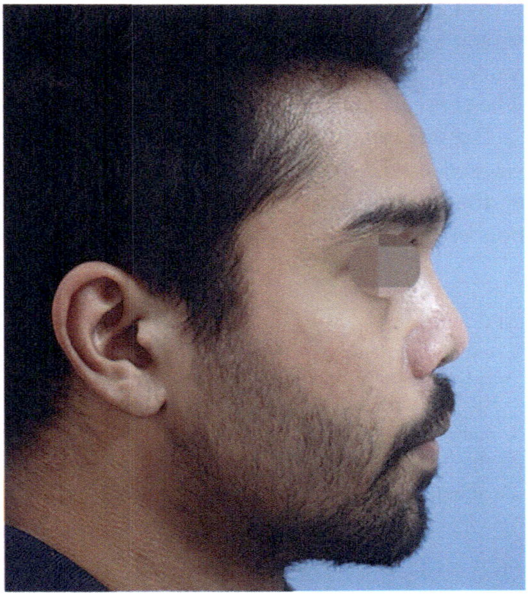

Fig. 6.28 Post-op lateral view

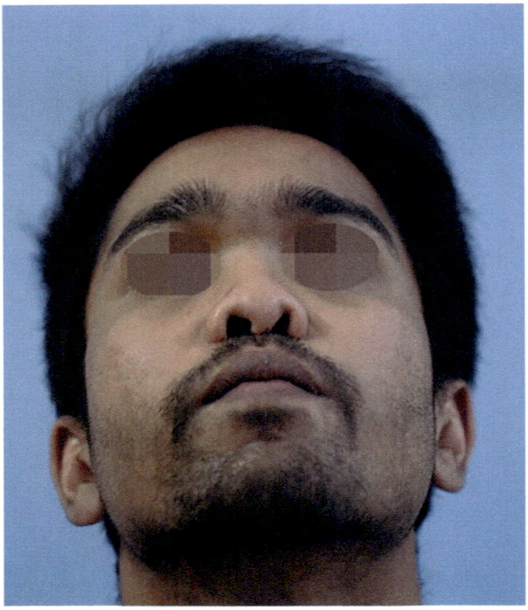

Fig. 6.29 Pre-op basal view

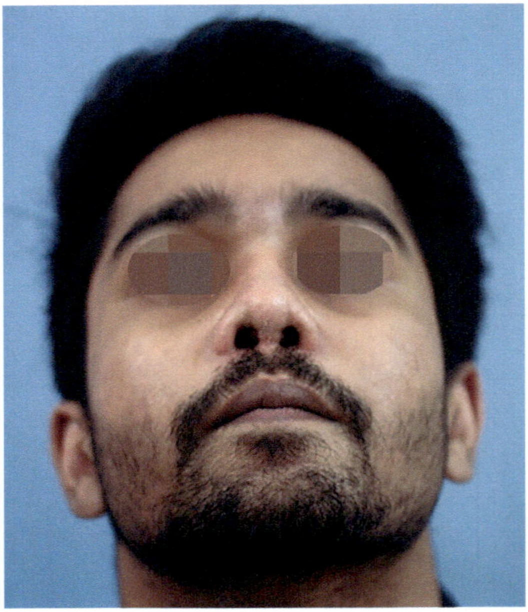

Fig. 6.30 Post-op basal view

SEG is preferred to columellar strut. SEG should be placed in front of ANS between middle crura up to the tip. SEG is a stronger support when compared to columellar strut.

Dorsal augmentation is achieved using stacked cartilage with/without fascia or diced cartilage fascia along with external valve bolstering.

SEG	Columellar strut
Fixed to septal cartilage mostly, can be fixed to alar cartilages (middle crus)	Fixed in between two medial crura of lower alar cartilage
Columella shape retained	Columella broadened
Stiffness of nasal tip	No stiffness
Used in facial asymmetry	Preferred while facial symmetry is maintained
Used if ANS is deviated	If ANS is in the centre
Very useful in Asian noses and in saddle noses	Useful in long Caucasian noses
May cause nasal obstruction if overlapping part is not trimmed adequately	It is placed in front of the septum; hence, this is not seen

E. *Type 4* (Figs. 6.31, 6.32, 6.33, 6.34 and 6.35) cases have large septal and bony valve defect. There is presence of columellar retrusion, overrotation and deprojection of the tip along with alar base widening and splaying. It invariably is associated with nasal lining along with external nasal valve compromise.

If the skin is necrosed or insufficient, a full-thickness grafting from the postauricular area is preferred to a V-Y plasty of columella:

- These cases require structural reconstruction with contoured solid costal cartilage with extended spreader graft (for lengthening) which are secured to nasal bones and stacked cartilage for augmentation. Most of the time, it cannot be managed by DCF alone.
- SEG is fixed to the anterior nasal spine and columellar strut is not preferred.
- Tip projection by dorsal onlay and shield grafts should be done.

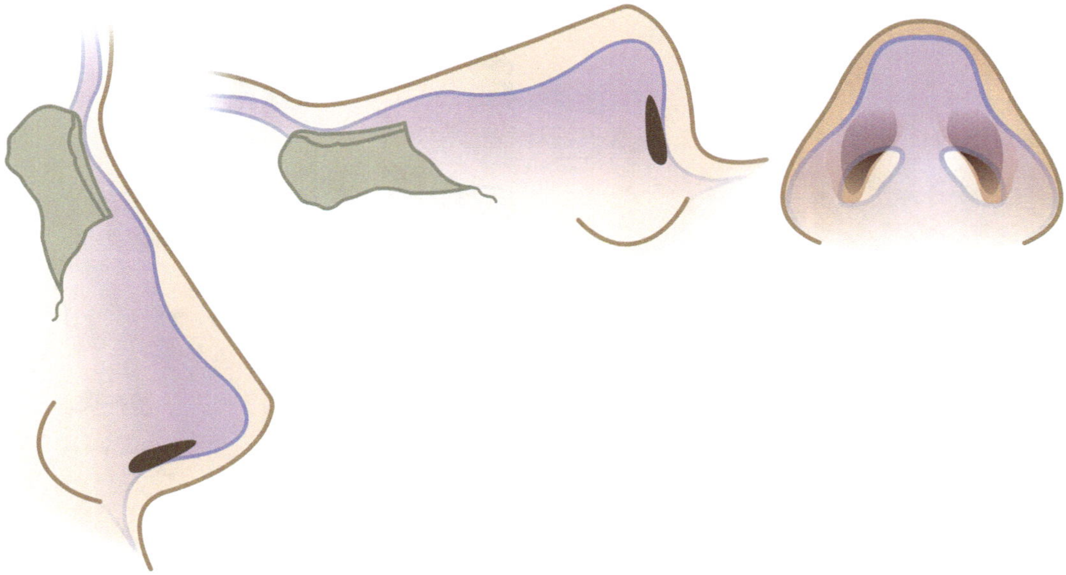

Fig. 6.31 *Type 4 deformity* showing columellar retrusion, overrotation and deprojection of the tip along with alar base widening and splaying

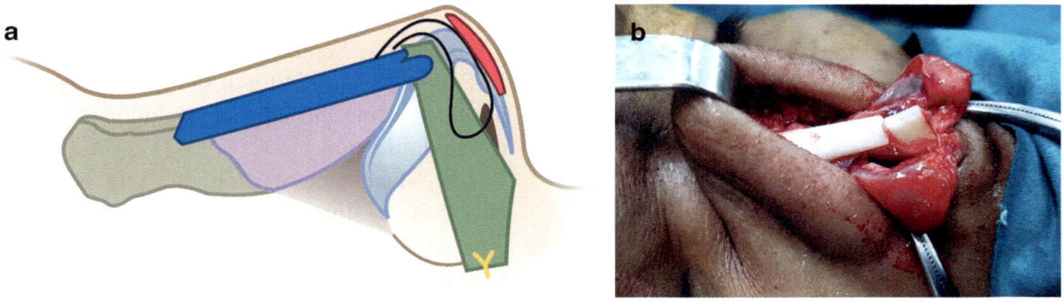

Fig. 6.32 (**a**, **b**) Structural reconstruction with contoured solid costal cartilage as an extended spreader graft

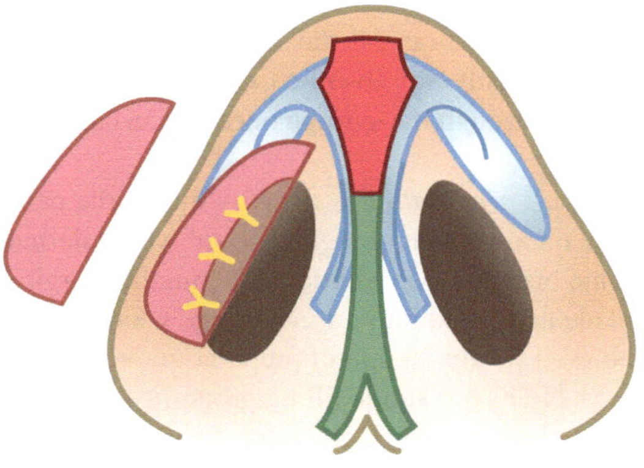

Fig. 6.33 SEG with shield graft with articulated rim grafts

- Lateral nasal wall reconstruction due to contracture of the skin is managed with articulated rim grafts.

F. *Type five* (Figs. 6.36, 6.37 and 6.38) deformity has complete collapse of bony and cartilaginous vault:

- It requires major reconstruction with extensive degloving and fixation with plates and screws of bony and cartilaginous supports. Tissues adjacent to the nose are also affected. *Solid rib cartilage* is used for augmentation.

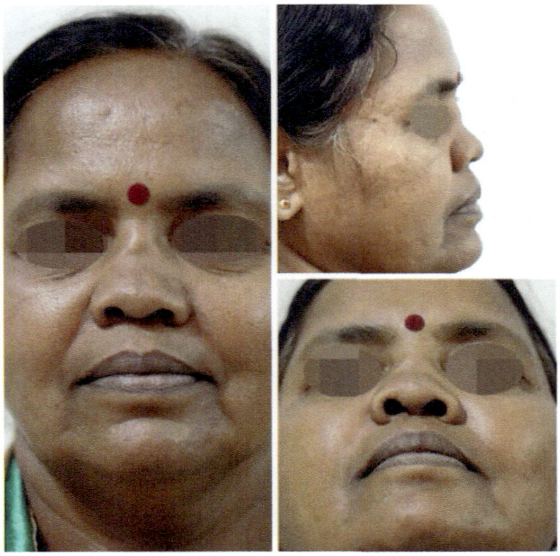

Fig. 6.34 Pre-op frontal, lateral and basal view

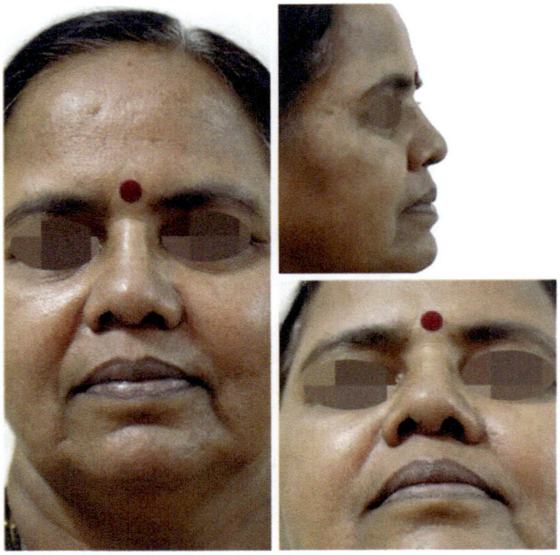

Fig. 6.35 Post-op frontal, lateral and basal view

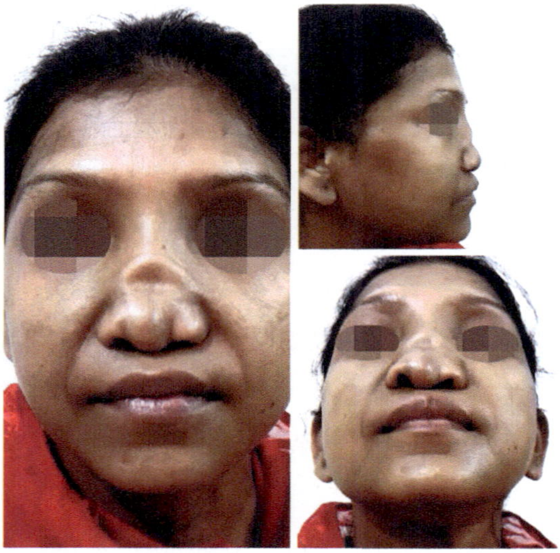

Figs. 6.36–6.38 (left: Fig. 6.36): Pre-op frontal; (right top: Fig. 6.37): Pre-op lateral; (right bottom: Fig. 6.38): Pre-op basal

6.4 Salient Features of Commonly Used Augmentation Techniques

Free Diced Cartilage (FDC) (Figs. 6.39, 6.40, 6.41, 6.42, 6.43 and 6.44) Free diced cartilage graft is an innovative technique with multiple applications. It is used for smoothening, augmentation or camouflaging of the nasal dorsum in primary or revision rhinoplasties.

Graft site—Septal, conchal or costal cartilage

Following harvesting of the graft, it has to be placed in saline and antibiotic solution for 30 min to avoid infection.

Size—Diameter of about 0.2 mm in size to ensure the facilitation of cartilaginous nutrition:

- As the size of the FDC graft (surface area) increases, there is possibility of compromise of cartilage viability and nutritional properties to the graft along with risk of easy palpation of the FDC.
- On the contrary, if the size is too small, they may easily get absorbed which might percolate through the syringe once squeezed.

Graft preparation is done by dicing the cartilage on a wooden or a glass board with a dermatome blade or a conventional 22 number surgical blade and is fed into a 1 cc syringe which should be used within 20 min of preparation preferably.

As FDC has subtle filling properties, it is considered as an ideal graft for finer refinements whereas corrections of large areas are usually benefitted from other types of grafts.

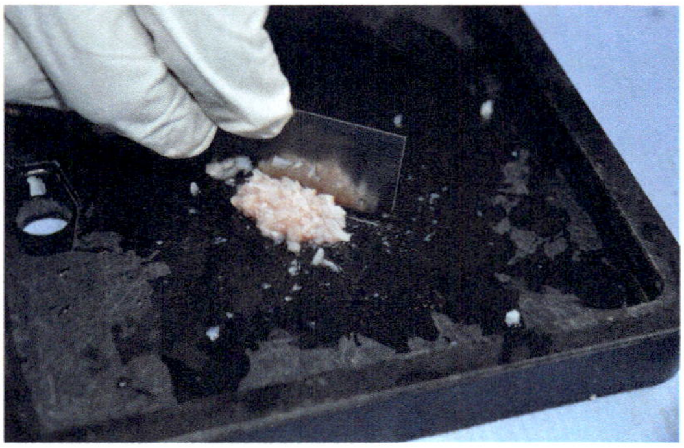

Fig. 6.39 Fine dicing of cartilage using dermatome blade

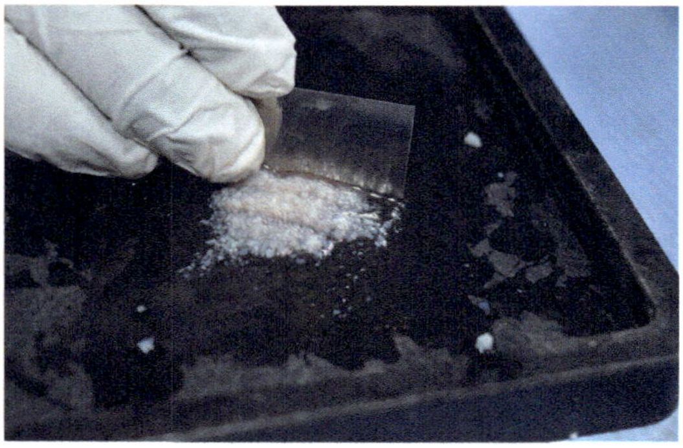

Fig. 6.40 Cartilage less than 0.2 mm in size

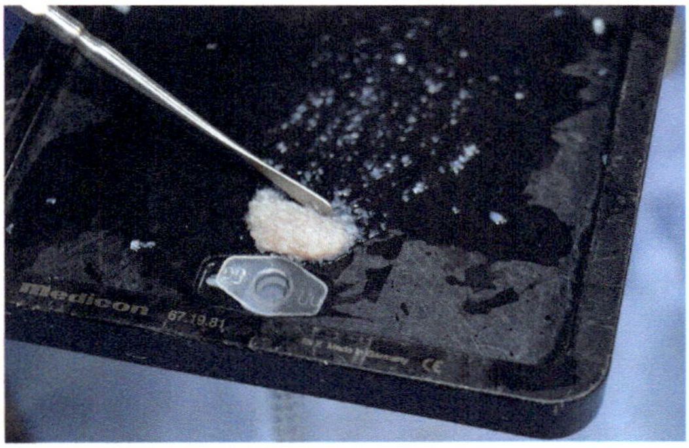

Fig. 6.41 Filling of the finely diced cartilage

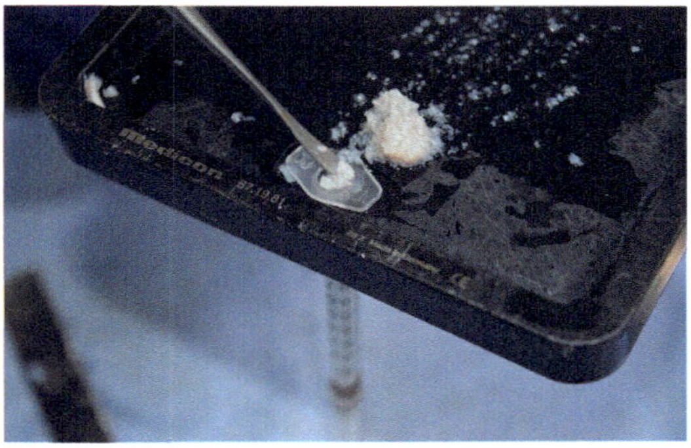

Fig. 6.42 A 1 cc syringe filled completely

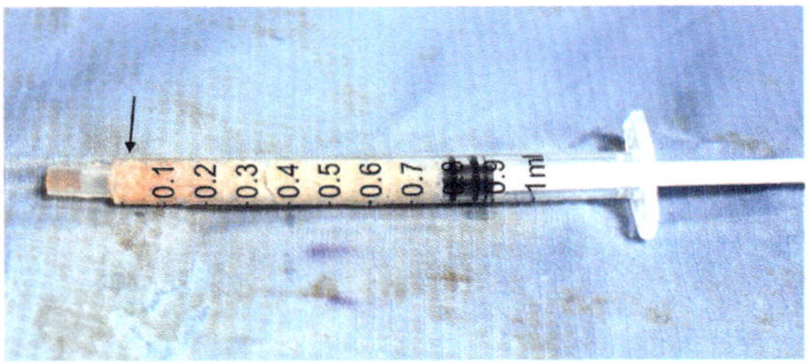

Fig. 6.43 A 1 cc syringe showing holes (arrow mark) at the advancing end for saline percolation

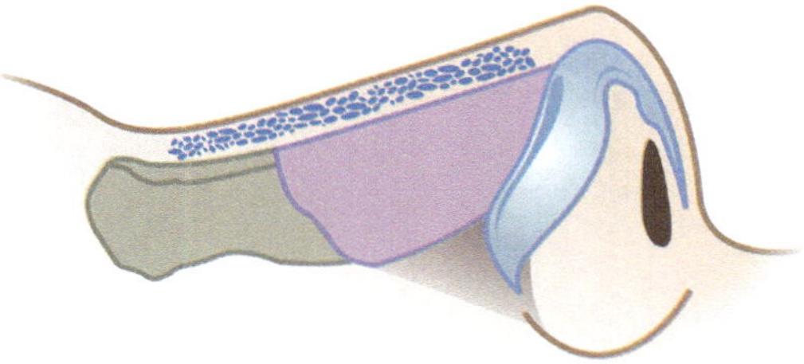

Fig. 6.44 FDC placed on the dorsum beneath the skin flap

Recently, fibrin glue is being used with FDC to ensure its better binding.

Finely diced cartilage filled in 1 cc syringe which has multiple holes in the advancing end for the saline to be squeezed out.

Arrow indicating the holes in the picture and explained in the picture.

Diced Cartilage with Fascia (DCF) (Figs. 6.45, 6.46, 6.47, 6.48, 6.49, 6.50 and 6.51) The concept of 'Turkish delight' which was given by Erol in 2000 *was revised by Daniel* where diced cartilage wrapped in surgical was used for augmentation rhinoplasty. Eventually diced cartilage with fascia is being used and is an ideal graft for dorsal aug-

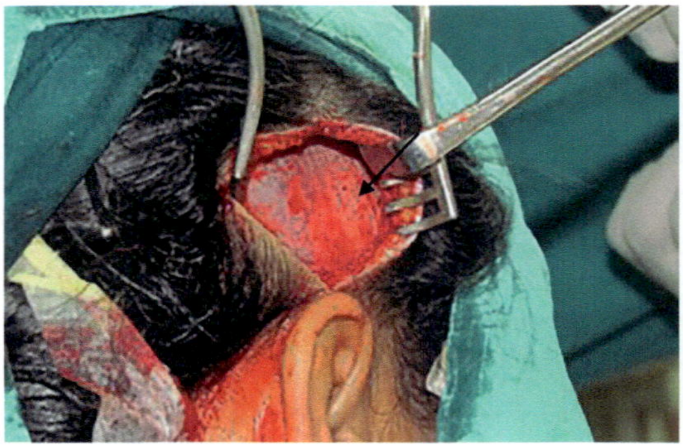

Fig. 6.45 Temporalis fascia graft harvesting

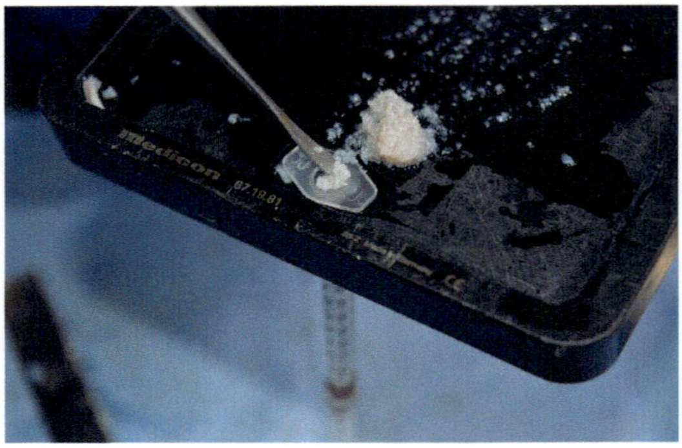

Fig. 6.46 Diced cartilage filled in a 1 cc syringe

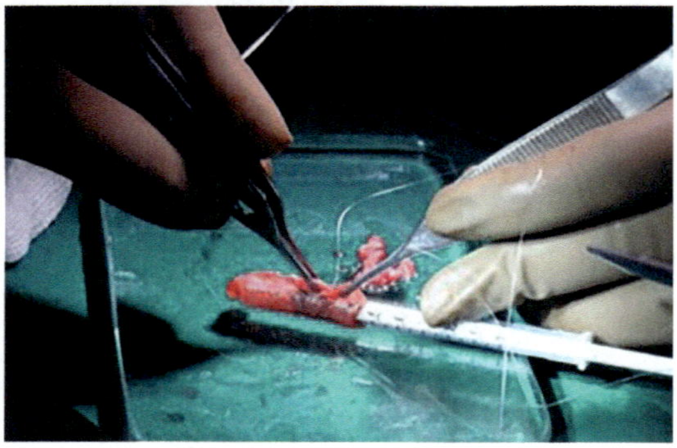

Fig. 6.47 Temporalis fascia used to make a bag by suturing the bag from the advancing to the non-advancing end which is kept open

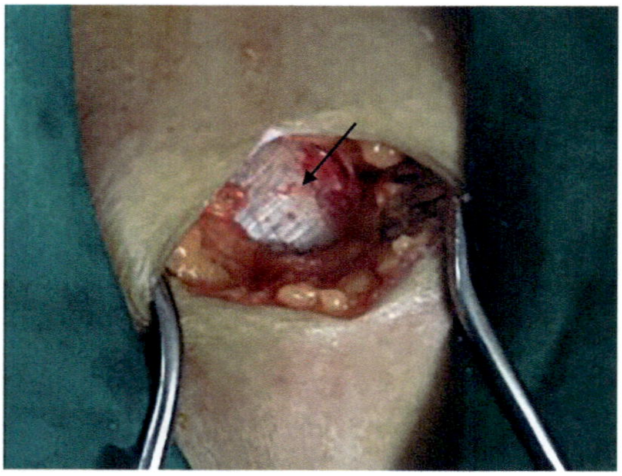

Fig. 6.48 Rectus fascia exposed to be harvested

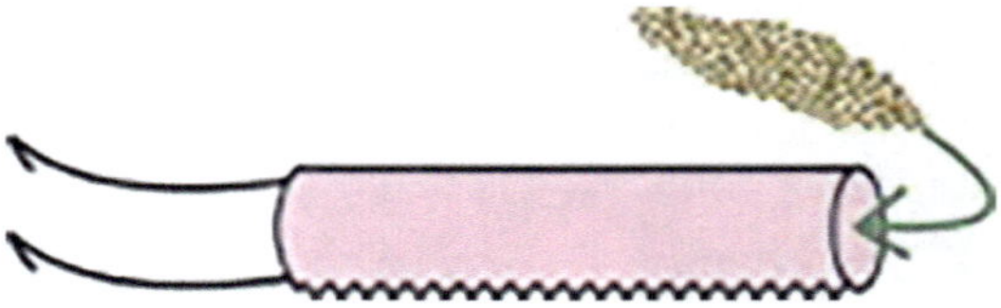

Fig. 6.49 FDC being introduced inside the fascial sheath

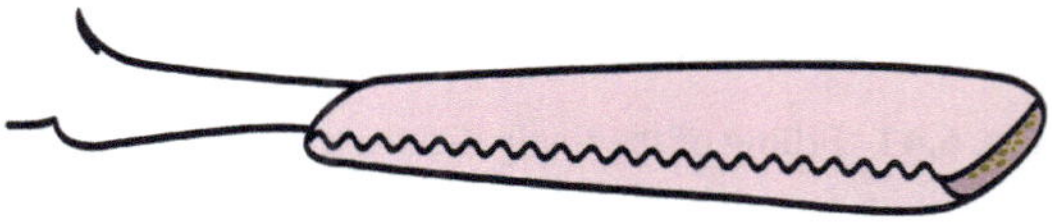

Fig. 6.50 Bag created

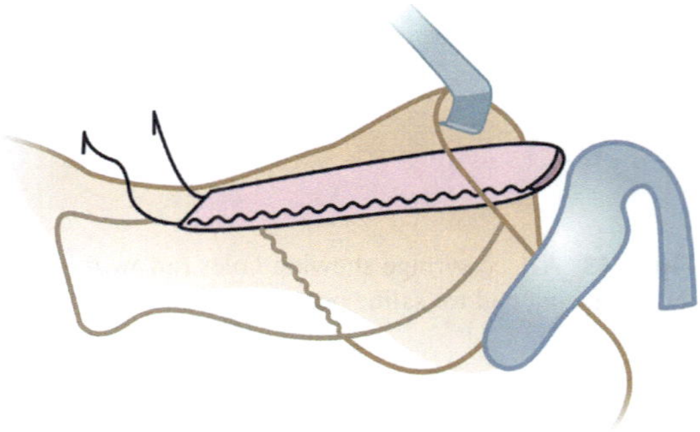

Fig. 6.51 DCF created and placed on the dorsum and the advancing end sutured at NFA

mentation, as it can be procured from the same site as graft harvesting, has lower complication rates and has minimal cartilage resorption while also providing a graft that has the ability to recreate the dorsal aesthetic lines in a natural and predictable manner.

Graft site—Conchal and septal cartilage with temporalis fascia and costal cartilage with rectus fascia.

Temporalis fascia—Vertical incision above the ear (to be careful not to injure superficial temporal artery) and temporalis muscle to be not dissected to prevent pseudo augmentation.

Rectus Fascia (Fig. 6.48) *We have to be aware of the fact that rectus fascia is relatively thicker medially when compared to laterally, and thinner laterally, so it is better to harvest the rectus fascia graft from the medial aspect.*

Size—Fascia of about 5 × 5 cm, rectangular shape and diced cartilage to

be lesser than 0.5 mm in size

Graft preparation:

The fascia is wrapped around the advancing end of the syringe, and the free margins of the fascia are sutured using 5-0 PDS, and the diced cartilage material is filled inside the bag of fascia by gradually pushing the plunger of the syringe. Once the bag is formed, it is placed on the dorsum beneath the skin and is fixed at the nasofacial angle.

DCF is fixed laterally to ULC in pinchable cases to avoid lateral displacement. The non-advancing end (caudal end) of fascial bag should be left open in the supratip area.

We recommend to overaugmenting by about 10% as there is a resultant 5–10% of volume reduction in the post-operative period.

Immediate taping has to be done to avoid lateral displacement.

Recent advances—Platelet-rich fibrin should be used to ensure reduced absorption and longevity of the graft placed.

Stacked Cartilage (Figs. 6.52, 6.53, 6.54, 6.55, 6.56 and 6.57) Dorsal deficiencies in nasal anatomy are particularly disharmonious.

Frequently associated with dorsal deficiencies are a low radix, poor tip projection and definition, a shortened columella and an obtuse nasolabial angle. So in situations where the availability of graft is not sufficient or if the expertise for dicing or DCF is not enough, stacked cartilage augmentation can be considered. Stacked cartilage is considered to DCF in cases where the skin pinch test is not easy suggesting tough underlying fibro-fatty tissue.

Graft site—concha, septum (even if a small amount is left) and costal cartilage.

Size—According to the size of the nose from nasofacial angle (NFA) to supratip area.

Unlike European patients, Indian patients do not prefer NFA obliteration.

Preparation—Two equal size grafts should be cut, stacked over one another and sutured using 5-0 PDS. Lateral aspects of the graft are carved and smoothened by fine knife or diamond burr. If NFA is deep, then the cranial part of cartilage

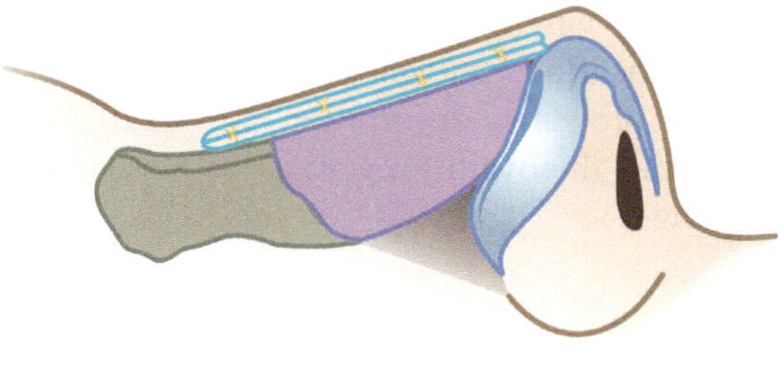

Fig. 6.52 Stacked cartilage without fascia on the dorsum

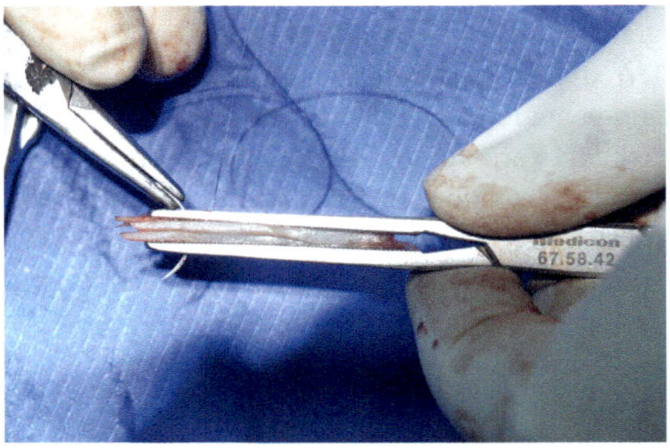

Fig. 6.53 Stacked septal cartilage—sutured using 5-0 PDS

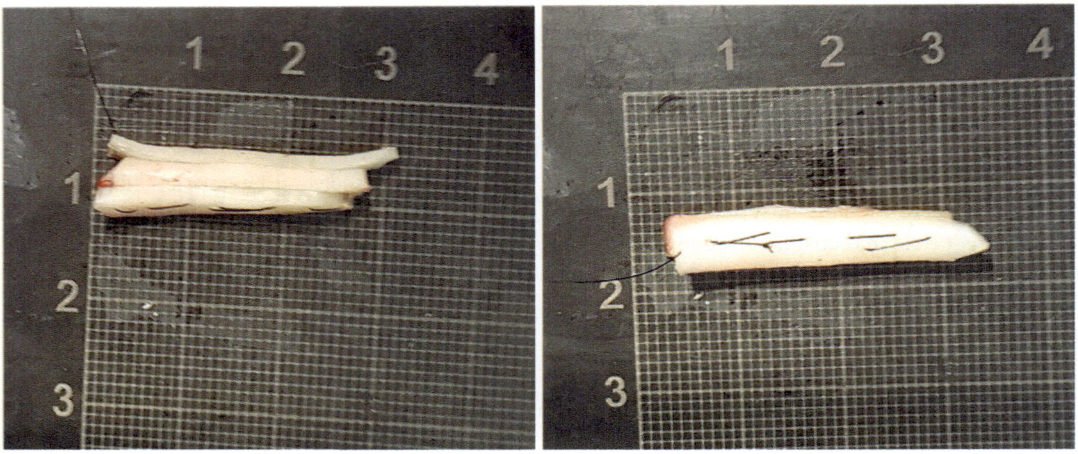

Fig. 6.54 (**a**, **b**) Stacked cartilage sutured from one end to another

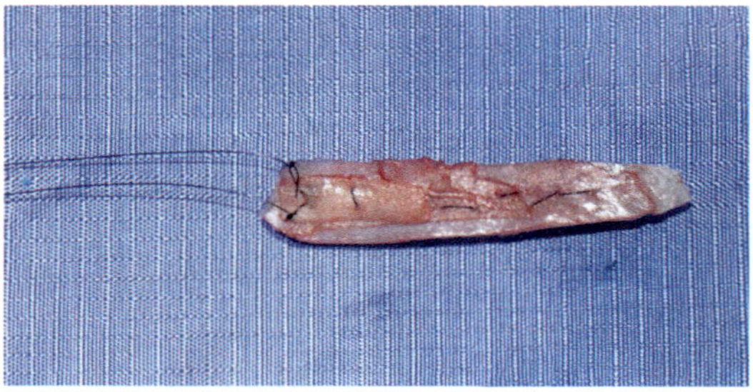

Fig. 6.55 The suture material kept long at the advancing end of stacked cartilage—ready for placing inside

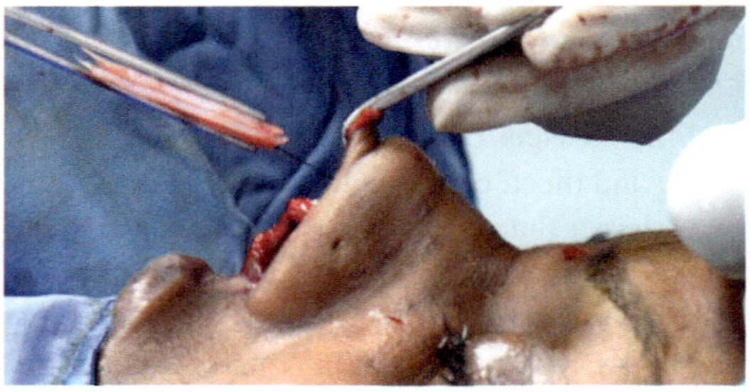

Fig. 6.56 Stacked cartilage being introduced on the dorsum

also has to be carved appropriately to fit in the deep nasofacial angle.

In some cases, if a single solid piece of cartilage is sufficient, solid rib cartilage is commonly used (Figs. 6.58 and 6.59). Sometimes, septum or conchal graft can be also be used. Solid cartilage grafting fills in a large dorsal defect and is a preferred graft technique where a large amount of augmentation is required but of course with the risk of warping, malalignment, resorption and nasal tip rotation. Fixing of solid cartilage with transosseous-transcutaneous cerclage (TTC) sutures to the bone and to the upper lateral cartilage with 5-0 PDS.

Stacked Cartilage Wrapped in Fascia (Figs. 6.60, 6.61 and 6.62) Dorsal grafting in rhinoplasty has been totally revolutionised. So the layered septal cartilage or stacked conchal cartilage or carved costal cartilage wrapped in a fascia is simpler to use, quicker and aesthetically superior to just solid rib grafting which helps in preventing warping and malaligning. Also, we have seen that the autogenous fascia may act as a perichondrium that promotes neovascularisation, prevents inflammatory reactions, prevents resorption of graft and maintains the overall regenerative potential of cartilage.

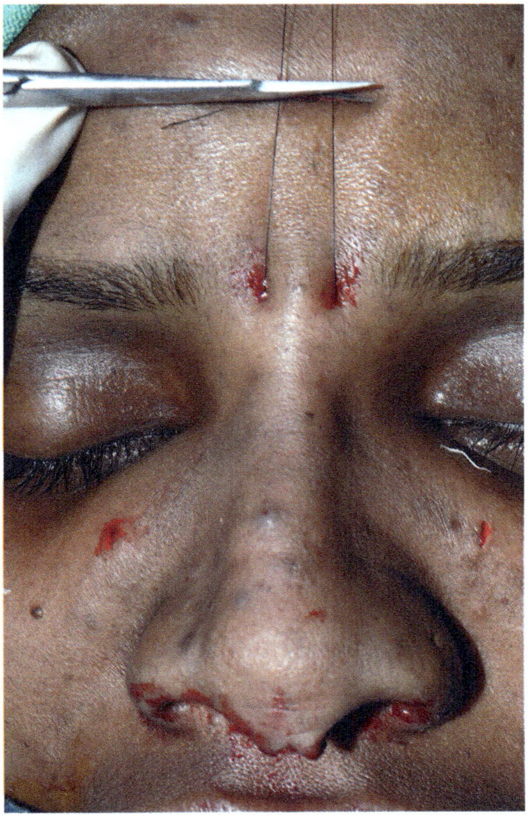

Fig. 6.57 Stacked cartilage placed on the dorsum and ends of suture brought outside at NFA and fixed

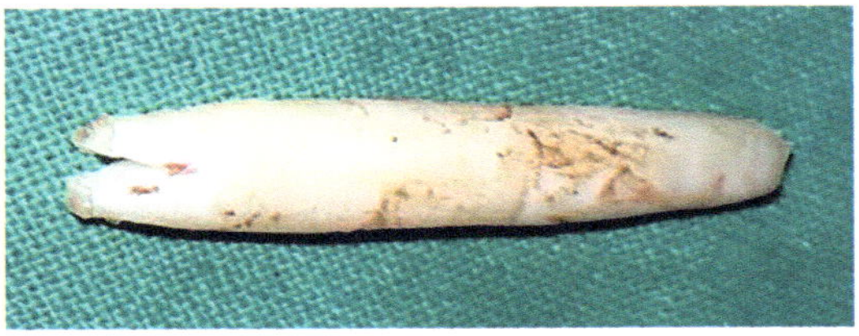

Fig. 6.58 Solid rib cartilage

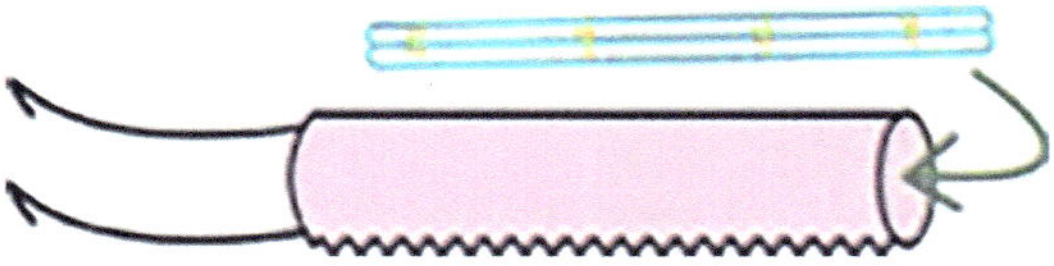

Fig. 6.59 Solid rib cartilage wrapped in fascia

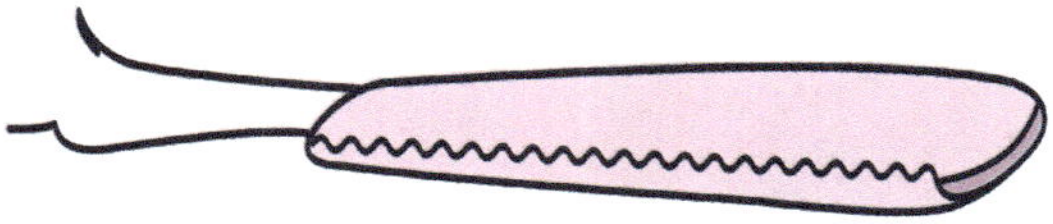

Fig. 6.60 Stacked cartilage

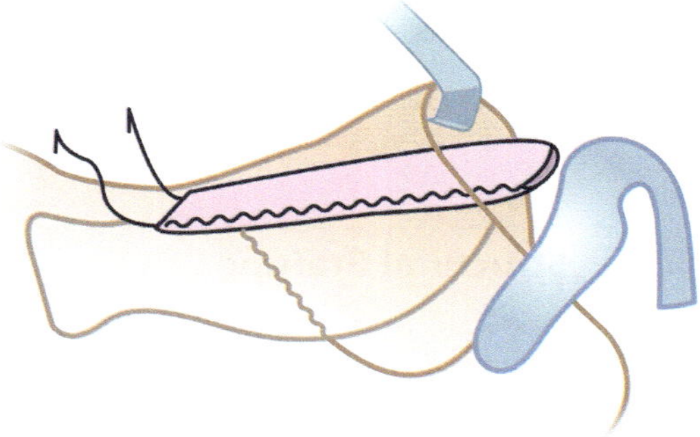

Fig. 6.61 Placed in a fascia bag

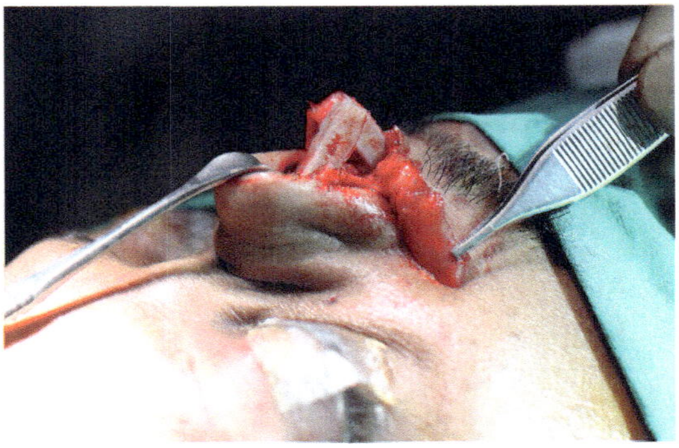

Fig. 6.62 Stacked cartilage wrapped in fascia placed on the dorsum

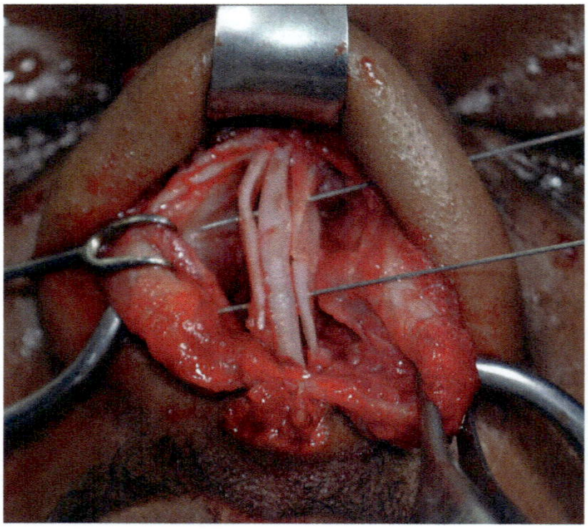

Fig. 6.63 Extended spreader with SEG which is fixed to the spine

6.5 Structural Grafting

Here the middle part of the costal cartilage is preferred where the cartilage cranially is fixed to nasal bones using TTC sutures and caudally is fixed to anterior nasal spine by drilling ANS using Lindemann's burr and fixing with 3-0 PDS (Fig. 6.63).

6.6 Spreader Grafts

Spreader grafts have got three main benefits:

1. To stabilise the nasal dorsum
2. To give dorsal aesthetic lines
3. To improve the nasal valve area

The cartilage length, used to form the spreader grafts, extends from just below the nasal bones to anterior septal angle sutured to upper lateral cartilage on either side and the septum in between (Fig. 6.64).

6.7 Extended Spreader Graft

These are used when the nasal lengthening needs to be done, and these extend from just below the nasal bones till the intermediate crus (Fig. 6.65).

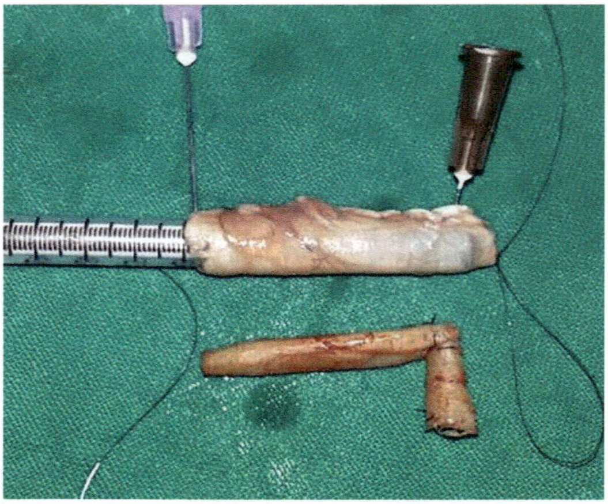

Fig. 6.64 Percutaneous fixation of spreader grafts on either side of the septum in between the ULC

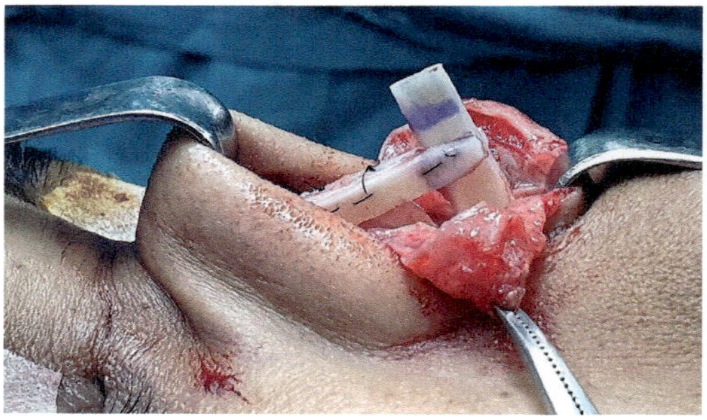

Fig. 6.65 Figure showing extended spreader grafts

6.8 Grafts

As the deformities become more complex, the need for restoration of structure and support becomes a must for the shape of the nose and to keep the airway open. For this purpose, according to me autologous cartilage is my first choice.

Costal cartilage is the only material with sufficient strength and volume to achieve the needed reconstructive goals, in cases where larger defects are present requiring bigger reconstruction, where the availability of septal cartilage and conchal cartilage is inadequate.

A brief overview of the commonly used autologous cartilages

	Donor site	Ease of harvesting	Quantity available	Advantages	Donor site comorbidities	Other aspects
1	Septal cartilage	Yes	May not be adequate	– Same incision – More rigid than auricular – Easier to shape as straighter – Can be used as single layered/sutured	Minimal	Not available for post-traumatic, secondary surgeries
2	Conchal cartilage	Yes	May not be adequate	Soft and ideal for tip grafts	Perichondritis	Brittle, more curved, less rigid, more difficult to carve, quantity available may be inadequate for extensive reconstruction, memory of cartilage
3	Costal cartilage	No	Adequate	The rib can also be harvested-composite graft-chondroosseous Most commonly right-sided 8/9 rib but sometimes fifth rib in females who want the scar to be hidden	Relatively long-lasting pain	– Pre-op CT of the thorax – Must be harvested prior to rhinoplasty – Surgical training required to minimize chances of pneumothorax – Unpredictable warping

Autologous bone grafts like iliac crest and calvarium and synthetic grafts like silicone are obsolete these days. I do not have much experience of use of Gore-Tex.

6.9 Post-Operative Period

Relative appreciable pain at the costal cartilage harvest site due to muscle pain is taken care of by infusion of bupivacaine administered every eighth hourly through epidural catheter placed at the wound site.

6.10 Complication

Post-op infection is rare but one of the most dreaded complications along with warping of cartilage, resorption and misalignment of the grafts which is explained in detail in *complication chapter*—Chap. 10.

6.11 Conclusion

Providing a good nasofrontal angle with a smooth nasal bridge and pleasing dorsal aesthetic lines and most importantly restoration of breathing through the provision of dorsal structural support and reconstitution of the nasal valves must be our aims of the results of dorsal augmentation rhinoplasty.

7 Dorsal Nasal Hump Deformity: Reduction Rhinoplasty

Main

A hump is a convexity of the nasal dorsum which may occur as a single deformity or in combination with various types of septal and pyramidal pathology. A hump alone usually only causes aesthetic complaints. These are the deformities which are very commonly seen in the northern part of our country. We have plenty of beautiful hump noses seen in people from Kashmir, where reduction rhinoplasty is not regularly requested by these patients solely for cosmetic purposes. However, patients with symptoms of nasal obstruction and/or old neglected childhood trauma causing dorsal hump deformity present for surgery.

Simplifying the hump noses to deal with their treatment and to understand a favourable outcome, the following classifications are useful (Figs. 7.1, 7.2, 7.3 and 7.4):

A. Cartilaginous hump
B. Bony and cartilaginous hump
C. Bony hump
D. Relative hump (pseudohump)

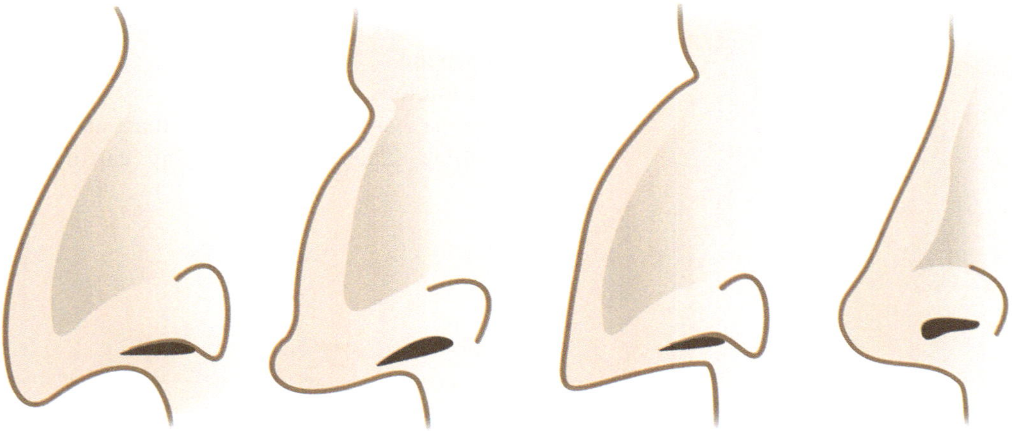

Figs. 7.1–7.4 (left: Fig. 7.1): Cartilaginous hump nose; (middle left: Fig. 7.2): Bony and cartilaginous hump nose; (middle right: Fig. 7.3): Bony hump nose; (right: Fig. 7.4): Pseudo-hump nose

V. Ghaisas, *Indian Ethnic Rhinoplasty*, https://doi.org/10.1007/978-981-16-2478-0_7

7.1 Cartilaginous Hump

The convexity here is limited to the cartilaginous dorsum. The cartilaginous complex is composed of the septum and the upper lateral cartilages (ULCs). This complex is the septum with bilaterally juxtaposed ULCs forming a single anatomical entity from a common embryologic origin (Fig. 7.5).

7.1.1 Treatment

Removal can be done in two parts:

1. *En bloc*—In this cartilaginous hump, part of the septum, upper lateral cartilage and a part of bony hump are removed at once. A 5 mm osteotome was introduced, and the three structures were removed en bloc. We used this technique previously. However, we do not prefer this now since it is historical and it is destructive technique (Fig. 7.6).

2. *Segmental*

We prefer segmental to an en bloc resection of the hump.

This is done in the following methodical steps called the split hump technique:

(a) Retraction of the skin flap in the avascular supraperichondrial plane.
(b) Meticulous elevation of the mucoperichondrial layers on both sides of the septum to avoid a mucosal injury when reducing the dorsum. This will result in a more controlled and faster healing process.
(c) A vertically positioned No. 11 blade is inserted underneath the cartilaginous vault, carefully avoiding trauma to mucoperichondrial flaps.
(d) Using paraseptal vertical incisions, the entire ULCs are bilaterally separate from the septum.
(e) Straight scissors or a No. 15 blade is used to reduce or shave the dorsal height of the septum.
(f) Judicious reduction of the bony dorsum is done using a rasp rather than an osteotome. Then, the underlying cartilage is

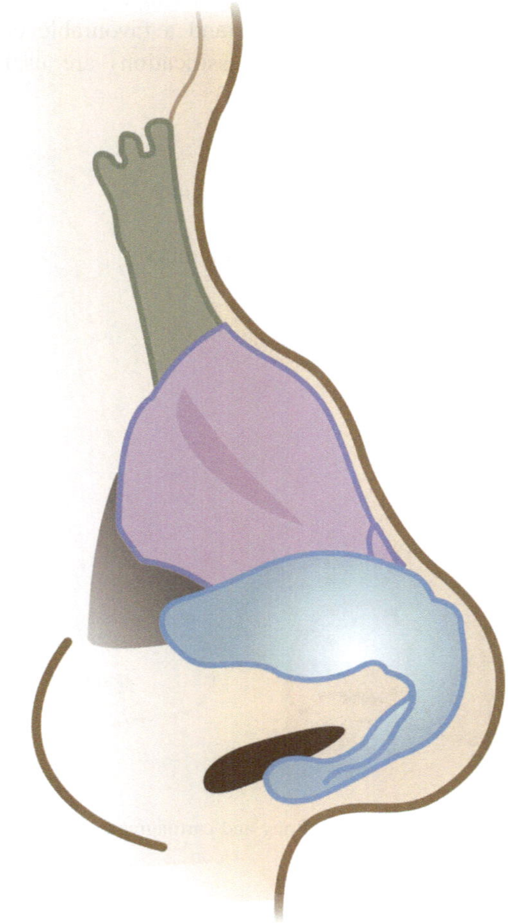

Fig. 7.5 Schematic diagram of cartilaginous hump deformity

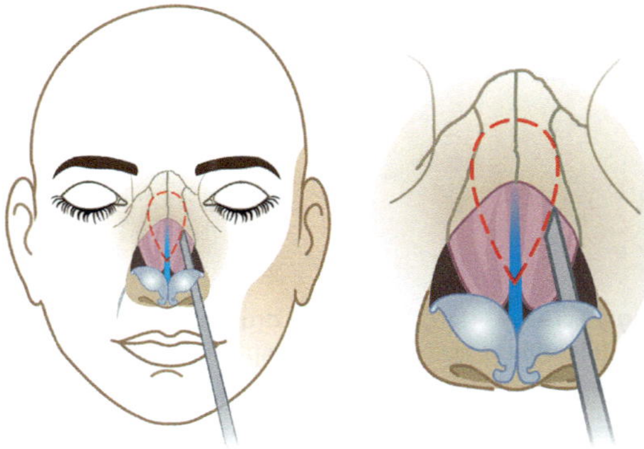

Fig. 7.6 En bloc excision of the bone and cartilage using a 5 mm osteotome

resected or repositioned in a controlled manner.

(g) Based on the nasal width and the length of the upper lateral cartilages, either:
- ULCs are aligned adjacent to the lowered septum.
- Spreader grafts placed on either side of the septum.
- If ULC >5 mm in height than the septum, then spreader flaps are created.

(h) Sharp instruments should be used for resection (Figs. 7.7, 7.8, 7.9, 7.10, 7.11 and 7.12).

Cartilaginous hump noses are usually associated with overprojected and downrotated tip for which a lateral crural sliding technique is done. This reduces the tip volume following which the tip rotates upwards, deprojects and becomes smaller (Figs. 7.13, 7.14, 7.15, 7.16, 7.17 and 7.18).

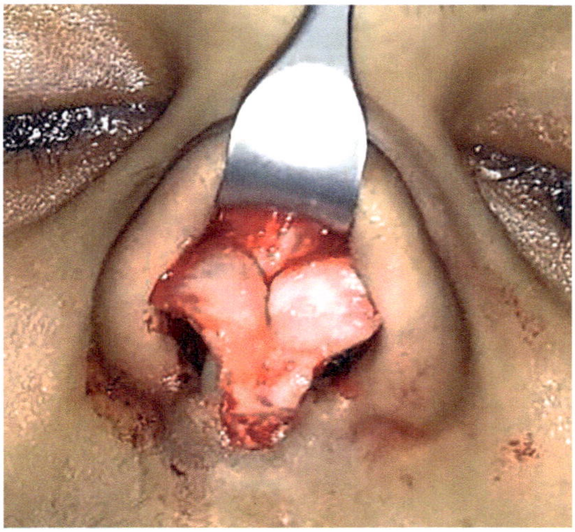

Fig. 7.7 Avascular supraperichondrial plane dissection

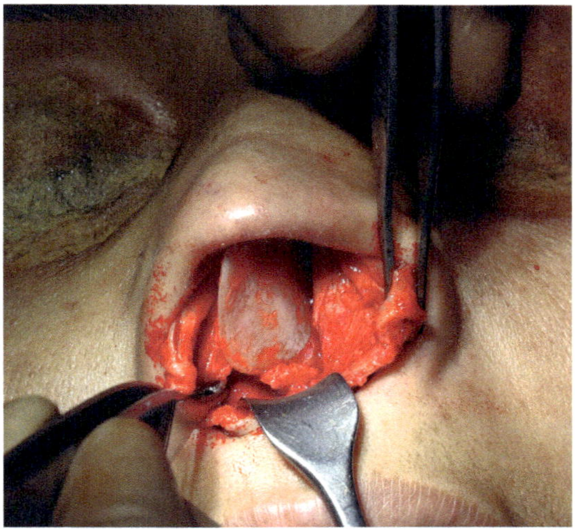

Fig. 7.8 Meticulous bilateral septal mucoperichondrial flaps elevated

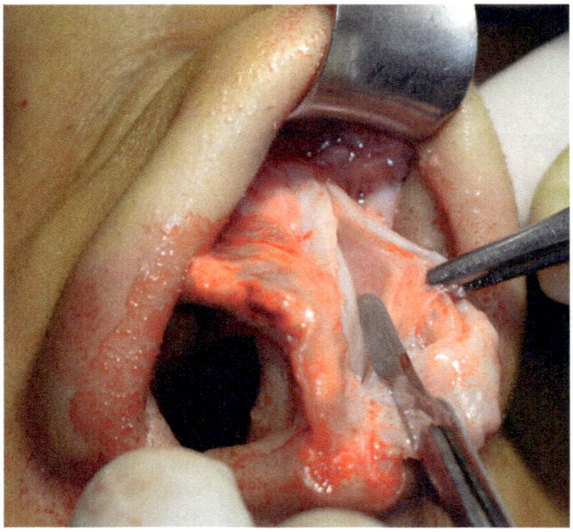

Fig. 7.9 ULC is cut in the paraseptal region with 11 No. blade

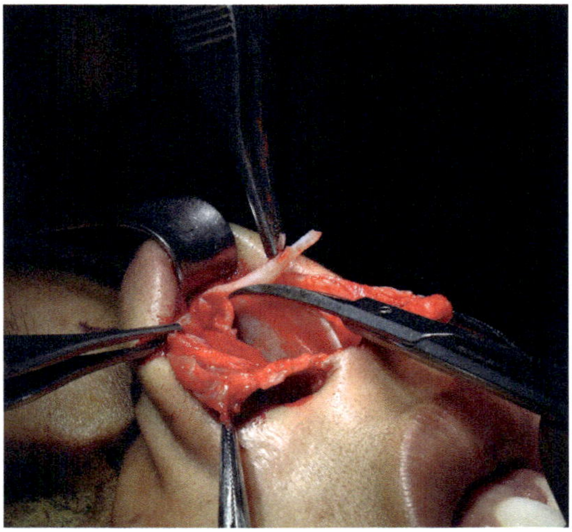

Fig. 7.10 The dorsal hump of the septum is resected using scissors

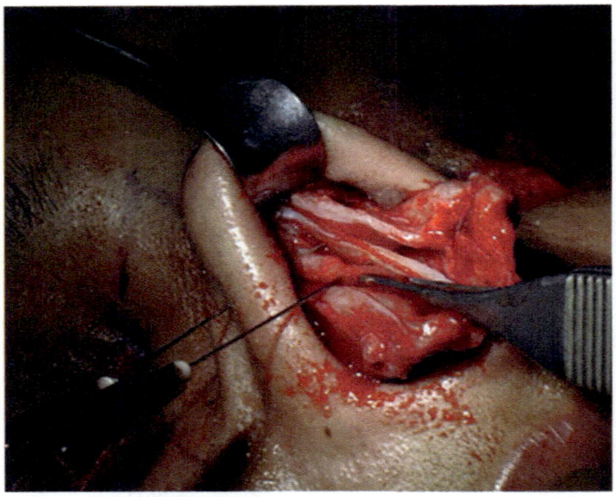

Fig. 7.11 Spreader grafts are placed on either side of the septum

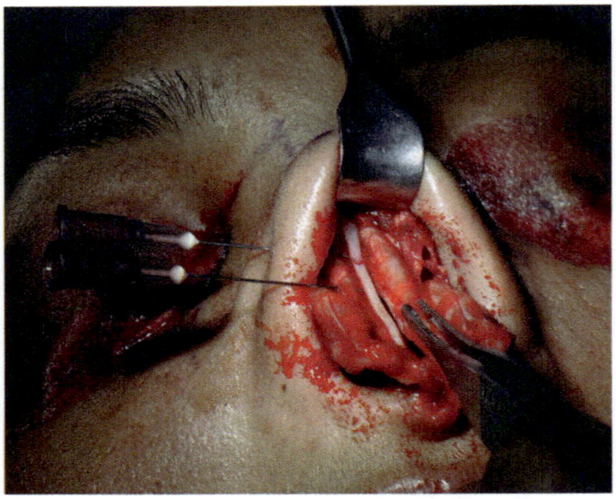

Fig. 7.12 Spreader flaps are formed

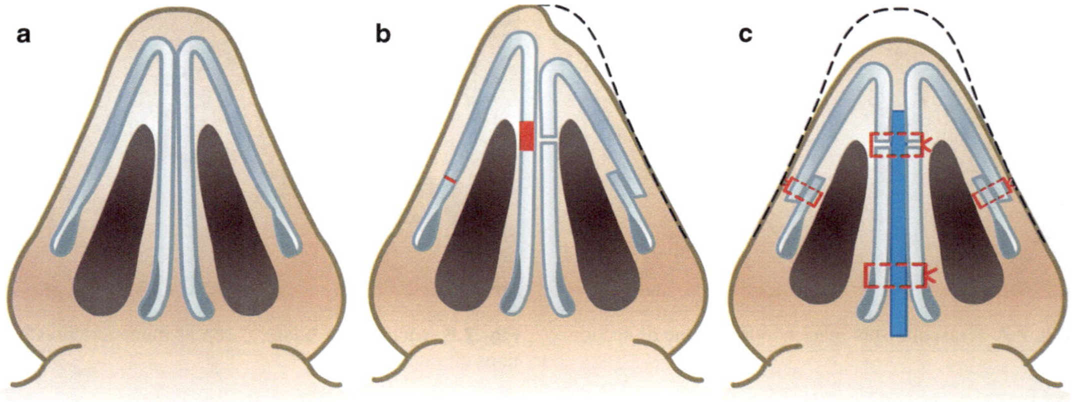

Fig. 7.13 (**a**, **b**, **c**) Schematic diagram of lateral crural sliding technique

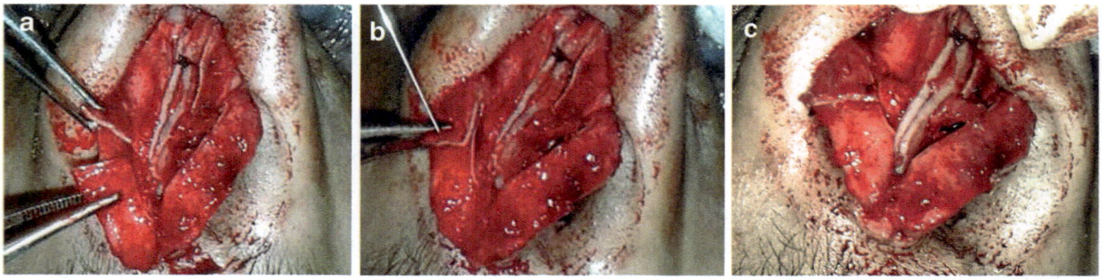

Fig. 7.14 (**a**, **b**, **c**) Corresponding pictures showing cutting of lateral crura, sliding over another and sutured with 5-0 PDS

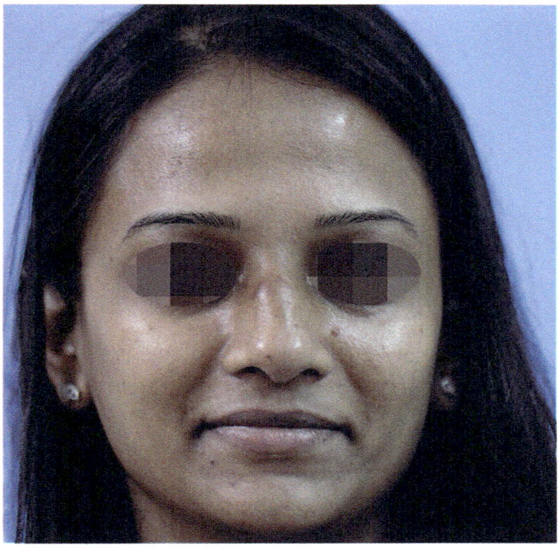

Fig. 7.15 Pre-op frontal view

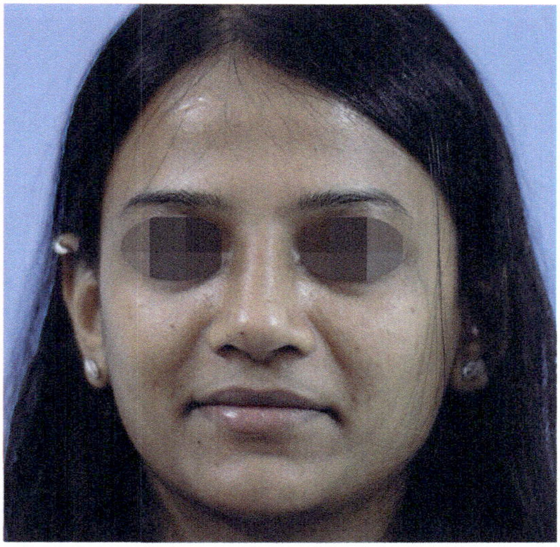

Fig. 7.16 Post-op frontal view

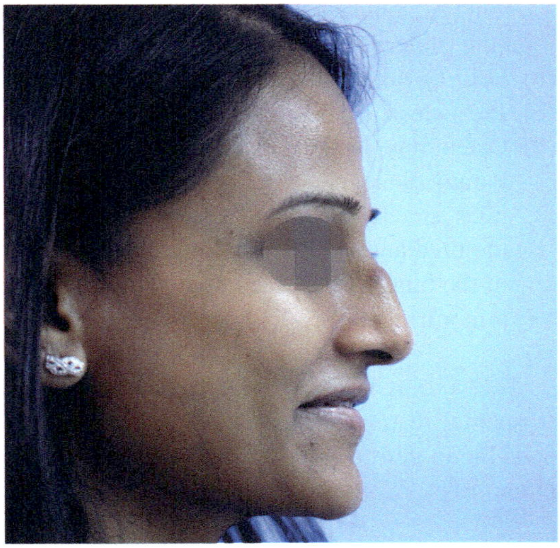

Fig. 7.17 Pre-op lateral view

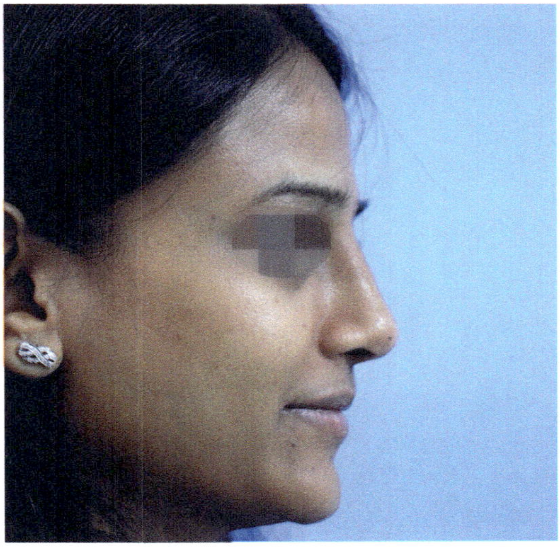

Fig. 7.18 Post-op lateral view

7.2 Bony and Cartilaginous Hump

Both the bony and the cartilaginous dorsa are convex (humped) (Fig. 7.19).

In this case both the bony vault and the cartilaginous vault reduction are done in a systematic manner:

1. Following the skin flap elevation.
2. Periosteum on the dorsal hump is cut and elevated.

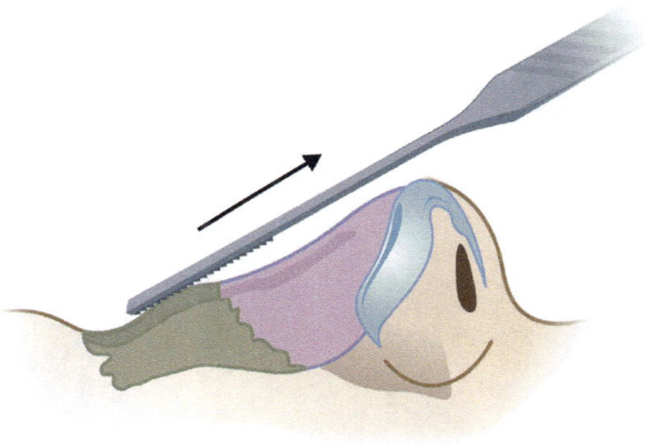

Fig. 7.20 Rasping of nasal bones

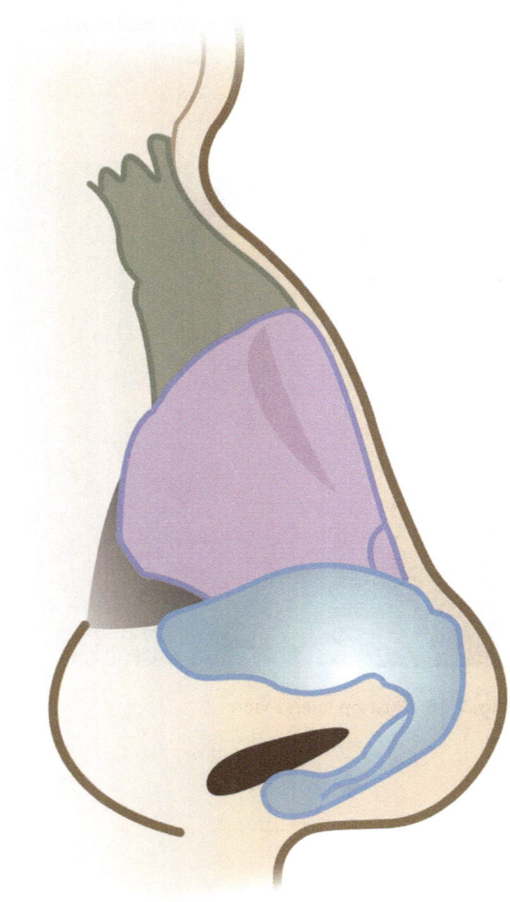

Fig. 7.19 Schematic diagram of both bony and cartilaginous deformities

Reduction of bony hump can be managed by:

(a) Rasping:
The beginner surgeon must remember that the rasp removes the bone only while being removed, unlike a file which removes the bone both while introducing and removal (Fig. 7.20).
(b) Drilling with a diamond burr.
(c) Piezoelectric device.
(d) Osteotomy using osteotomes and realigning. Paramedian, lateral and transverse osteotomies are done. Bony vault is mobilised as required and modified depending on the size of the hump. Free diced cartilage is used for minor irregularities.

The cartilaginous hump is then reduced in a segmental manner as described in the cartilaginous hump deformity using the split hump technique (Figs. 7.21 and 7.22).

7.3 Only Bony Hump

Here the convexity is confined only to the bony pyramid (Fig. 7.23).

Rasping, drilling or piezoelectric device is used to reduce only bony hump deformities. Osteotomy is performed depending upon the nasal width. Sometimes, smoothening of the hump helps in small bony deformities, and this

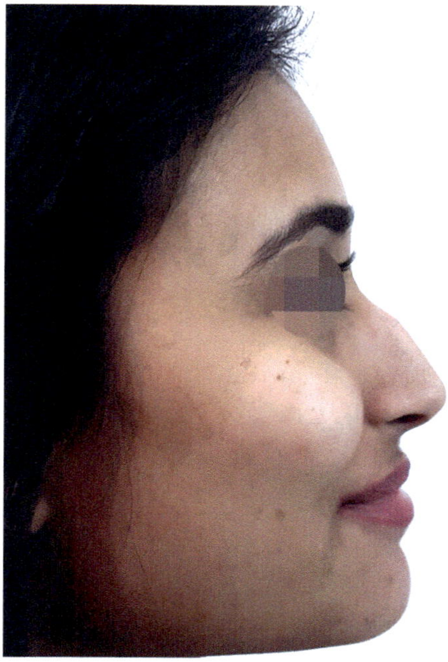

Fig. 7.21 Pre-op lateral view

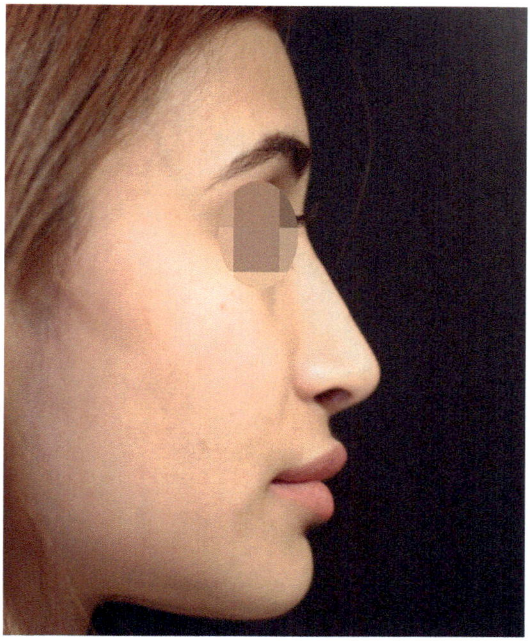

Fig. 7.22 Post-op lateral view

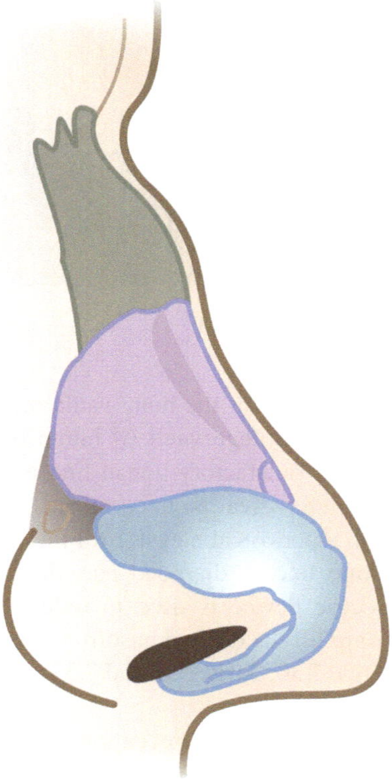

Fig. 7.23 Schematic diagram of only bony hump

can be achieved by filing. This step must be paid attention to avoid the post-operative irregularities encountered if proper smoothening of the hump is not done. Bone dust is removed and washed with cold saline. In case of small irregularities, free diced cartilage will help. As an additional advantage, it helps to prevent adherence of the skin to the bone and prevent pain, which occasionally patients complain of during the post-operative period, especially where the skin adheres to bony irregularities (Figs. 7.24, 7.25, 7.26 and 7.27).

7.4 Relative Hump (Pseudohump)

A pseudohump refers to a nose in which the radix is underdeveloped, which leads to a profile in which the tissue below the radix appears even fuller and underprojected than it really is. Pseudohump can be produced by either soft tissue fullness or bone. The pseudohumps are generally appreciated by many. However, beauty lies in the eye of a beholder, and Indian patients prefer to have a deep nasofrontal angle (Fig. 7.28).

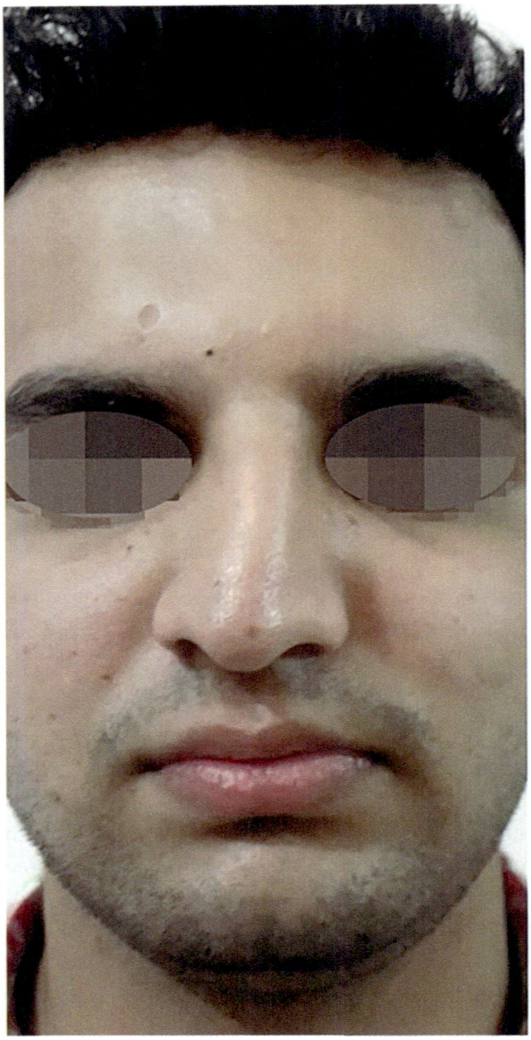

Fig. 7.24 Pre-op frontal

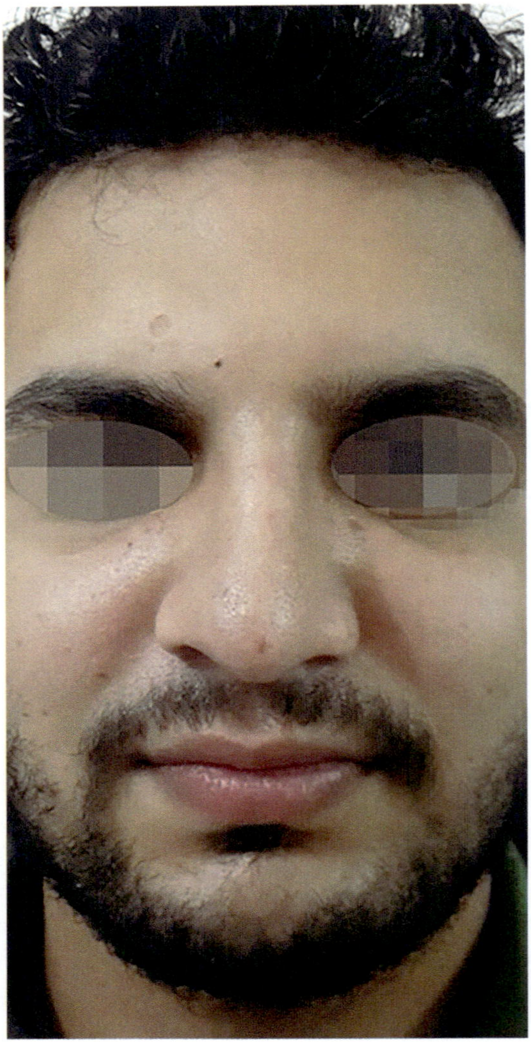

Fig. 7.25 Post-op frontal

Two ways to reduce radix are:

(a) *Soft tissue radix reduction*: Care should be taken to assess both the soft tissue fullness that blunts the nasofrontal angle and the width of the medial orbital lines that continue into the dorsal lines. Excision of the soft tissue fullness is done in these cases. *Procerus muscle needs to be trimmed* (Fig. 7.29).

(b) *Bone reduction*: En bloc excision of the dorsal bone is avoided. The dorsum is reduced using rasps for the bony vault and a scissor for the cartilage vault (if hump is present). Once a satisfactory dorsal line is produced, the radix area is undermined extensively with a periosteal elevator till the nasofrontal suture line. A diamond burr drill or piezoelectric device is used to reduce the bony hump till the desired nasofrontal is achieved (Figs. 7.30, 7.31, 7.32 and 7.33).

Steps to ensure the prevention of excess hump removal (Figs. 7.34, 7.35 and 7.36):

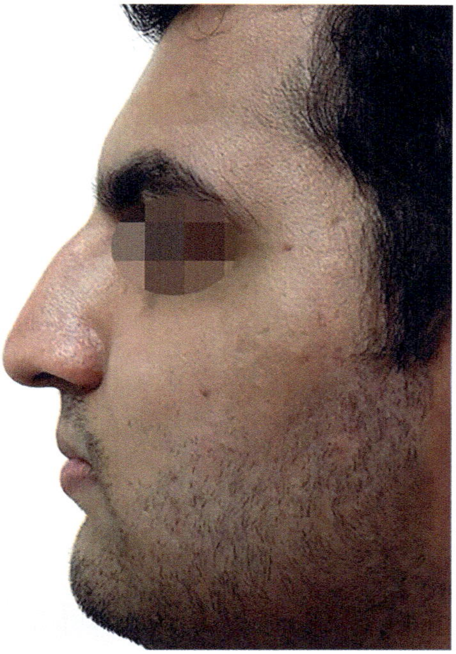

Fig. 7.26 Pre-op lateral

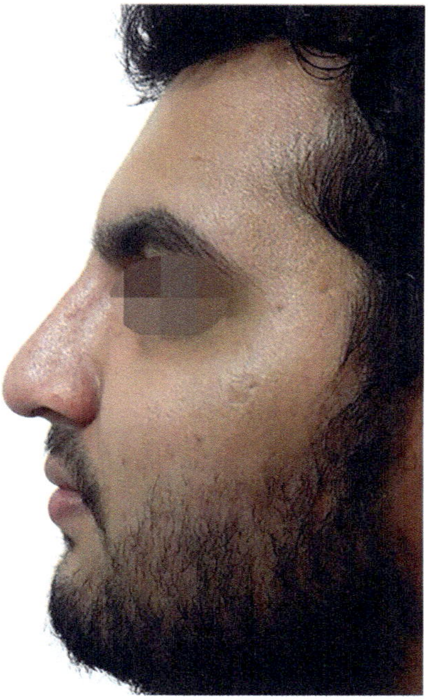

Fig. 7.27 Post-op lateral

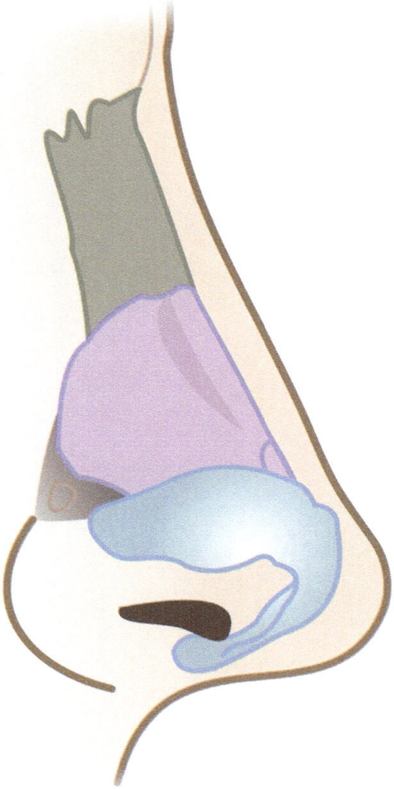

Fig. 7.28 Schematic diagram of pseudo-hump deformity

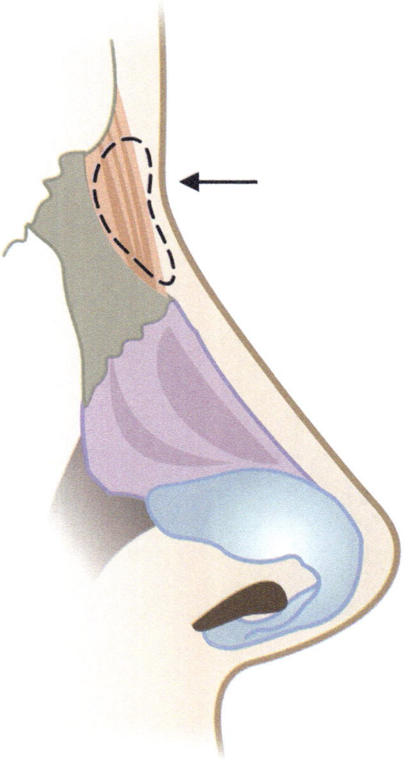

Fig. 7.29 Procerus muscle at the radix

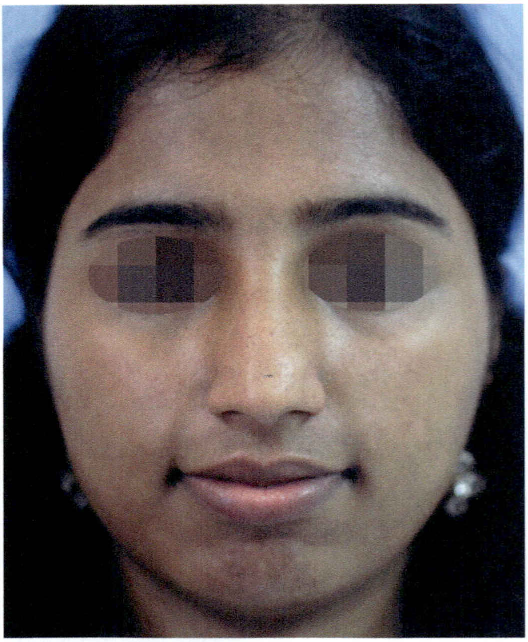

Fig. 7.30 Pre-op frontal

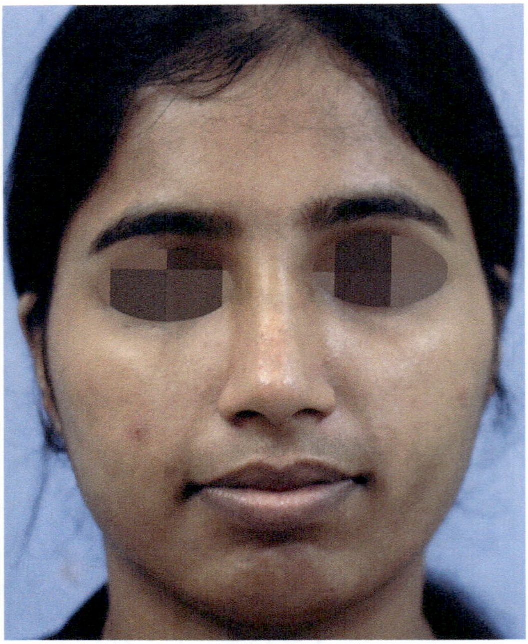

Fig. 7.31 Post-op frontal

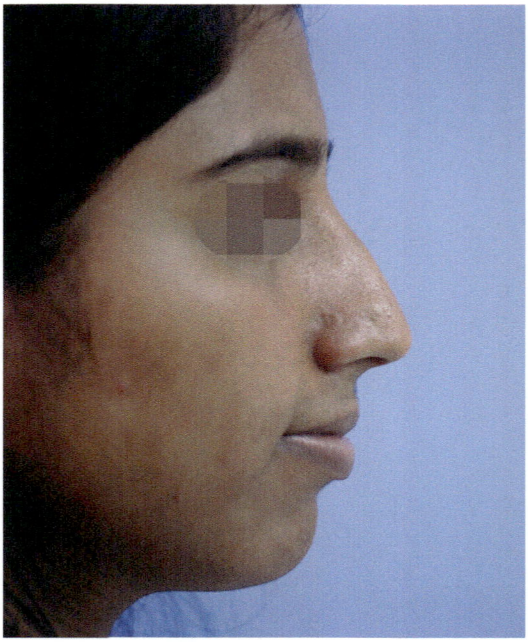

Fig. 7.32 Pre-op lateral

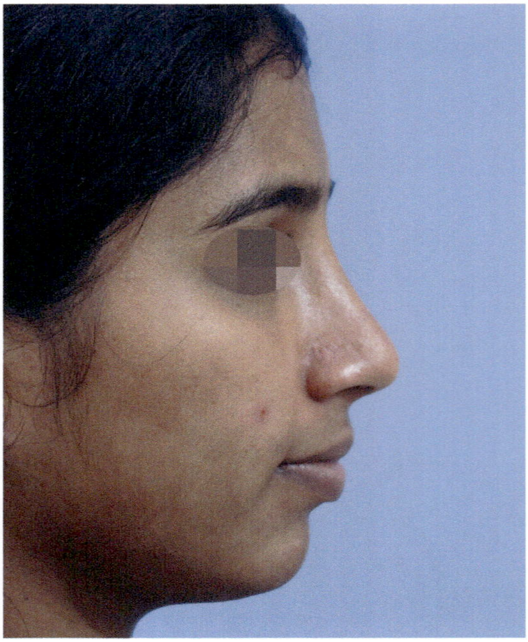

Fig. 7.33 Post-op lateral

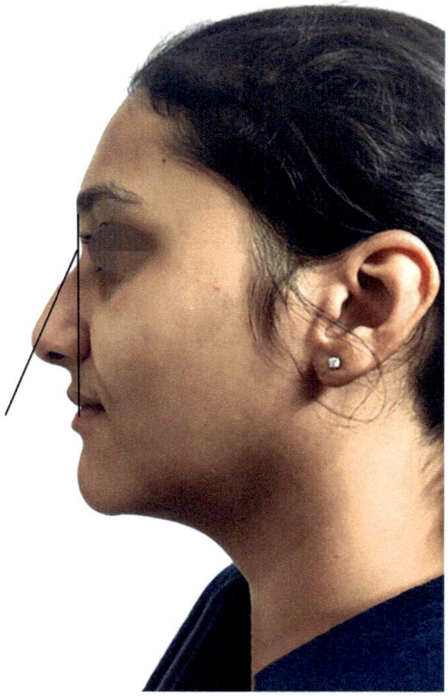

Fig. 7.34 Lateral view of bony and cartilaginous hump nose and resection is planned above the line drawn on the nose

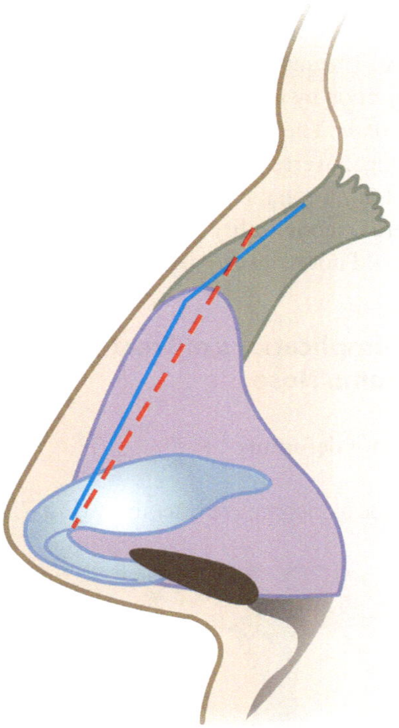

Fig. 7.35 Hump reduction. Blue line—ideal line for hump reduction. Red dotted line—to be avoided

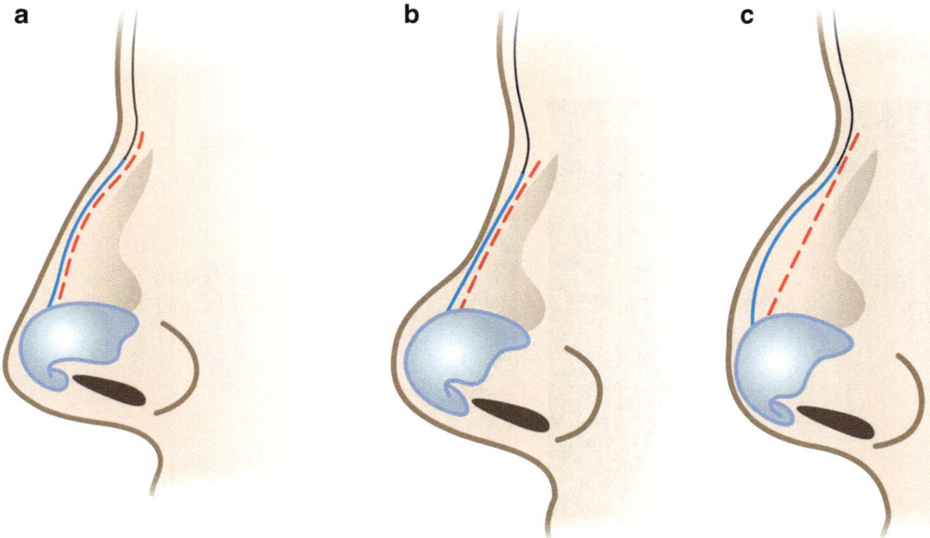

Fig. 7.36 (**a**, **b**, **c**) The line of excision should be slightly convex. (**a**) Allowing for differential skin thickness. This produces a straight external, lateral profile. Straight-line excision leads to inadequate dorsal height relative to tip projection (**b**, **c**)

- *Marking to be done from the tip to NFA*: Defines the extent of removal
- *Preserve*: The underlining mucosa and the rhinion projection by not excising in a straight line.
- *Nasal bones*: The caudal part of nasal bones is thin; hence, overresection is avoided there. On the contrary, cephalic part is generally thicker, and there is a possibility of underresection and this should not be overlooked.

7.4.1 Complications of Treating Hump Nose

(a) Open roof deformity

This is due to incomplete osteotomy (Fig. 7.37).

(b) Ski slope nose the open roof is due to insufficient reconstruction of the dorsum by spreader flaps

This is a commonly seen deformity involving both the bony and cartilaginous parts as a result of excessive hump removal, especially in the K area. To some extent, inadequately supported caudal septum can also be responsible for this deformity. This can be prevented by paying attention to the reduction of the lower bony dorsum and not forgetting to fix the cartilaginous septum to the anterior nasal spine. Grafting with DCF in 'K' area also must be done. Hence, during reduction rhinoplasty, along with hump reduction, tip reduction is done to deproject the nose (Figs. 7.38 and 7.39).

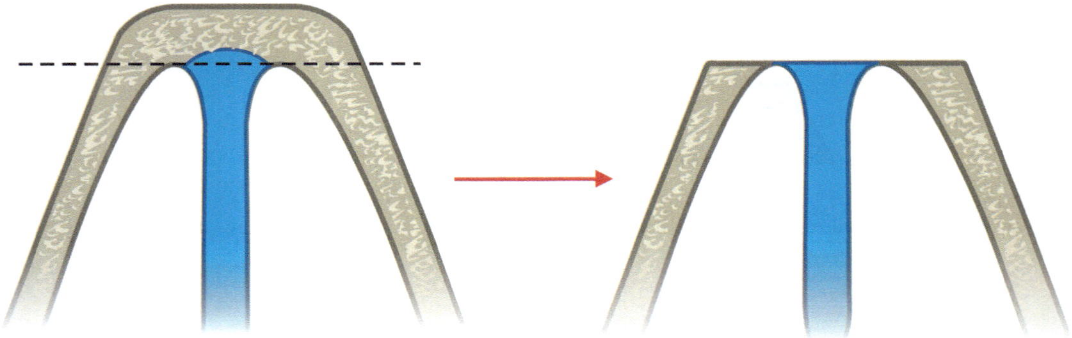

Fig. 7.37 Open roof deformity

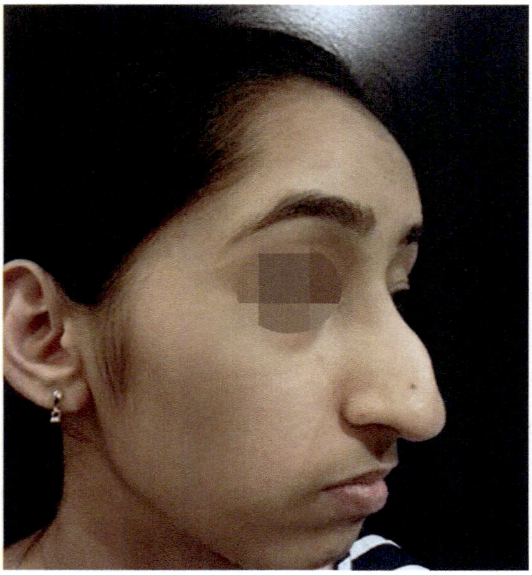

Fig. 7.38 Pre-op picture of cartilaginous and hump nose

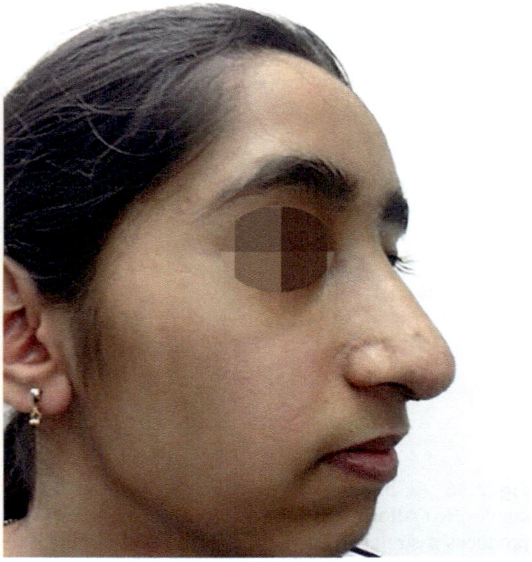

Fig. 7.39 Post-op picture—ski slope nose

(c) Spontaneous bone growth

This can be prevented by removing the bone dust thoroughly following drilling and rasping.

(d) Inverted V deformity

Inverted V deformity can be prevented by placing spreader grafts to prevent the loss of stability at the "K" area to retain the smooth contour of the pyriform aperture.

(e) Small irregularities/localised irregularities

This can be filled with free diced cartilage. In patients from South India, a thicker skin can help to mask the small irregularities.

7.5 Preservation Rhinoplasty

Conventional hump resections are a hallmark of rhinoplasty; there has been a rekindled interest in dorsal preservation, which claims to have superior functional and aesthetic results.

What Exactly Happens in Preservation Rhinoplasty?

- Dorsal preservation allows for mobilisation of the osseocartilaginous nasal vault as a single unit and thereby prevents disruption of the natural keystone area.
- Osseous nasal vault is managed with transverse osteotomy and either bilateral single or bilateral bony wedge resection.
- The septum is resected based on the location of cartilage. Subdorsal, *high septal*, mid-septal and inferior septum resections are different techniques which result in pleasing dorsal aesthetic lines.
- Patency of the internal nasal valve is improved with dorsal preservation techniques.

High septal resection technique does suggest positive functional and cosmetic outcomes.

Deviated Noses or Crooked Noses 8

Main

Deviated or crooked noses are one of our favourite deformities and contribute to nearly 60% of our rhinoplasty practice. We have always loved tackling and treating crooked noses because each case is different and beautiful in its own way. It is certainly a challenging problem as a beginner, and a lot of time is needed to analyse and consider the various techniques needed to provide good results. The terms deviated nose, crooked nose and scoliotic nose encompass a multiplicity of deformities that require specific manoeuvres to be corrected precisely.

8.1 Presentation

Unlike other nasal deformities, most of the patients are symptomatic, the main presentation being nasal obstruction, in addition to the cosmetic deformity. Associated nasal septal deviation is common. The commonest cause of revision surgery in such cases is a failure to pay adequate attention to the treatment of nasal obstruction, especially in the nasal valve area.

8.1.1 Causes of Deviated Nasal Septum

The surgeon's first task is to elucidate the aetiology of the obstruction and then plan surgical correction, which can range from placement of spreader grafts to support the internal nasal valve to radical decisions like extracorporeal or partial extracorporeal septal reconstruction:

1. *Trauma*: Severe nasal septal deviations usually arise as a result of nasal trauma. Trauma can be frontal, fronto-lateral or lateral. Unrecognised birth trauma or early childhood trauma disrupts the growth centres of the septum and results in marked abnormal development that manifests at puberty. In most of the post-traumatic cases, usually there is displacement of the caudal septum from the groove of the maxillary crest, correction of which is of paramount importance for the successful straightening of the septum and, consequently, the external nose. The severe form of post-traumatic nasal deformity sometimes presents with cartilage and bony septal deformities in all three levels of the nasal septum. If the cartilage is torn or fractured and if it heals in the wrong position, angled deformities often appear that are difficult to correct using classic techniques. Consequently, as many as 50% of cases of post-traumatic nasal deformities require subsequent revision septorhinoplasty.
2. *Previous surgery*: Rohrich and Adams reported that the incidence of post-septoplasty deformity requiring subsequent septorhinoplasty ranges from 14% to 50%. They attributed this high revision rate to unrecognised or uncorrected septal deviation.

V. Ghaisas, *Indian Ethnic Rhinoplasty*, https://doi.org/10.1007/978-981-16-2478-0_8

3. *Congenital malformations*, like cleft noses, have very typical septal deviations in the mid-portion to the cleft side and caudally to the normal side.
4. *The diseases of the septum and internal nose* like septal abscess and granulomatous disease of the nose may cause resorption of the supporting structures leading to collapse of nasal valves and deviation. These cases are characterised by a massive deformation/deformities in all levels of the septum with consequent blockage of one or both nostrils.

8.1.2 Internal Nasal Valve

The morphology of internal nasal valve is given in detail in Chap. 5—Septum. The internal nasal valve is a crucial regulator of nasal airflow dynamics and must be preserved and/or reconstructed during every septorhinoplasty. Anterior septal deviations, particularly if high on the septum, are often accompanied by a narrow valve angle. Even small anterior deviations cause significant nasal obstruction because they are located exactly in the narrowest portion of the nasal cavity, the nasal valve. Studies (carried out by Grymer et al.) used pre- and post-operative acoustic rhinometry measures to prove that the nasal obstruction impact caused by minimum anterior nasal septum deviations is much greater than the one caused by large posterior deviations.

Injury and destabilisation of this complex, by either surgery or trauma, may result in collapse and subsequent nasal airway obstruction. So, special attention must be given to internal nasal valve during pre-operative examination, especially in cases of high septal deviations, where the valve appears closed or collapsed. Also, special attention must be given intraoperatively to the internal nasal valve region very meticulously. Even after removal of a large septal spur, posterior deviation and relocation of caudal septum over nasal spine, if the internal nasal valve still doesn't open up, then a more aggressive approach is generally required to relieve the obstruction. Patient does not get satisfaction of breathing unless the air current passes through the internal nasal valve. So, if the internal nasal valve doesn't open up at the end of septal surgery, there is a very high probability that the patient may not benefit from surgery.

8.1.3 Classifications of DNS

Various classifications of septal deviations are proposed like Baumann classification, Mladina classification, Jang classification and Bahman Guyuron. Yet, there is no universally accepted classification of the septal deviation till now for guiding the surgeon to do proper intervention in treating the problem. However, majority of the currently published classification systems for internal nasal septal deviations can be summarised as C-shaped or reverse C-shaped, S-shaped or reverse S-shaped deviations in the anteroposterior and cephalo-caudal dimensions (Figs. 8.1, 8.2, 8.3 and 8.4).

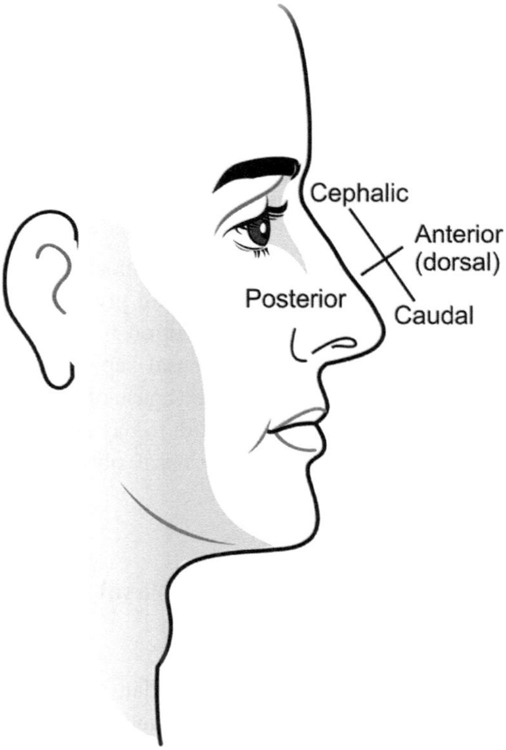

Fig. 8.1 Nose: understanding the dimensions

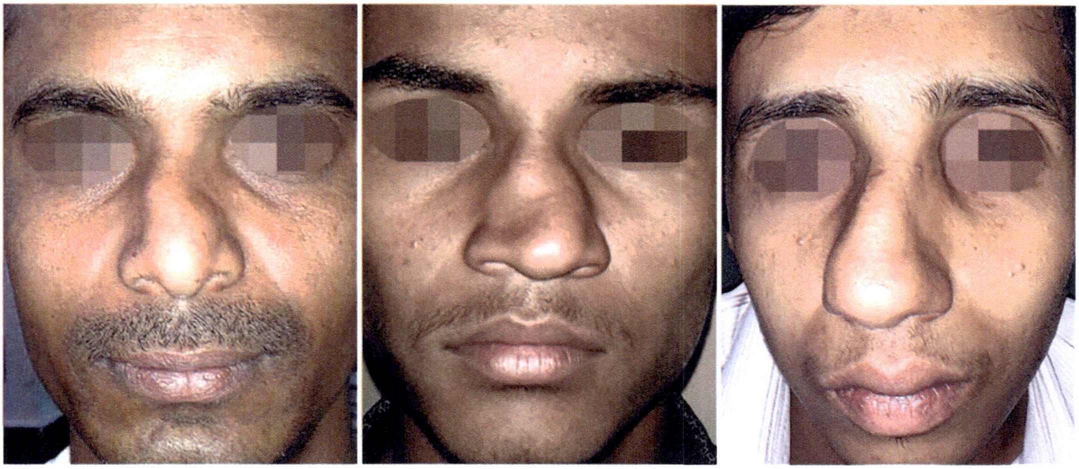

Figs. 8.2–8.4 (left: Fig. 8.2): S-shaped deviation; (middle: Fig. 8.3): Reverse S-shaped deviation; (right: Fig. 8.4): C-shaped deviation

So, for the purpose of surgical considerations, classification proposed by Bahman Guyuron is the most appropriate, which proposes six classes of septal deviation.

1. *Septal tilt* (Fig. 8.5): The most common type of septal deviation is a septal tilt, in which the septum itself has no significant underlying curvature but is tilted to one side because the caudal septum is dislodged to one side of the vomer bone. In most cases of septal tilt, the internal dislodgement of the septum is to one side, and the external deviation of the nose is to the opposite side.
2. *C-shaped anteroposterior (caudal) deviation* (Fig. 8.6) is usually associated with deviation of the vomer plate. External reflection of the anteroposterior C deviation is often similar to the septal tilt.
3. *S-shaped anteroposterior (caudal) deviation* (Fig. 8.7) is defined by two opposite curvatures in continuity in the anteroposterior direction. Externally, the anteroposterior deviation will present with a shift of the nose to the left or right. Rarely, the anterior portion of the nose may look totally straight.
4. *C-shaped cephalo-caudal (dorsal) deviation* (Fig. 8.8) is similar to the previous type except that the curvatures are in cephalo-caudal direction. The external nose follows the pattern of the septal deviation.
5. *S-shaped cephalo-caudal (dorsal) deviation* (Fig. 8.9) is defined by two opposite curvatures in continuity in the cephalo-caudal direction. The external nose follows the pattern of the septal deviation.
6. *Localised deviation or spur* (Fig. 8.10) is the last type of septal deviation. This is a purely functional problem and has no translation to the external shape of the nose.

Typically, a septoplasty suffices in addressing an isolated spur, but on occasions where there are severe septal deviations, more than 30 degrees from the axis, it warrants a single-stage septorhinoplasty. The C- or S-shaped curvatures are difficult to correct surgically or will frequently return post-operatively. C- and S-shaped deformities are sometimes surgically scored on the convex side to silence the cartilaginous memory. One must remember that whenever scoring is done, it's always advisable to splint it with cartilage or perpendicular plate of ethmoid with multiple drill holes.

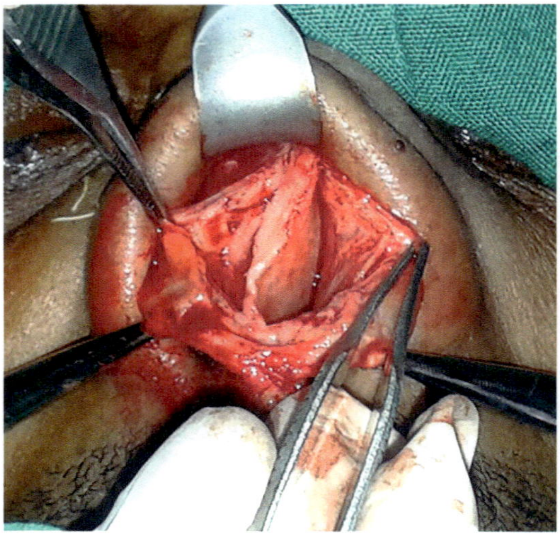

Fig. 8.5 Septal tilt

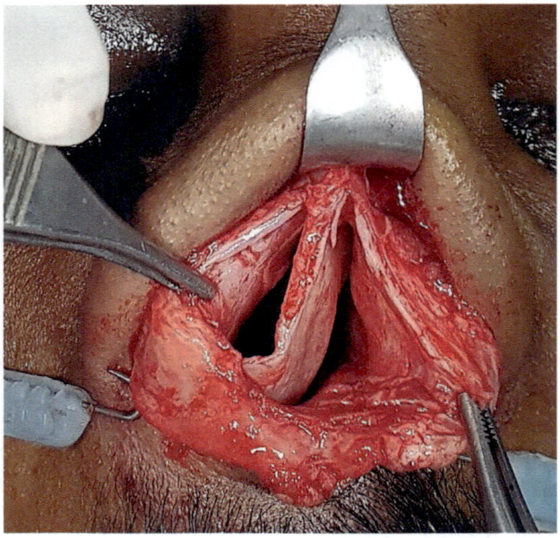

Fig. 8.6 C-shaped caudal (anteroposterior) deviation

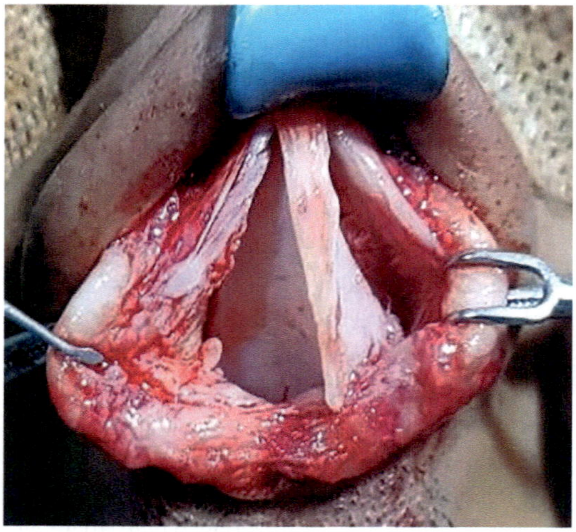

Fig. 8.7 S-shaped caudal (anteroposterior) deviation

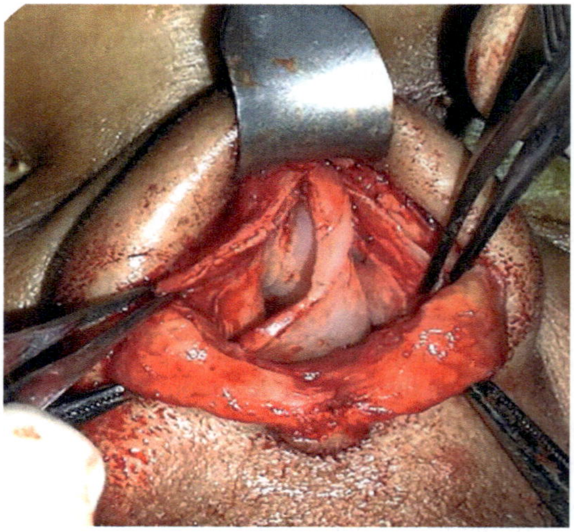

Fig. 8.8 C-shaped dorsal (cephalo-caudal) deviation

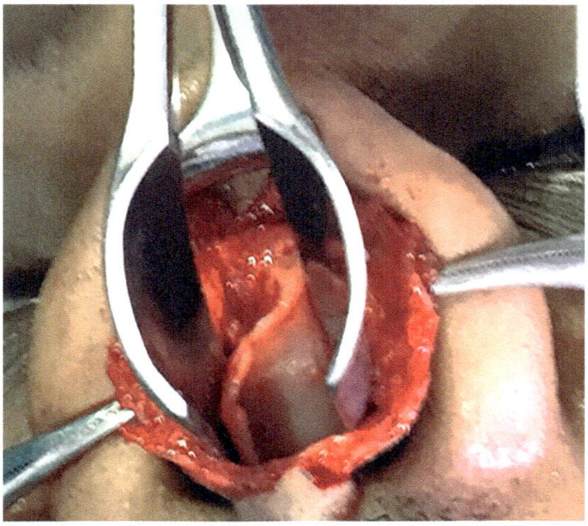

Fig. 8.9 S-shaped dorsal (cephalo-caudal) deviation

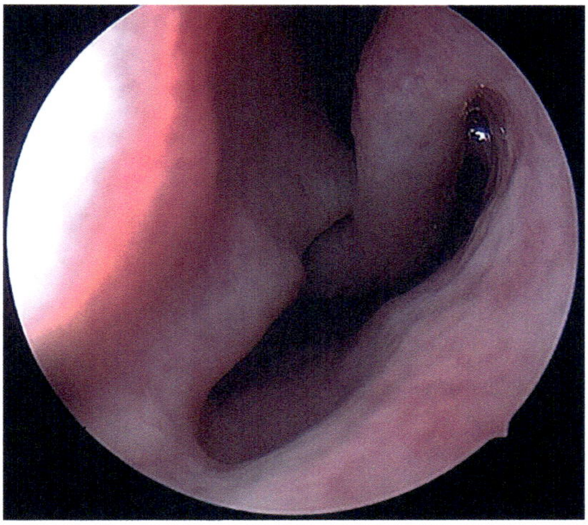

Fig. 8.10 Isolated septal spur

8.1.4 Patient Assessment

A comprehensive assessment of the nasal septum serves an essential role in pre-operative planning, re-establishing function and overall cosmetic appeal. At the end of patient assessment, the surgeon must be able to make an accurate diagnosis of the deformity so as to formulate an appropriate surgical plan considering various factors like balance, proportion, symmetry and correction of nasal function.

8.1.5 Examination

With a thorough examination, the surgeon should be able to define the deformity of the nasal septum in essentially two dimensions, i.e. in cephalo-caudal (along the dorsum) and the anteroposterior (along the caudal margins). *The deformities can be divided into septal tilt, C-shaped or S-shaped.*

This should be aided by actual palpation of the dorsal septum and the caudal septum with the help of the thumb and forefinger to appreciate the curvature and thickness of the septum. During examination, the identification of the C and S shapes remains crucial to identifying potentially complex surgeries compared to less technically challenging operative interventions such as septal tilts. Tip recoil of the septum during palpation will also help you to get an overall idea about the strength of the anterior septal cartilage. Cottle's test to check the involvement of the internal nasal valve has been explained in Chap. 3—Evaluation of Indian Ethnic Rhinoplasty Patient.

8.2 Types of Septal Deviations

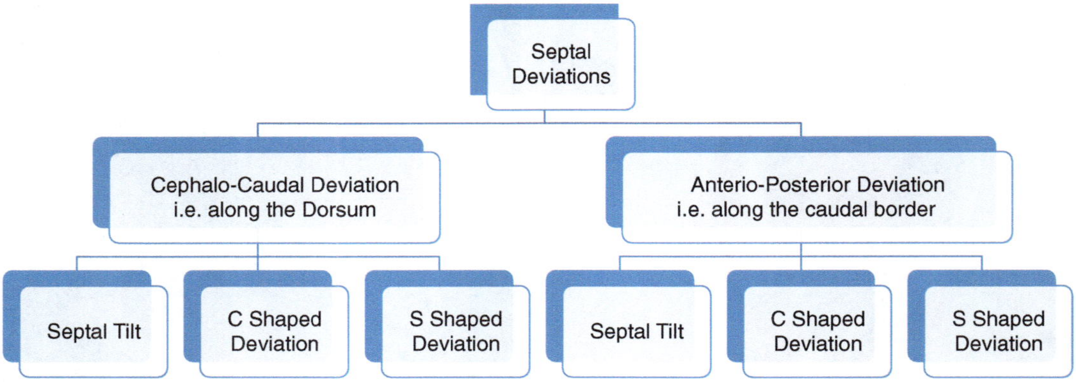

8.2.1 Facial Asymmetry

In crooked nose rhinoplasty, it is very crucial to identify if there is any significant facial asymmetry. This can easily be done by photographic analysis. The prerequisite is a proper front view photograph taken from a minimum of 5 ft distance with both ears of the patient equally seen on the sides, in a Frankfurt horizontal plane. Then, a straight vertical line passing through the midpoint between the centre of the eyebrows is drawn vertically downwards, and the surgeon should note if it passes through the centre of the philtrum. If it does, then the face is symmetrical, and if doesn't, then there is a definite facial asymmetry. Asymmetry, if any, should be brought to notice of patient, and guarded prognosis should be given in such cases of facial asymmetry (Figs. 8.11, 8.12 and 8.13). In cases of facial asymmetry, the nose should be aligned straight from the root of the nose to camouflage the deformity maximally.

8.2.2 Rhinomanometry (Fig. 8.14)

8.2.3 Formulation of Surgical Plan

After detailed clinical examination and photographic analysis, the surgeon should be able to arrive at a diagnosis of the deformity and should

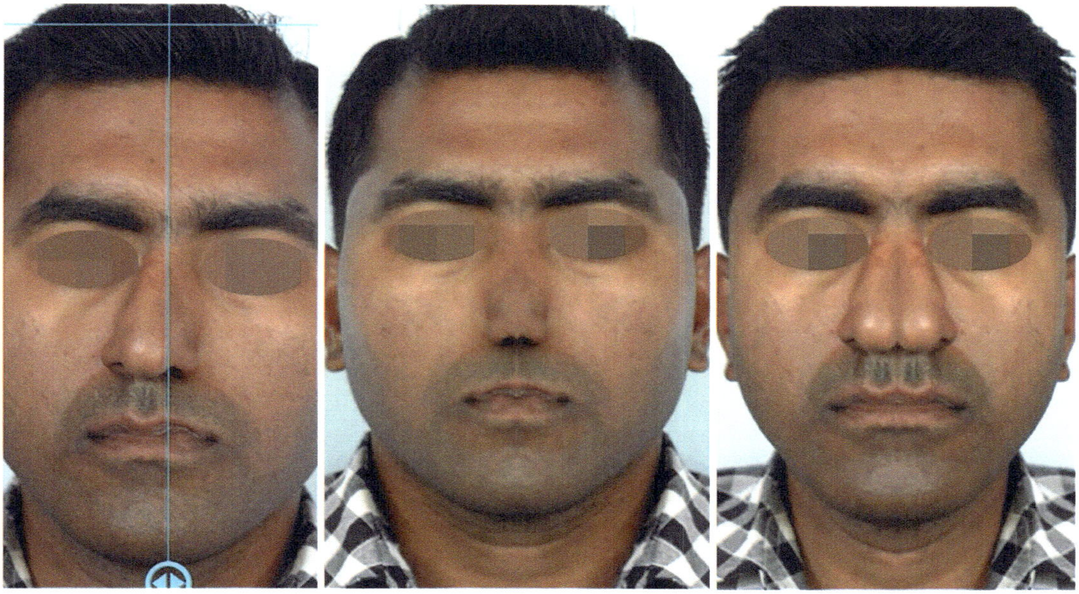

Figs. 8.11–8.13 (left: Fig. 8.11): Vertical line drawn through the centre of the forehead doesn't pass through the centre of the philtrum; (middle: Fig. 8.12): Duplicating the left side of the face; (right: Fig. 8.13): Duplicating the right side of the face

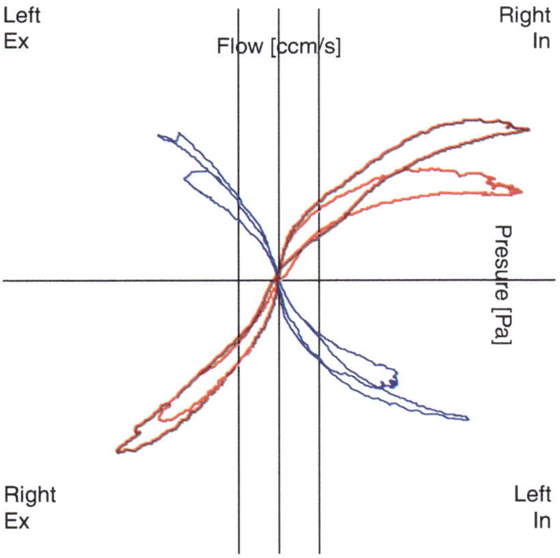

Fig. 8.14 Four-phase rhinomanometry showing typical valve phenomenon with loops on inspiration as well as expiration

be able to formulate a tentative surgical plan regarding the choice of technique of septoplasty that needs to be employed. The final surgical plan should be formulated only after opening the nose and separating the septum from the upper lateral cartilages. The points to be considered after this step are the position of the septum at the keystone area (whether it lies in the centre or in the paramedian position in relation to the centre of the eyebrow) and the position of nasal spine (whether it lies in the centre or in paramedian position in relation to the philtrum). It is prudent to mark these points intraoperatively at the centre point of the forehead between the eyebrows and the centre of the philtrum. The alignment of the same should be checked and confirmed by holding a straight instrument like a straight elevator between these markings.

8.3 Surgical Planning for Deviated Noses

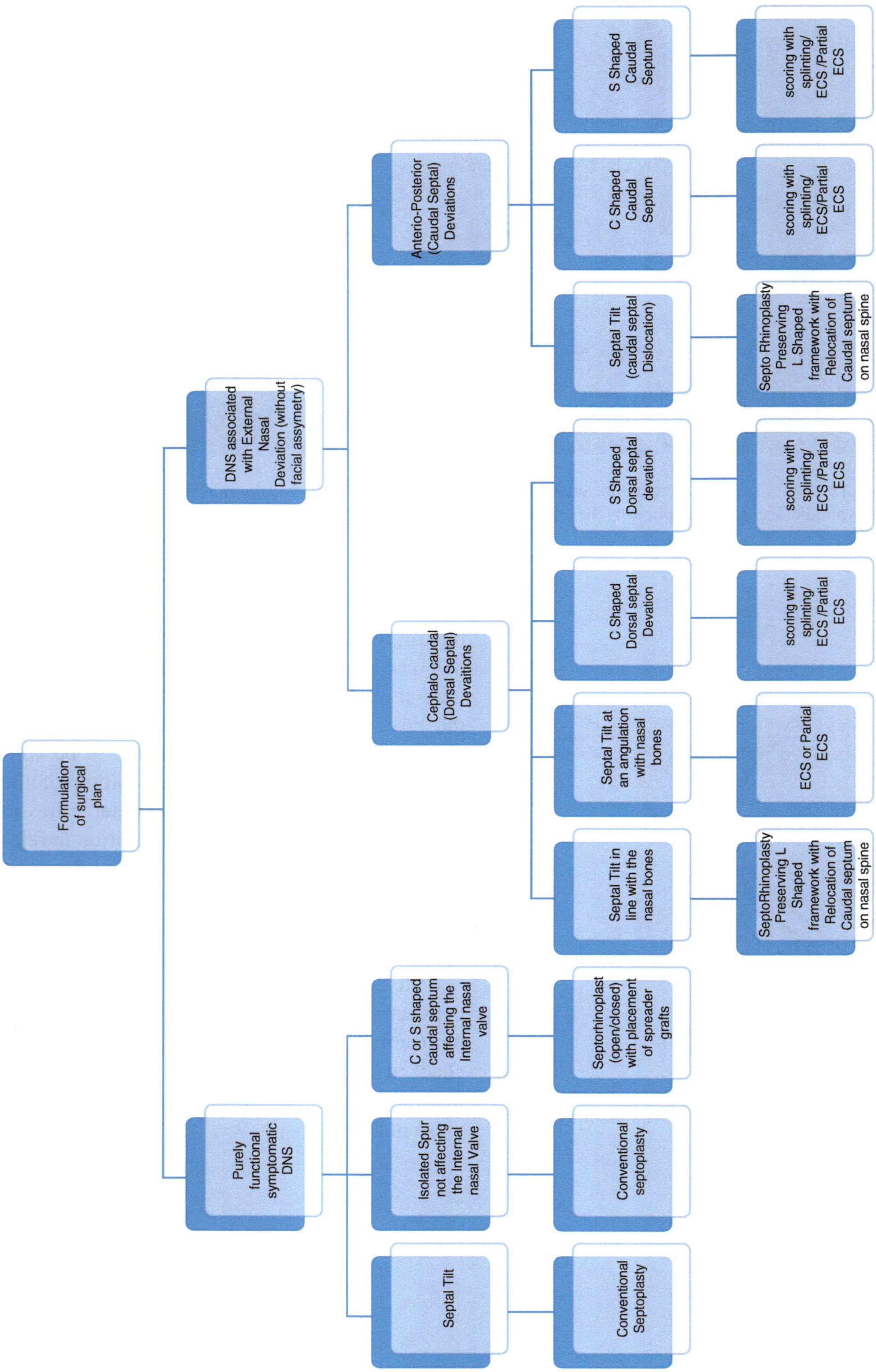

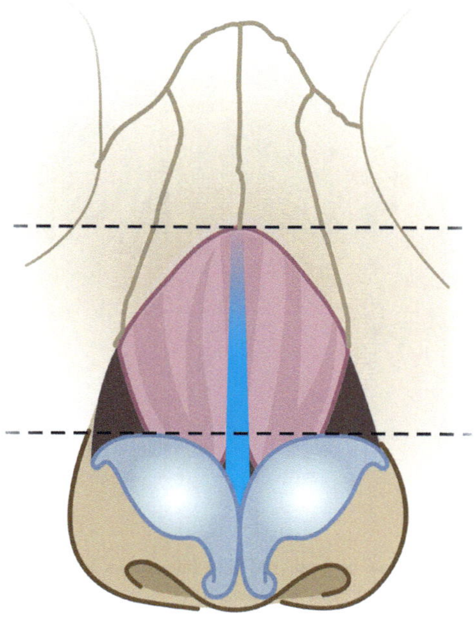

Fig. 8.15 Divisions of the nose

8.3.1 Surgical Treatment of the Deviated Nose

The surgical management of the deviated nose is a challenging problem even for an experienced rhinoplasty surgeon as the aesthetic and functional failures in correcting this problem are not uncommon. The septum and the nasal bones control the direction of the nose. Thus, deviation of the nose can result from misalignment of one or the other, or a combination of both. Often, the nasal bones follow the direction of the deviated septum. However, these structures may move independently.

For easier understanding of the management strategy and to simplify the complexity of the treatment, I like to divide the nose into three divided horizontal segments (Fig. 8.15).

8.4 Correction of Upper 1/3rd (Bony Vault) Deviations

The upper one-third of the nose is composed of nasal bones and ascending process of maxilla. So, mobilisation of the bony dorsum with osteotomies needs to be done. Osteotomy, according to us, is the most difficult technique to master. Beginners have to understand the anatomy of the bones and the right technique to fracture the bone completely and align it further is fundamental (explained in detail in basic rhinoplasty surgery). We always prefer paramedian, low to low lateral and transverse osteotomy (Figs. 8.16 and 8.17) in most of the cases of deviated noses as it mobilises the bony pyramid completely and then nasal bones can be repositioned at a desired position. To avoid return of nasal bones to its previous position, spreader grafts can be very useful.

In cases of convex nasal bones, it is sometimes prudent to do osteoplasty either by rasping or by powered instruments like a drill or a Piezotome. The second option, in such cases of convex nasal bones, is to do an intermediate osteotomy, which has to be done before doing the lateral osteotomy.

In cases of concave nasal bones, one can use morselized cartilage or diced cartilage to camouflage the defect after doing osteotomy.

8.5 Correction of Middle and Lower 1/3rd Deviations

A long-standing shift of the midline structures cannot be simply corrected with an osteotomy and forceful repositioning. It requires component separation and realignment of all the structures individually, including the nasal bones, the septum and the upper lateral cartilages.

The majority of the techniques, which have been traditionally described to correct nasal septum deviations, only remove more posterior portions of the cartilage, sparing the anterior deviated portion. Doing more conservative procedures such as mobilisations, sutures or weakening this portion, although does not cause any cosmetic harm, the resultant septum deviation correction being inadequate causes the possibility of persistent nasal obstruction post-operatively.

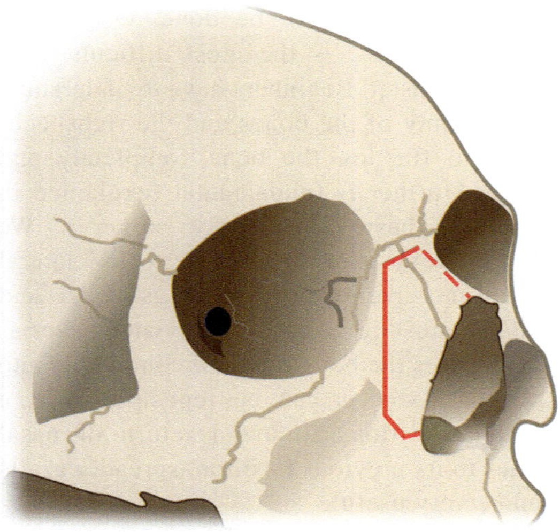

Fig. 8.16 Medial, transverse and lateral osteotomy

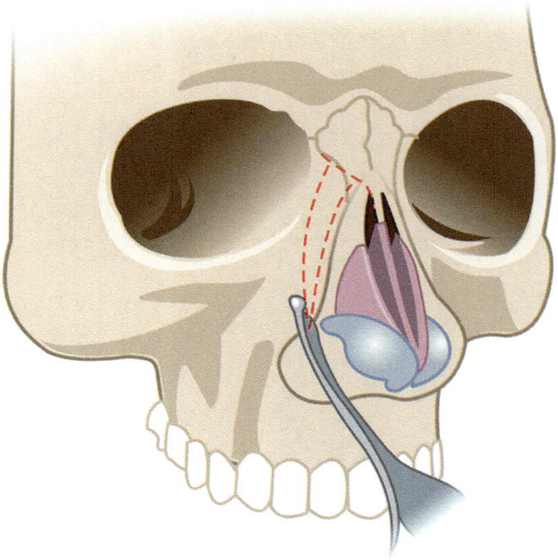

Fig. 8.17 Low to low (red line lateral) vs low to high lateral osteotomy (red line medial)

8.5.1 Correction of Caudal Septal (Lower 1/3rd) Deviations

For the ease of understanding, let's consider the correction of lower 1/3rd first. The functional problems with caudal septum can be deviations and deformities, which are treated by resection, relocation or replacement—the *three Rs* of caudal septal surgery.

8.5.2 Correction of Septal Tilt (Relocation by Swinging Door Technique)

Septal tilt can be corrected by removing the deviated cartilage, leaving an L-shaped strut behind of 1.5 cm of dorsal and caudal septum. A cardinal step is the separation of the dislodged caudal and posterior portion of the L strut from the vomerine groove and anterior nasal spine. Another crucial step is the removal of the small piece of redundant portion of the caudal septal cartilage to provide a 'swinging door'-type free movement of this cartilage (Figs. 8.18 and 8.19). It is imperative to reposition and fix the septum to the anterior nasal spine. We believe in transosseous fixation of this posterior caudal septum to nasal spine by making 2–3 horizontal drill holes in the nasal spine with the help of Lindemann's burr and fixation with a permanent non-absorbable suture like 4-0 Nylon with at least 2–3 passes.

Prior to repositioning of the septum, it is essential to ensure that the anterior nasal spine is in the midline. Otherwise, the free caudal septum will be fixed to a deviated foundation. This can be accomplished by palpation of the anterior nasal spine and comparing its position with the point marked on the centre of the philtrum and another point marked on the centre of the forehead. If the anterior nasal spine is deviated, it is greenstick-fractured and repositioned. The second option for this is fixation on posterior-caudal septum to the other side of the deviation of nasal spine. Sometimes, for proper fixation of the posterior-caudal septum over the nasal spine, one may have to make a groove on the nasal spine with the help of a drill.

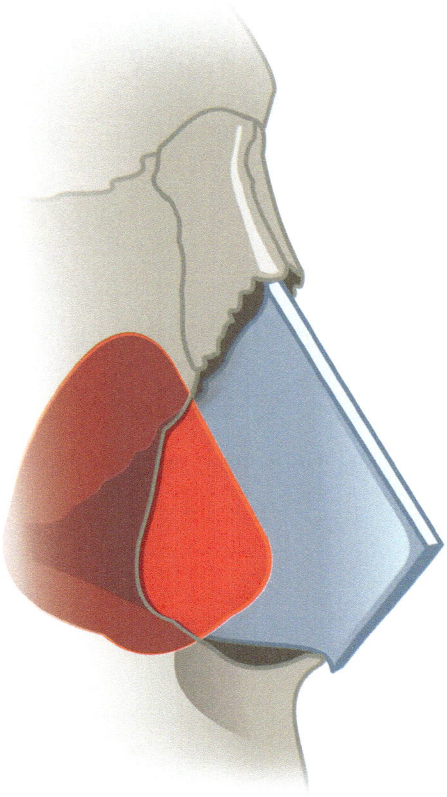

Fig. 8.18 Removal of the small piece of redundant portion of the caudal septal cartilage

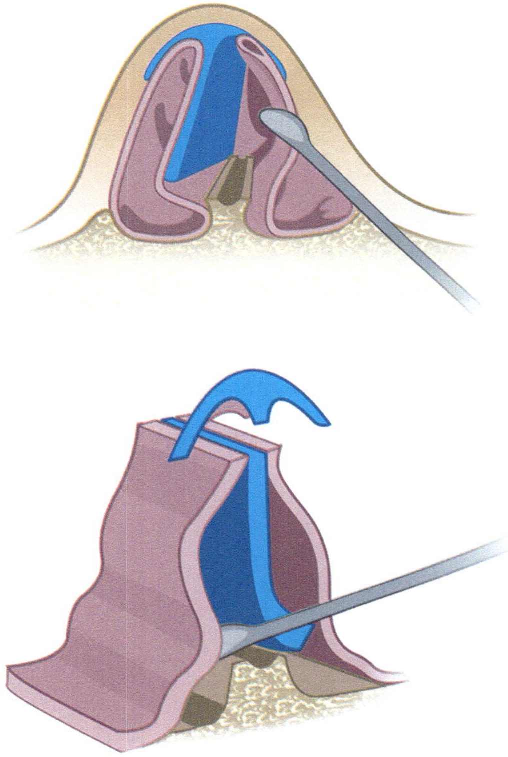

Fig. 8.19 Swinging door technique

Resection If excess caudal septum is present, then excision of the caudal septum or scoring of the septum must be done.

Replacement In some patients, the cause of nasal airway obstruction includes a narrow valve angle and high septal deflection, which are generally not treated with standard septoplasty techniques. In more extreme septal deformities when the septum is deviated off the nasal spine at an angle of greater than 30° in the axial plane, it can be difficult to address the septum by conventional open or endonasal methods, and thus a more aggressive approach may be required like an extracorporeal septoplasty or partial extracorporeal septoplasty and will be discussed in the following section (Figs. 8.20, 8.21, 8.22 and 8.23).

8.5.3 Correction of Dorsal Septal (Middle 1/3rd) Deviations

Dorsal septal deviations can be either a septal tilt, C-shaped or S-shaped cephalo-caudal deviations. Solving these problems needs addressing the specific defects of the various components of the entire osseocartilaginous vault and septum.

Mild degree of C- or S-shaped dorsal septal deviations (>30 degree off the axis) can be corrected by scoring on the concave side (Figs. 8.24 and 8.25) and then splinting with plate of ethmoid bone by making multiple drill holes (Figs. 8.26 and 8.27) and passing multiple through-and-through sutures for straightening and stabilisation.

Use of grafts like spreader grafts a powerhouse graft used in rhinoplasty being useful in numerous

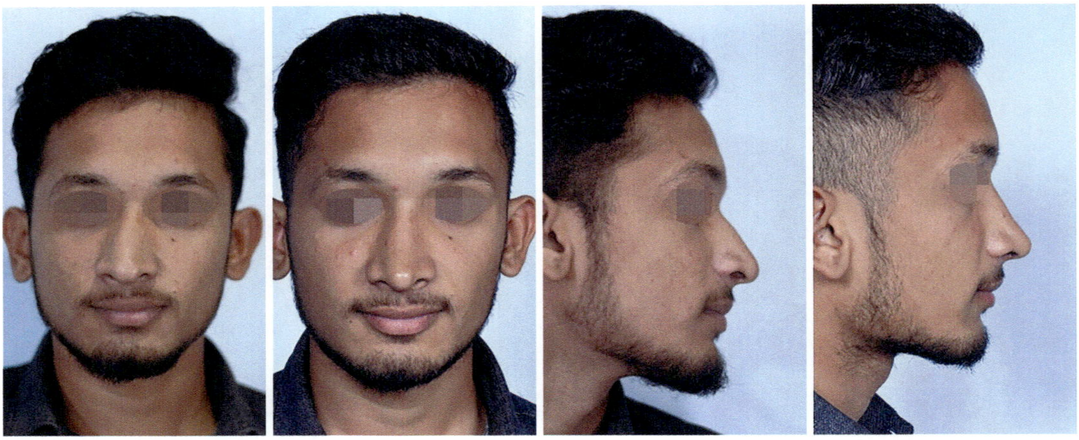

Figs. 8.20–8.23 (left: Fig. 8.20): Pre-op frontal view; (left middle: Fig. 8.21): Post-op frontal view; (right middle: Fig. 8.22): Pre-op lateral view; (right: Fig. 8.23): Post-op lateral view

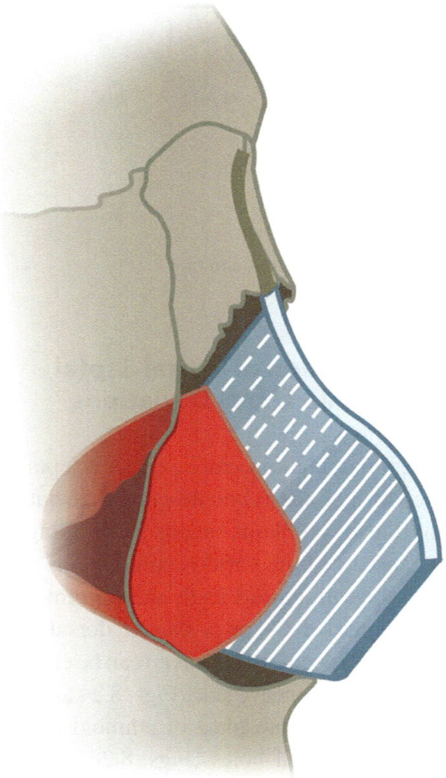

Fig. 8.24 Scoring S-shaped dorsal deviation >30 degrees off the axis

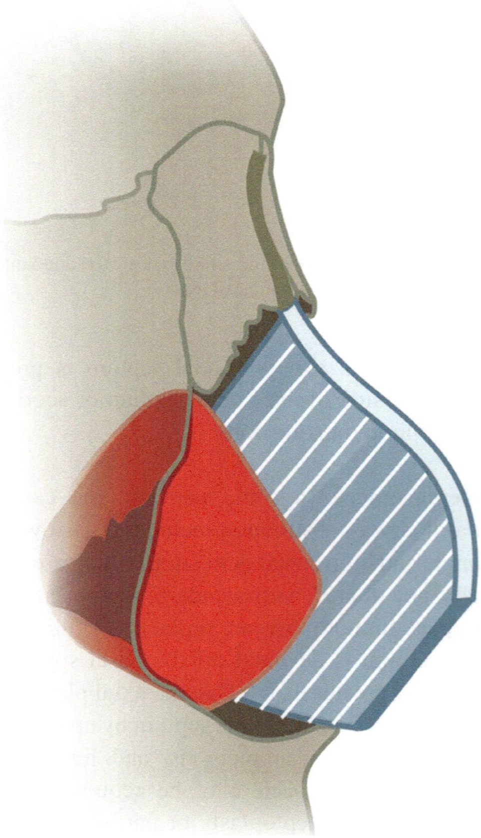

Fig. 8.25 Scoring the C-shaped deviation >30 degrees off the axis

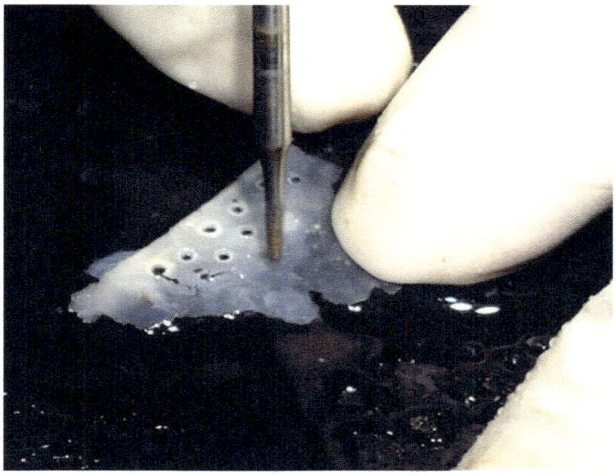

Fig. 8.26 Making drill holes in perpendicular

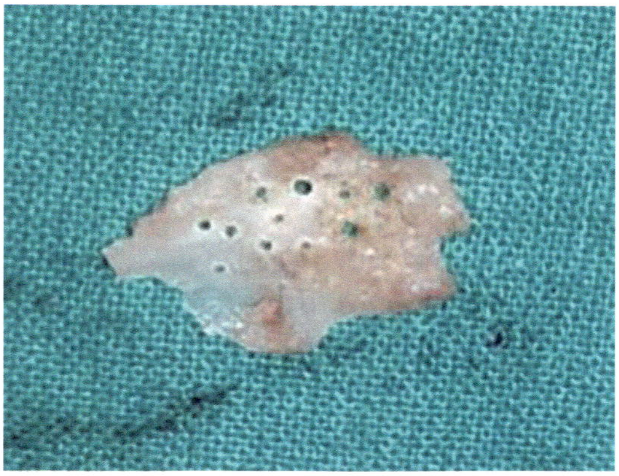

Fig. 8.27 Ethmoid bone with holes plate of ethmoid bone with Lindeman's burr

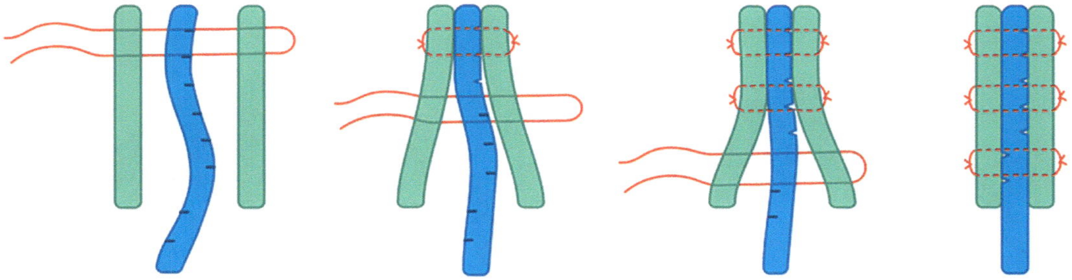

Fig. 8.28 Suturing the spreader grafts to control the curvature >30 degrees off the axis

ways. These are rectangular pieces of cartilage placed on both sides of the nasal septum acting as laminating grafts. The approximate length of the cartilage is 1.5–2 cm length and 1–3 mm in width depending on the patient's deformity. It is inserted submucosally, with its cephalic end extending below the bony pyramid. They are sutured in place as shown below (Figs. 8.28, 8.29 and 8.30).

Advantages include functionally opening the internal nasal valve, providing dorsal stability, helping to achieve straight and parallel dorsal aesthetic lines and preventing 'inverted V deformity' post-operatively.

This is followed by suturing the upper lateral cartilages to this assembly by 2–3 running sutures making it a five-layer sandwich graft.

Figures 8.31, 8.32, 8.33 **and** 8.34**: C-shaped Dorsal (Cephalo-caudal) Deviation**

Figures 8.35, 8.36, 8.37 **and** 8.38**: S-shaped Dorsal (Cephalo-caudal) Deviation**

8.5.4 Extreme Septal Deviations (>30 Degrees Off the Axis)

In cases of more extreme septal deformities when the axis of septal deviation is greater than 30° off the nasal spine or the keystone area, these extreme C- or S-shaped deviations or angulations of dorsal or caudal septum are difficult to address by conventional open or endonasal methods, and

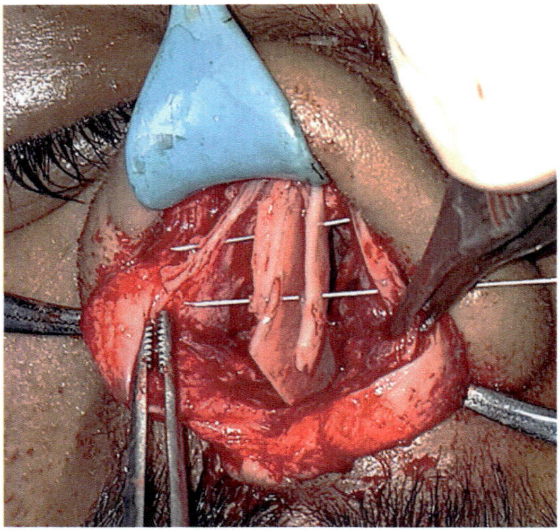

Fig. 8.29 Percutaneous fixation of spreader grafts

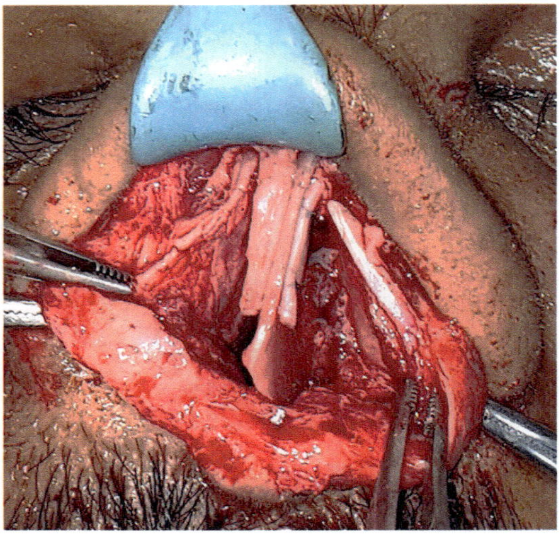

Fig. 8.30 Suturing after scoring the cartilage

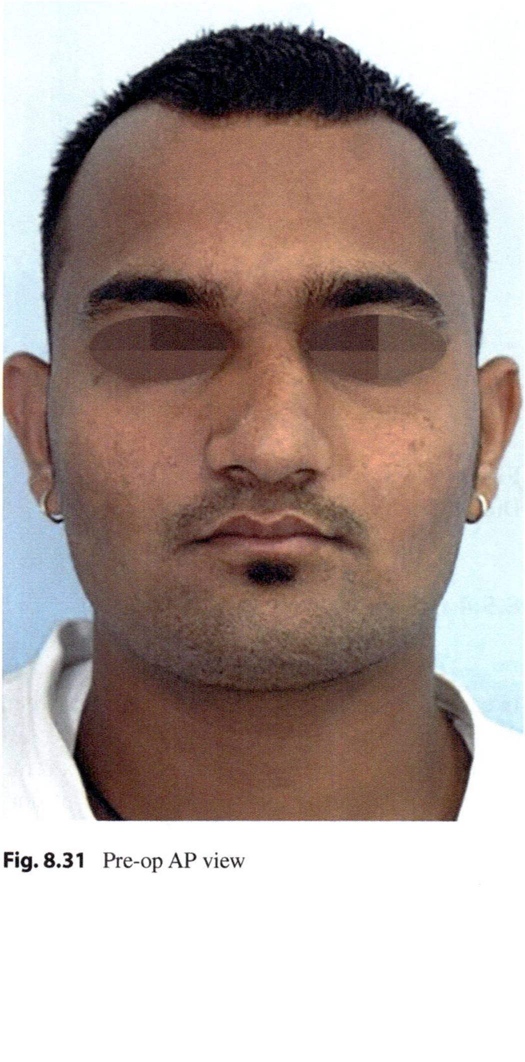

Fig. 8.31 Pre-op AP view

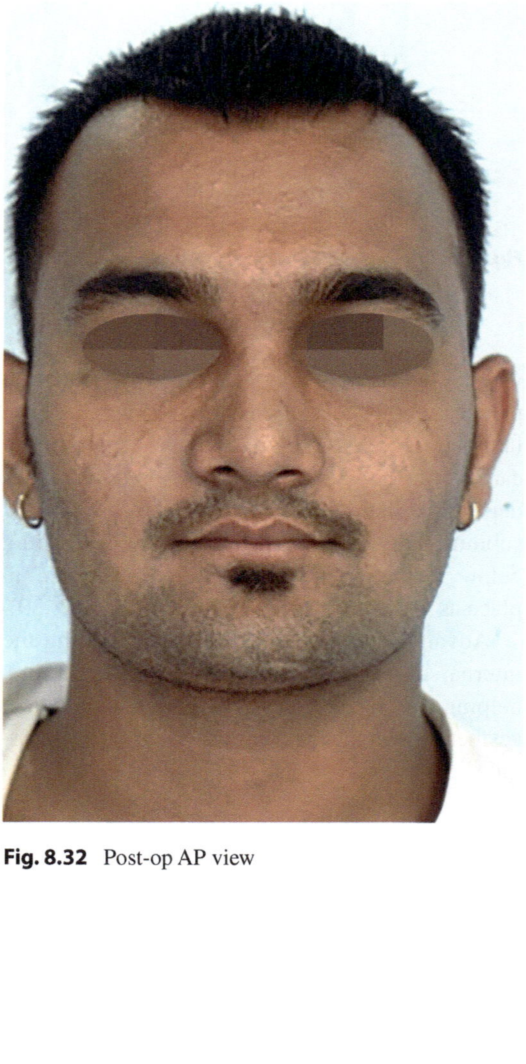

Fig. 8.32 Post-op AP view

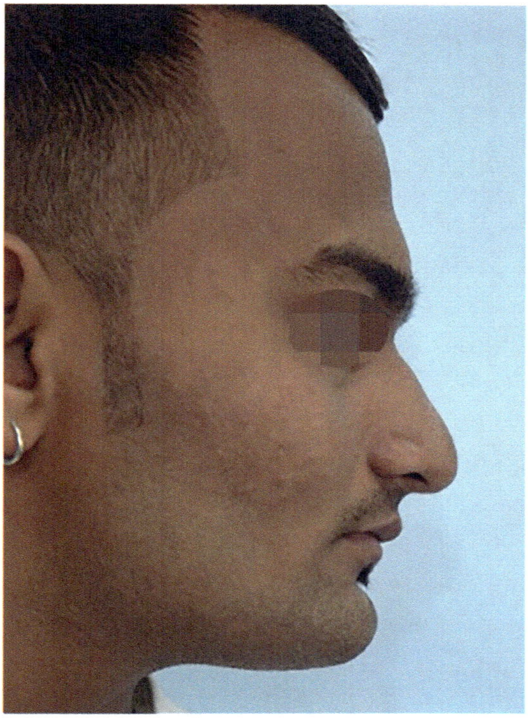

Fig. 8.33 Pre-op lateral view

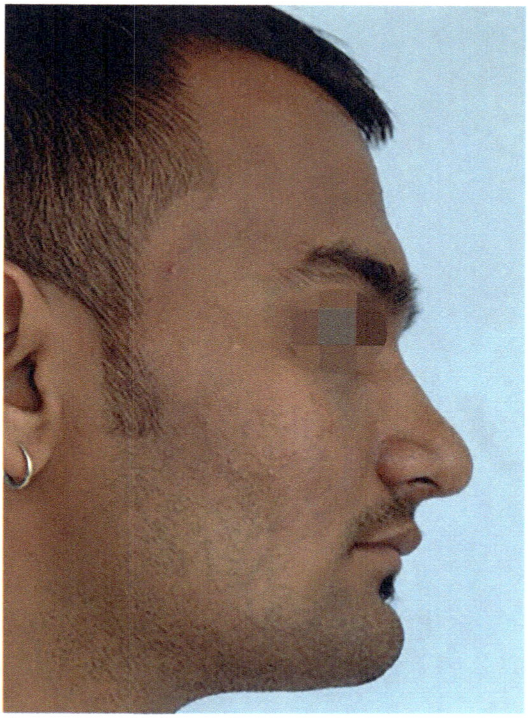

Fig. 8.34 Post-op lateral view

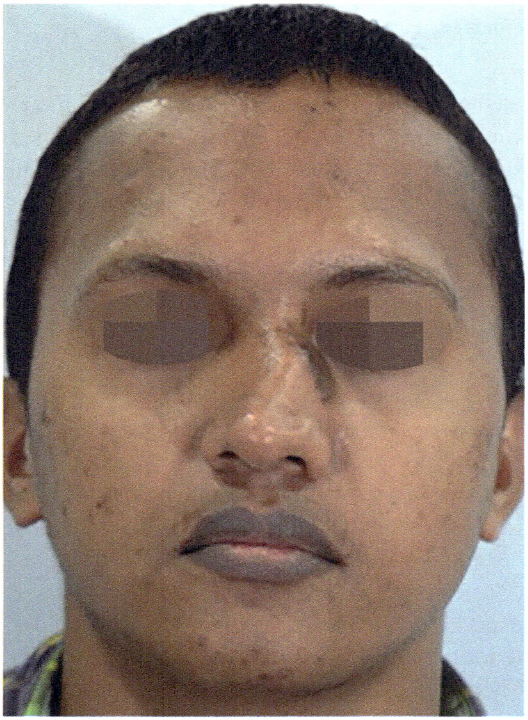

Fig. 8.35 Pre-op AP view

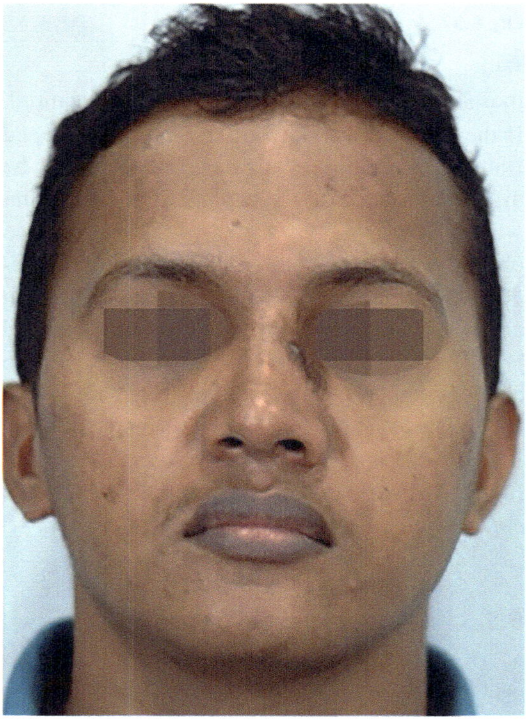

Fig. 8.36 Post-op AP view

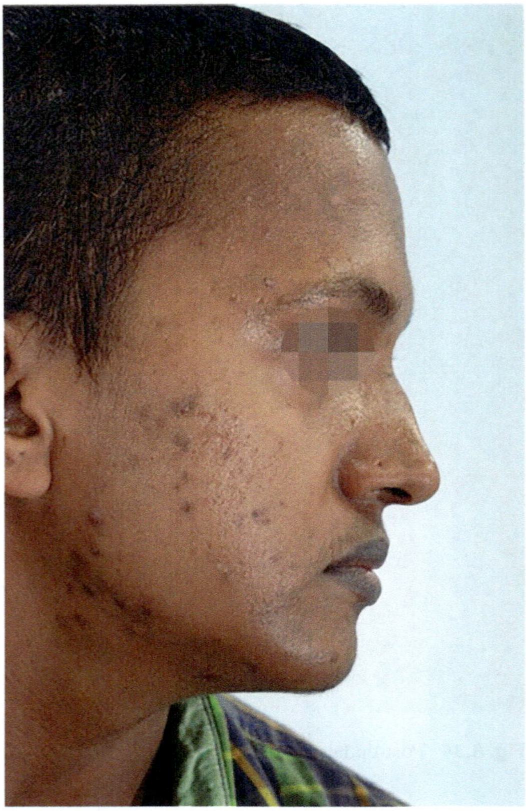

Fig. 8.37 Pre-op lateral view

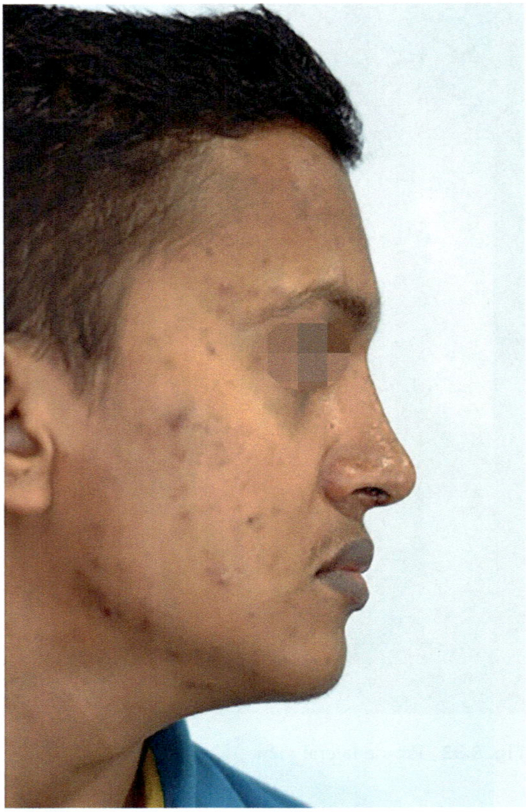

Fig. 8.38 Post-op lateral view

thus a more aggressive approach may be required. If the dorsal or caudal cartilage of the L-shaped framework is bent or angulated, then it may be difficult to achieve a complete straight septum without reconstructing the L strut. There are two options for this problem, the less difficult procedure that preserves the straight part of septum and takes out only the deformed segment is called *partial extracorporeal septoplasty*, and the more challenging procedure that involves taking out the entire septal framework and its reconstruction is called *extracorporeal septoplasty. Corporeal (body)—extracorporeal means to remove the entire septum outside, correct and place it back.*

8.5.5 Extracorporeal Septoplasty

As the name suggests, extracorporeal septoplasty means complete removal of the cartilaginous septum along with bony septum in one piece and then reinsertion of a straight L-shaped framework, which is a replica of original septal dimensions. At first glance it seems excessive and fraught with risks, but the long-term results are excellent and the complications are few. Prof. Gubisch (2006) has summarised his 35 years of experience with extracorporeal septoplasty in a lucid manner in his publications.

8.5.5.1 Operative Technique

Exposure We always prefer an open approach for severely deviated noses especially extracorporeal septoplasty. Anterior septal angle is exposed, the upper lateral cartilages are detached from the dorsal septum, and a top to down dissection is done beginning on the easier concave side first to expose the body of the septum followed by a posterior-to-anterior elevation for ease of dissection. Then, mucoperichondrium and mucoperiosteum are elevated on the more complex convex side having sharp septal angulations and spur.

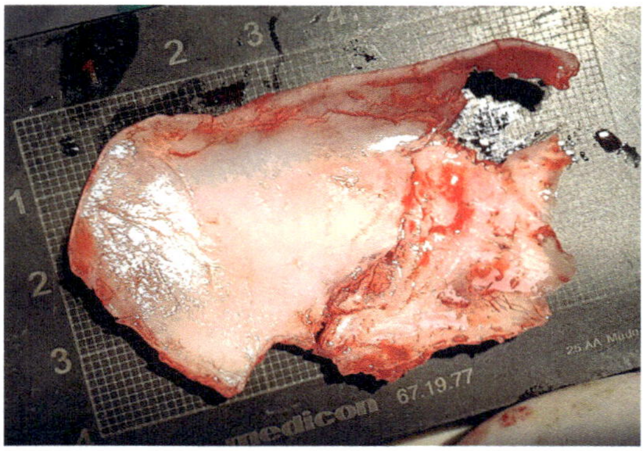

Fig. 8.39 Entire septum removed with bone and the dimensions of dorsal and caudal septum noted

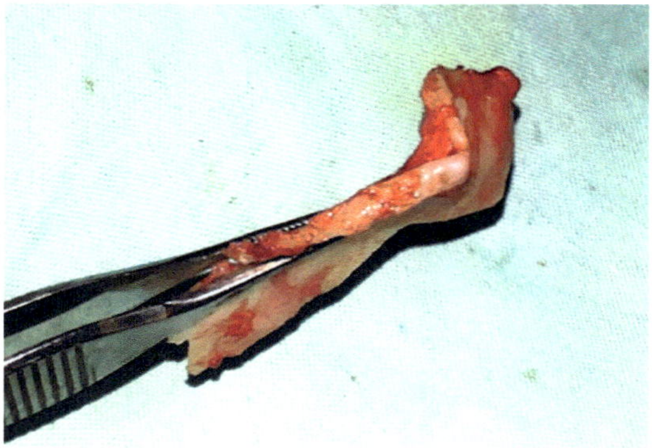

Fig. 8.40 Sharp angulation more than 30 degrees off the axis

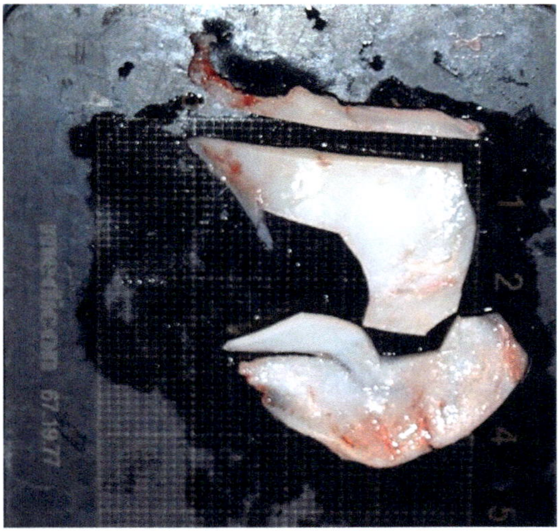

Fig. 8.41 Straight L-shaped cartilage fitting into original dimensions cut from deformed cartilage

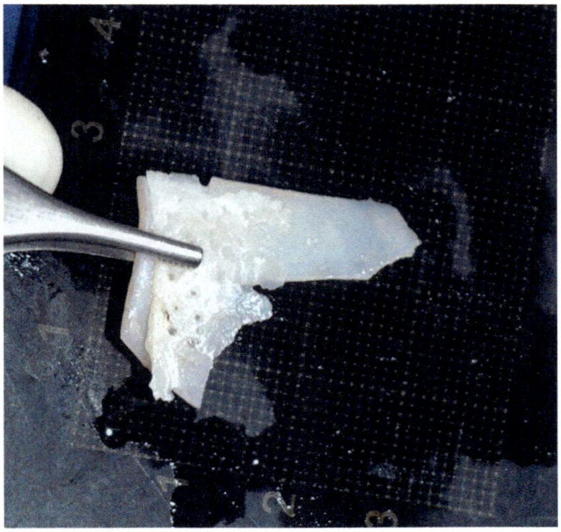

Fig. 8.42 Curvatures if any can be splinted with ethmoid bone with through-and-through sutures

Excision Once the septum is completely exposed, we reassess the deformity and operative plan. Cartilaginous septum is separated from the bony spur and the anterior nasal spine. Then, the perpendicular plate of ethmoid is fractured, and lastly the septum is detached from the keystone area. And thus the entire septum, along with perpendicular plate of ethmoid, is removed completely (Figs. 8.39, 8.40 and 8.41).

Shaping the Graft The cartilage is then placed on a Sheens grid and its outline traced. The dimensions of dorsal and caudal septum are noted along with the angle between them. The dorsal septum generally measures around 30–35 mm, and the caudal septum measures 20–25 mm in extracorporeal septoplasty. It is prudent to mark and draw the exact dimensions of original septum on a towel, which helps in the reconstruction of neo-septum. Typically, a straight piece fitting into these dimensions is located at bony cartilaginous junction. If a straight segment with the required dimensions is not available, the bent segment can be stariaghtened by scoring followed by splinting with perpendicular plate of ethmoid bone with multiple drill holes and taking through-and-through sutures (Fig. 8.42). In extra-

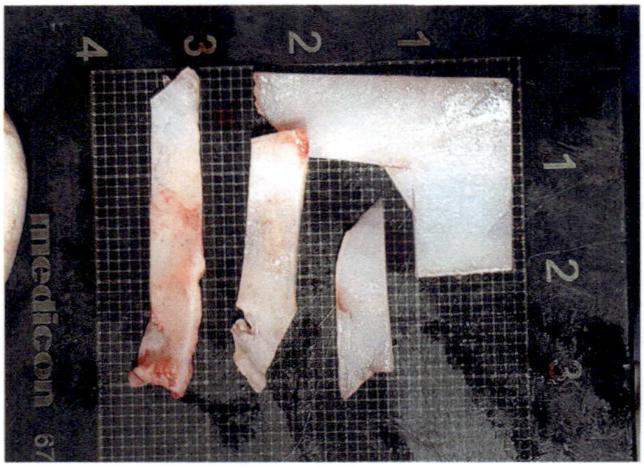

Fig. 8.43 Straight L framework with spreader grafts

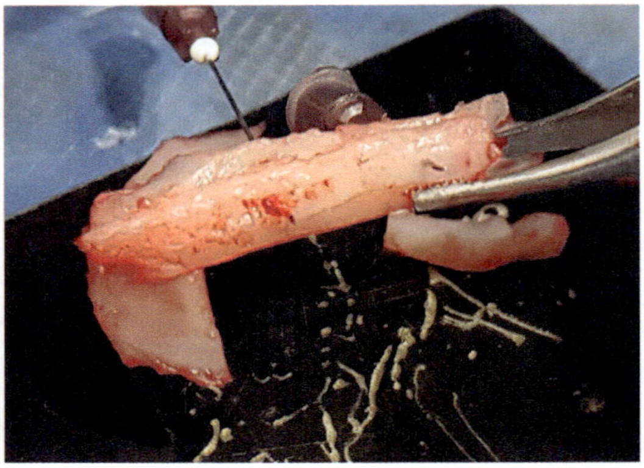

Fig. 8.44 Spreader grafts fixed to the dorsal septum

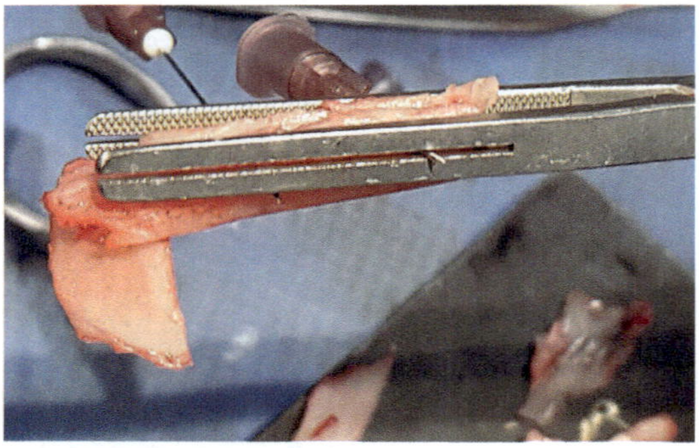

Fig. 8.45 This assembly held with Gubisch-Aiach forceps

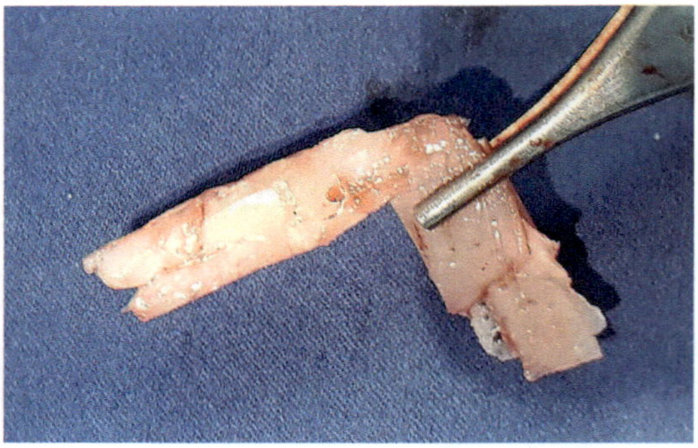

Fig. 8.46 Straight L-shaped neo-septum with spreader grafts along dorsal septum

corporeal septoplasty, spreader grafts are always sutured to the dorsal septum to keep the dorsum straight and also support the internal nasal valves (Figs. 8.43 and 8.44). This is done by fixing the spreader grafts on either sides of dorsal septum with needles. This assembly is held with a special Gubisch-Aiach forceps (Fig. 8.45) with continuous slit in it to aid suturing. Then, either through-and-through sutures or multiple sutures are taken, preferably with a straight needle.

Nowadays, in most of the cases of extracorporeal septoplasty, we prefer to use a septal extension graft (SEG) to support the tip cartilages assembly instead of putting a separate columellar strut and has a more reliable result as far as tip positioning is concerned (Fig. 8.46). Whenever using SEG, the length of dorsal septum has to be longer (cephalocaudal length) by about 1 cm more than the length of the original septum around 40–45 mm.

Reinsertion and Fixation of Neo-septum with TTC Technique—Transcutaneous-Transosseous-Cerclage Technique

Neo septum-Reinsertion and fixation A precise fixation of the replanted septum is essential for the success of the procedure. First it is essential to fix the neo-septum to the upper lateral cartilages and the nasal bones as well. For suturing the neo-septum to the nasal bones, drill holes are made on each side of the nasal bones. I prefer to pass permanent 4-0 Nylon suture passing the needle through this drill hole on the right side which comes out through the upper lateral cartilage on the left side. This is followed by passing the same suture through the hole on the left side which comes out from the upper lateral cartilage on the right side. This is called a *criss-cross technique*.

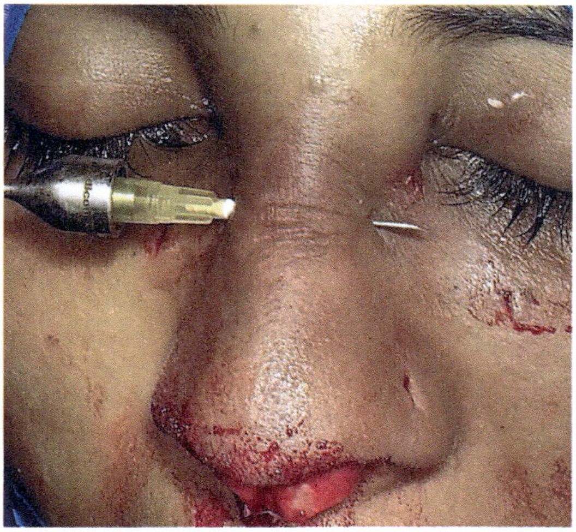

Fig. 8.47 18 Gauge needle mounted on Haack adaptor and used to make percutaneous hole passing through skin-right nasal bone-neo-septum-left nasal bone-skin on opposite side

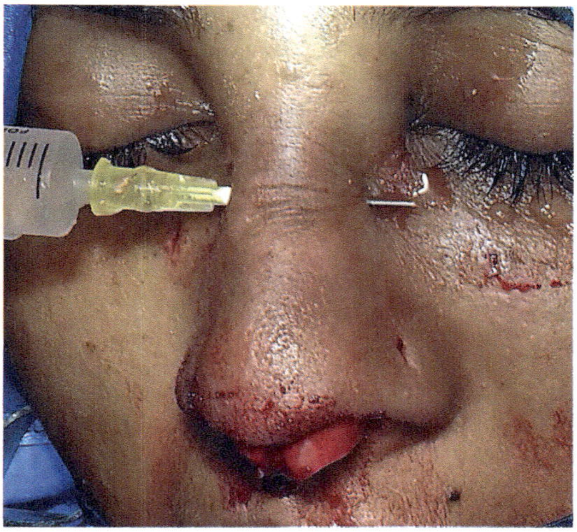

Fig. 8.48 This needle is flushed to clean the bone dust in the needle

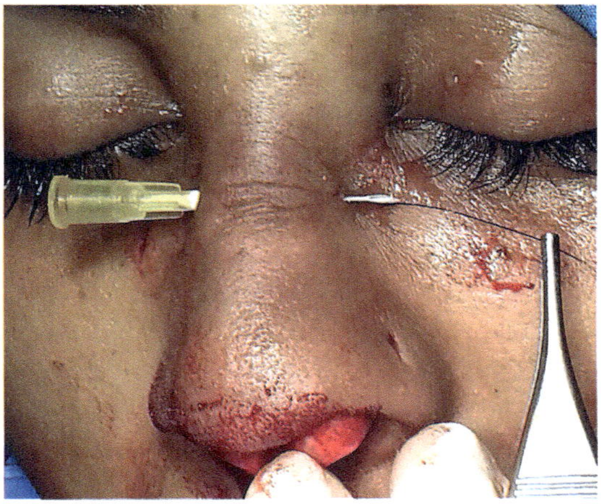

Fig. 8.49 4-0 Nylon passed through this needle

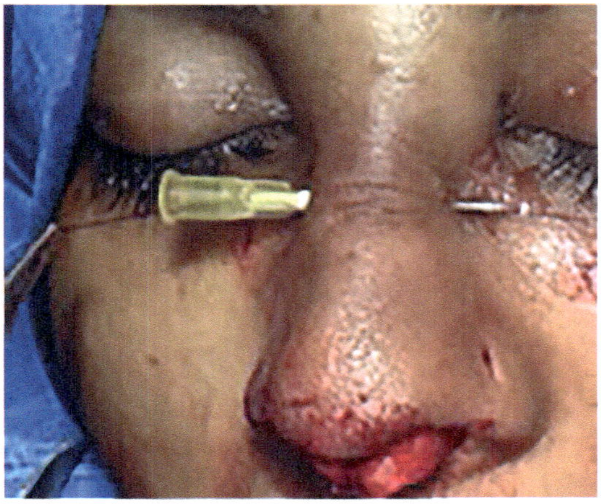

Fig. 8.50 Nylon coming out from the needle hub

If the nasal bones are short, then another technique called *TTC technique—transcutaneous-transosseous-cerclage technique* (Figs. 8.47, 8.48, 8.49, 8.50, 8.51 and 8.52)—is used. In this technique, the hub of 18 gauge needle is mounted on a cylindrical drill or a specially designed Haack adaptor and is used to make a drill hole in the nasal bones. This needle is passed through the skin over the nasal bones, then the nasal bone on right side, the neo-septum and nasal bone on left side and finally comes out from the skin on the left side. This needle is then left in position and disconnected from the drill. The bone dust in the needle is flushed with a syringe, and a permanent suture 4-0 Nylon is fed retrograde through the needle tip until it comes out of the needle hub. Then, the needle is removed leaving behind the suture in place. A small hook is passed to retrieve the two ends of this suture beneath the skin flap. A suture is then tied over the bony dorsum to firmly fix and immobilise the dorsal end of neo-septum to the keystone area, and the suture remains buried subcutaneously.

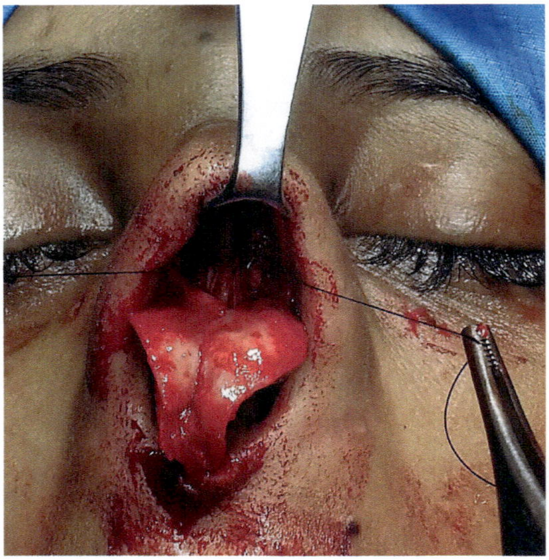

Fig. 8.51 Needle removed and both the ends of this suture taken out with a hook and tied over nasal bones percutaneously

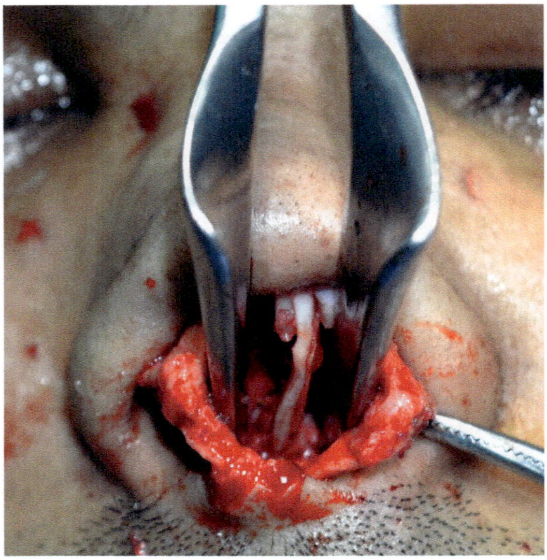

Fig. 8.52 Posterior-caudal end of neo-septum fixed over the groove made over nasal spine by making a drill hole in nasal spine (transosseous fixation)

The caudal septum is then fixed to the nasal spine by passing a suture through the drill hole made in the nasal spine fitting onto the groove made on it. Quilting sutures are taken and Doyle splints are then sutured on either sides of the septum and left for 10 days.

Although this technique is highly effective for straightening a deformed septum and replacing it in the nose to restore nasal function, it has been criticised for being very technically demanding to execute. There is also a risk of aesthetic complications, especially in the area of transition from the bony dorsum to the reconstructed cartilaginous dorsum.

8.5.5.2 Indications of Extracorporeal Septoplasty (Figs. 8.53, 8.54, 8.55, 8.56, 8.57, 8.58, 8.59 and 8.60)

Prerequisite for partial extra corporeal septoplasty is: is a straight dorsal septum til the keystone area

- Gross septal deviations >30 degrees parallel to the dorsal septum with saddling
- Post-traumatic noses with saddling
- Crooked noses with hump
- Revision rhinoplasty
- Total septal reconstruction

8.5.5.3 Advantages of Extracorporeal Septoplasty

- This is the only technique that gives an exact straight post-operative septum.
- It gives excellent functional and aesthetic results, if executed properly.
- It is the only technique that can be used where total septal reconstruction is indicated in severely damaged septum like total resorption of cartilage in septal abscess and many revision rhinoplasties.

8.5.5.4 Disadvantages of Extracorporeal Septoplasty

One drawback of this technique is destabilisation of the junction of the quadrangular cartilage and nasal bones (keystone area), with resultant requirement for unique forms of fixation, such as TTC percutaneous sutures, or criss-cross sutures through nasal bones, which is a challenging procedure and requires a certain amount of expertise. In case destabilisation occurs, it is better to identify it on the table and put grafts like free diced cartilage (FDC) or other camouflaging grafts over the keystone area.

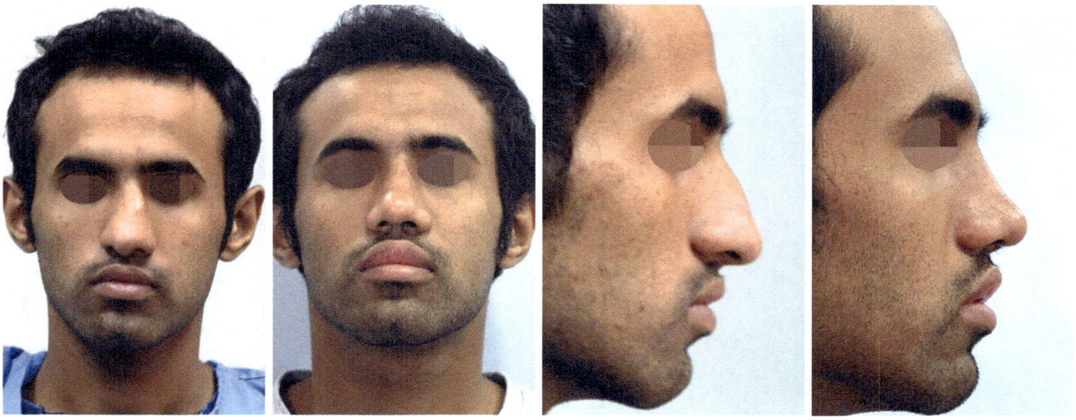

Figs. 8.53–8.56 (left: Fig. 8.53): Pre-op AP view; (left middle: Fig. 8.54): Post-op AP view; (right middle: Fig. 8.55): Pre-op lateral view; (right: Fig. 8.56): Post-op lateral view

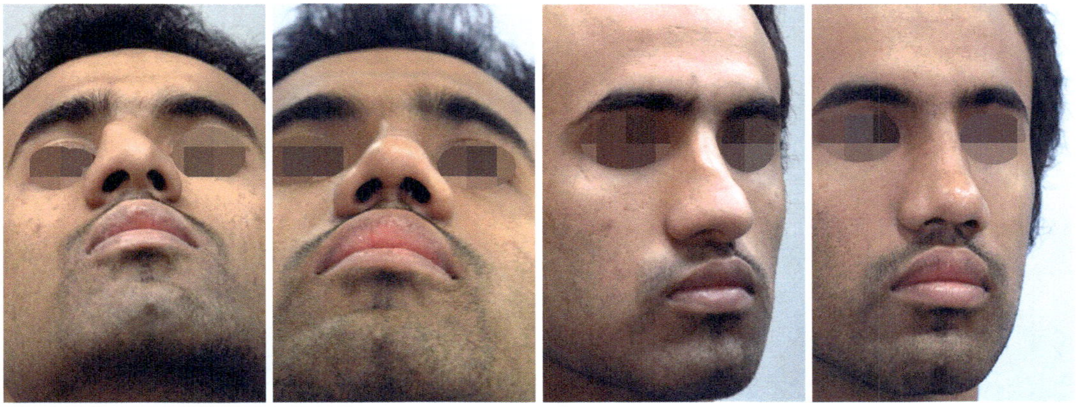

Figs. 8.57–8.60 (left: Fig. 8.57): Pre-op basal view; (left middle: Fig. 8.58): Post-op basal view; (right middle: Fig. 8.59): Pre-op oblique view; (right: Fig. 8.60): Post-op oblique view

8.5.6 Partial Extracorporeal Septal Reconstruction

Thus, to minimise the destabilisation of the keystone area, the less difficult procedure for severely deviated noses is a modification of extracorporeal septoplasty called *partial extracorporeal septoplasty*, in which the straight part of septum is preserved and only the deformed segment is taken out and reconstructed. When only anterior part of septum is deformed, this technique can be termed as *anterior septal reconstruction* or a *septal exchange technique.*

8.5.6.1 Operative Technique

Exposure and Excision After adequate exposure, the septum is released from all its attachments except the keystone area. Attachment of the dorsal septum to keystone area is assessed by comparing the reference point marked on the centre of the forehead between the eyebrows and also with the nasal spine and the point marked on the centre of the philtrum. The position of attachment of dorsal septum to keystone area can be in the centre or in a paramedian position.

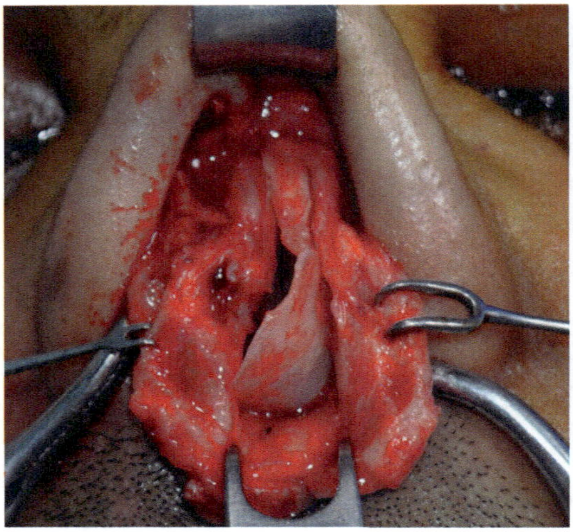

Fig. 8.61 Extreme C-shaped dorsal deviation <30 degrees off the axis with septum arising from centre of keystone area

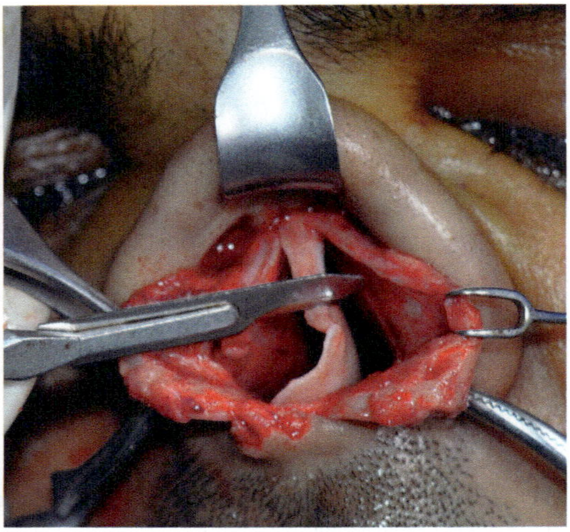

Fig. 8.62 10 mm cut made just above the point of deviation leaving straight dorsal strut attached to keystone area

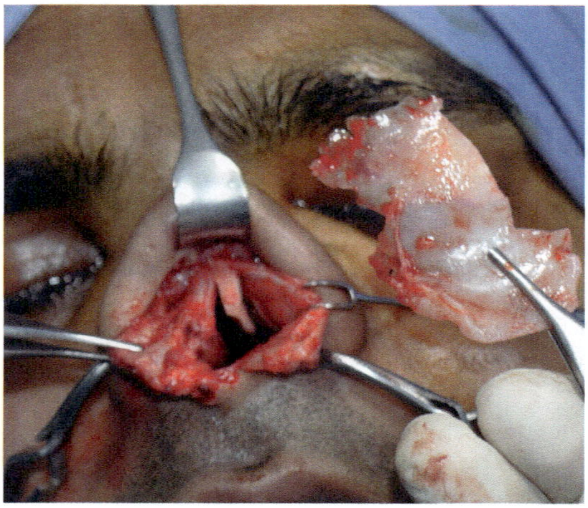

Fig. 8.63 Rest of the septum removed along with bone preserving this dorsal strut

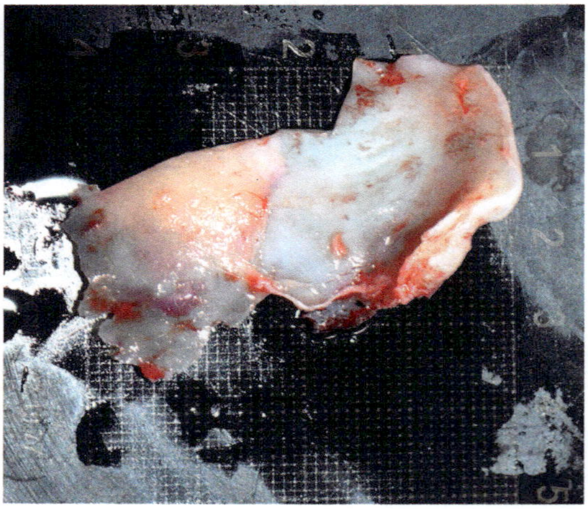

Fig. 8.64 Dimensions of the dorsal and caudal septum noted

A) *When Dorsal Septal Attachment to Keystone Lies in the Centre* (Figs. 8.61, 8.62, 8.63, 8.64, 8.65, 8.66, 8.67, 8.68, 8.69, 8.70, 8.71, 8.72, 8.73, 8.74, 8.75, 8.76, 8.77 and 8.78)

When the dorsal septum lies in the central position, then the point of deviation along the dorsal cartilaginous septum is defined, and then a vertical cut 10 mm in height is made just above the point of deviation. This is followed by a cut made parallel to the dorsal septum extending towards the ethmoid plate, leaving 10 mm dorsal septal strut attached to keystone area. Then, the remaining part of septum is released from the ANS, premaxillary and vomerine grooves and is removed along with perpendicular plate of ethmoid and vomer, preserving this straight dorsal strut attached to keystone area.

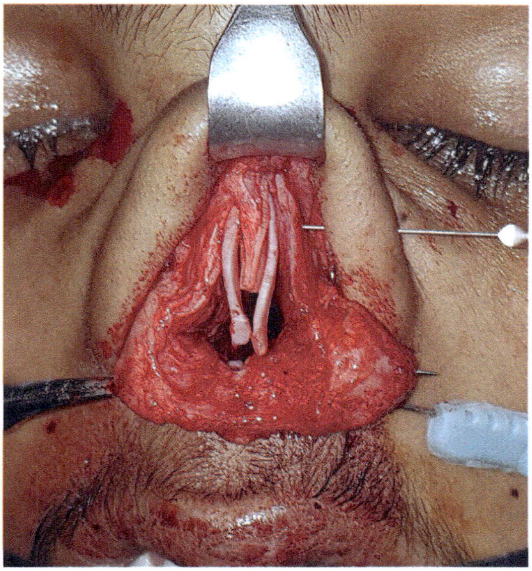

Fig. 8.65 Spreader grafts attached to the dorsal strut with percutaneous needles

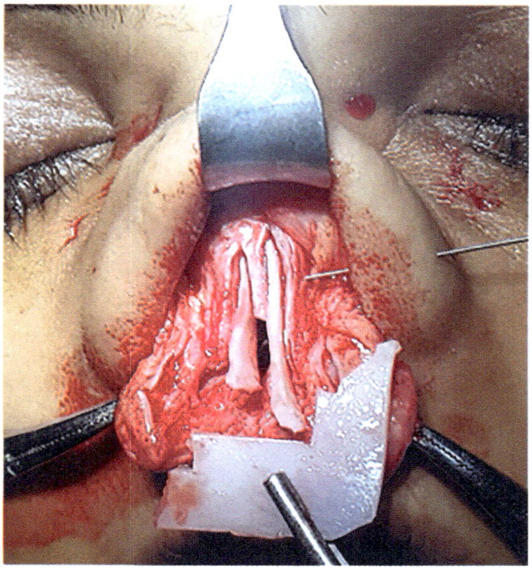

Fig. 8.66 L-shaped anterior septal replacement graft along with SEG with notch for ANS

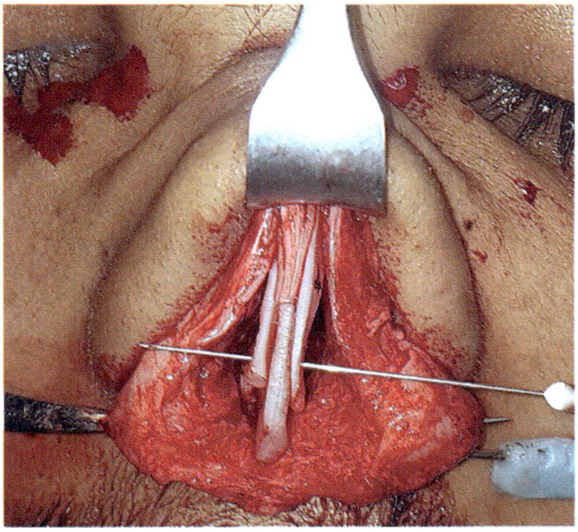

Fig. 8.67 End-to-end fixation of the anterior septal

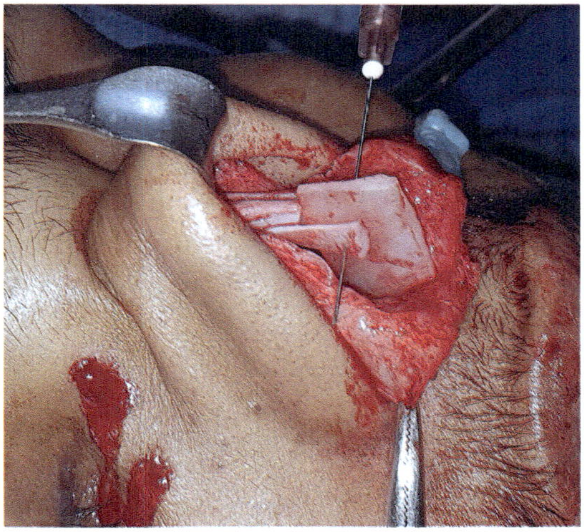

Fig. 8.68 Caudal dimensions with needle replacement graft of excessive length

Shaping of the Graft The harvested cartilage is then placed on a Sheens grid, and the dimensions are noted of original dorsal and caudal septum along with the angle between them. Generally, in partial extracorporeal septoplasty, septal extension graft—SEG—is used instead of a separate columellar strut, which has more stability supporting the tip assembly. When SEG is used, the total dorsal length has to be about 10 mm more than the original septum. So, depending upon the length of the dorsal septal strut preserved, this has to be subtracted from the total dorsal length of SEG planned, and the length of the replacement graft is determined. The vertical length of caudal

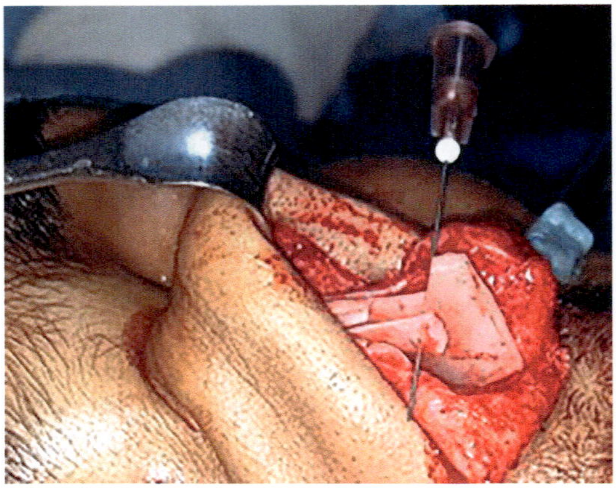

Fig. 8.69 Trimming of this excess cartilage as per aesthetic requirements

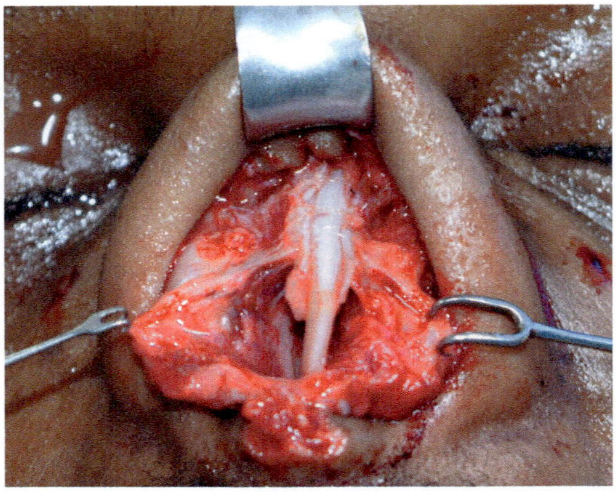

Fig. 8.70 Upper lateral cartilages sutured to this assembly of neo-septum with running sutures and tip cartilages advanced over SEG

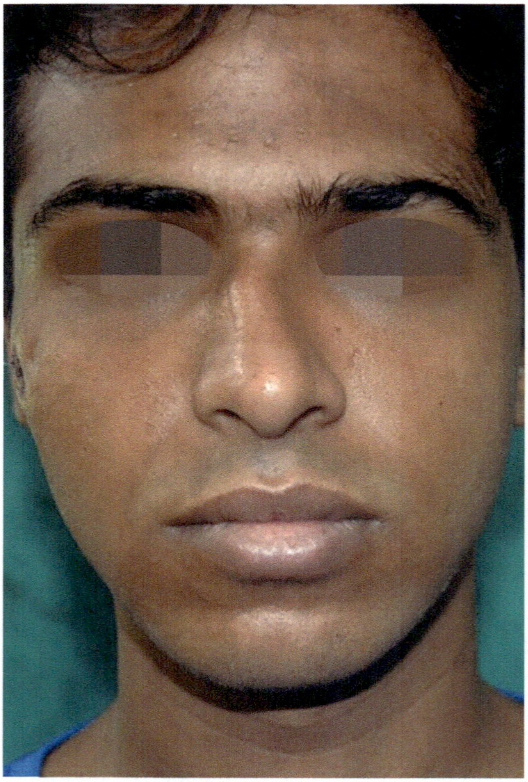

Fig. 8.71 Pre-op AP view

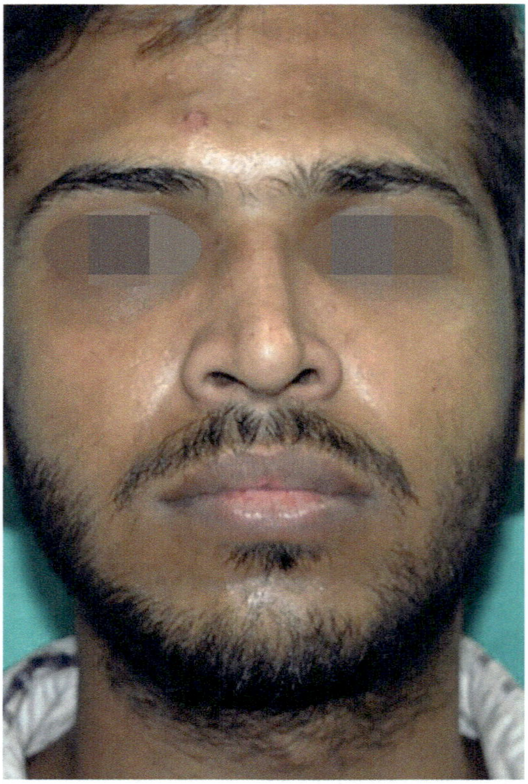

Fig. 8.72 Post-op AP view

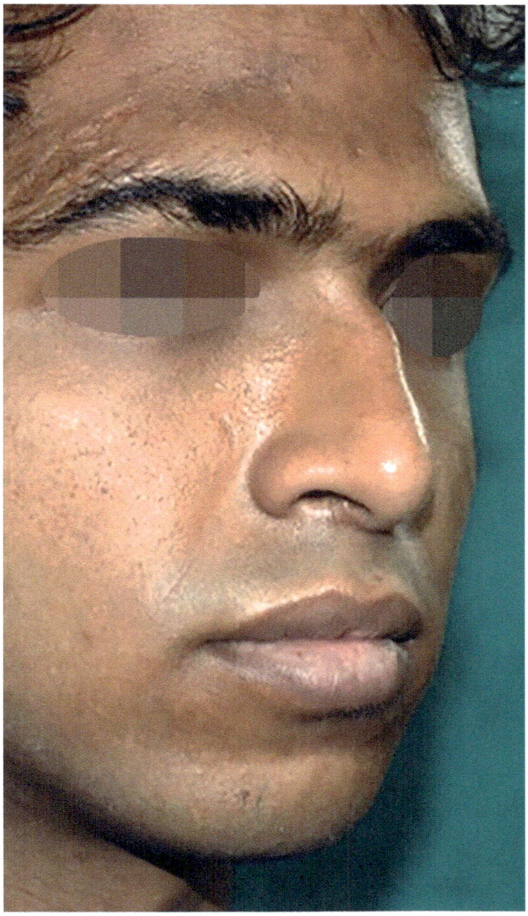

Fig. 8.73 Pre-op oblique view

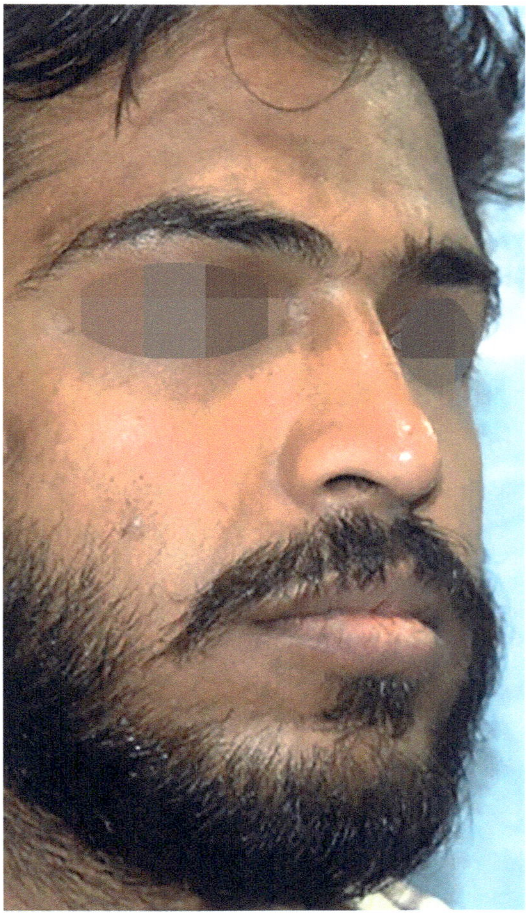

Fig. 8.74 Post-op oblique view

septum may be kept 5 mm higher than original dimensions of the caudal septum, depending upon the availability of the graft material.

Fixation of the Graft First spreader grafts are fixed to the dorsal strut attached to keystone area by percutaneous needles and secured with 5-0 PDS. Then, the replacement graft is inserted between the free ends of these spreader grafts, and an end-to-end fixation is done with the dorsal strut. This is achieved by initially fixing with percutaneous needles and then with sutures. Needles are then removed after sutures are secured. After this the posterior part of the caudal septum is relocated onto the groove made on nasal spine, and a transosseous fixation is achieved by passing the suture through the drill hole made in the nasal spine.

At this point reassessment is made regarding the dimensions of neo-septum. Any excess of the septal length can be marked and trimmed. Lastly, the upper lateral cartilages are approximated to this assembly of septal replacement graft and spreader grafts with percutaneous needles and secured using running sutures to aid opening the internal nasal valves even more.

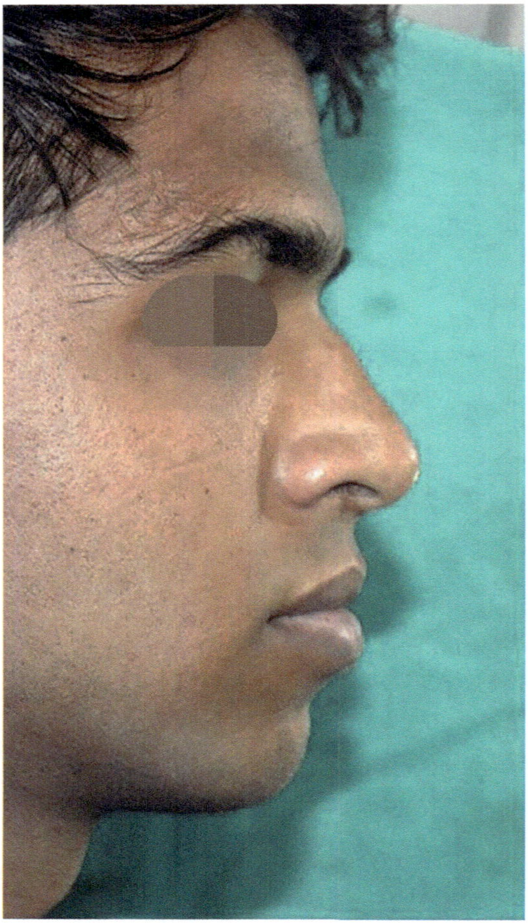

Fig. 8.75 Pre-op lateral view

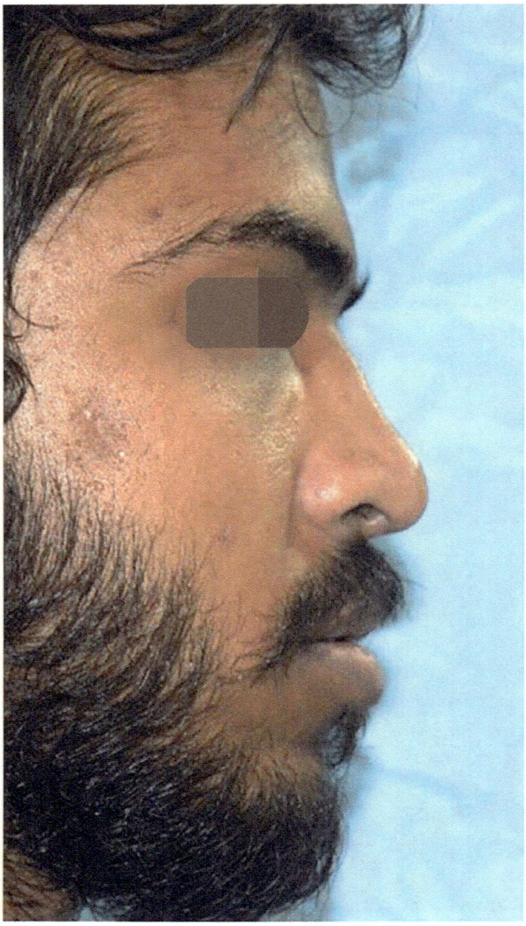

Fig. 8.76 Post-lateral view

B) *When Dorsal Septal Attachment to Keystone Lies in Paramedian Position* (Figs. 8.79, 8.80, 8.81, 8.82, 8.83, 8.84, 8.85, 8.86, 8.87, 8.88, 8.89, 8.90, 8.91, 8.92, 8.93 and 8.94)

When the dorsal septum lies in the paramedian position, then this portion of septum can be utilised as a spreader graft on one side, and the neoseptum can be designed accordingly. In such a situation, the point of deviation along the dorsal cartilaginous septum is defined, and then a vertical cut 4 mm in height is made just above the point of deviation. Then, a cut is made parallel to the dorsal septum extending towards the ethmoid plate leaving 4 mm dorsal septal strut attached to the keystone area. Then, the remaining part of septum is released from the ANS, premaxillary and vomerine grooves and is removed along with perpendicular plate of ethmoid and vomer while preserving this straight dorsal strut attached to keystone area. The only difference is this dorsal strut is 4 mm in width when used as a spreader graft.

Neo-septum planned should be 10 mm more in length than original septum so that it can be used as a SEG. This L-shaped strut is attached to medial side of this retained piece of cartilage to be used as a spreader graft on one side. Then, another piece of spreader graft is attached to this L strut on lateral side with the help of percutaneous needle. This is then secured with 5-0 PDS and the needles are removed. The posterior end of caudal septum is secured onto the ANS by 4-0 Nylon passing the suture through the drill hole made in ANS (transosseous fixation).

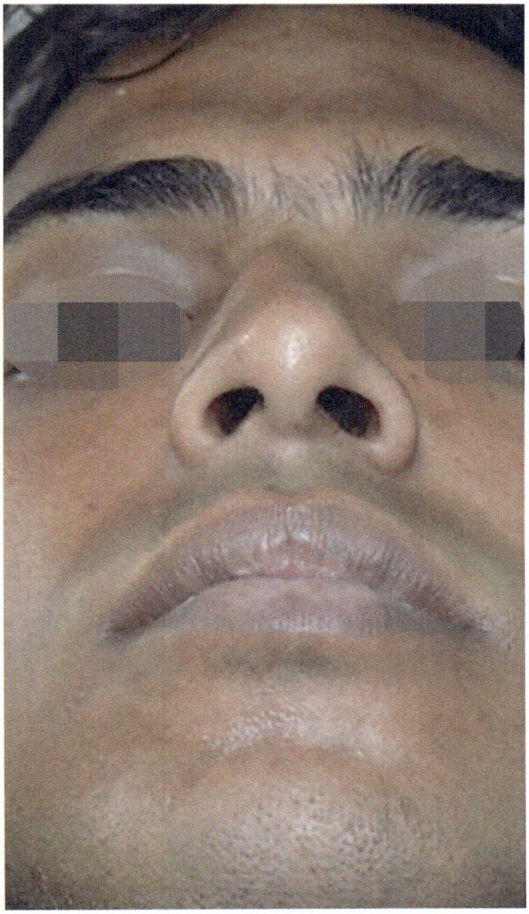

Fig. 8.77 Pre-op basal view

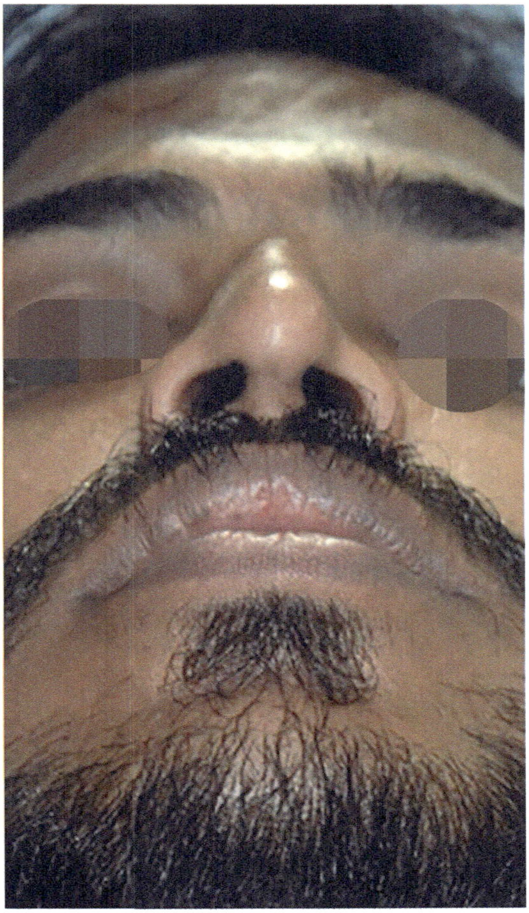

Fig. 8.78 Post-op basal view

8.5.6.2 Indications of Partial Extracorporeal Septoplasty

Prerequisite for partial extra corporeal septoplasty is : is a straight dorsal septum til the keystone area:

- Gross septal deviations <30 degrees off the axis
- Crooked noses with hump
- Revision rhinoplasty
- Unilateral cleft lip noses

8.5.6.3 Advantages of Partial Extracorporeal Septoplasty

- This technique gives an exact nose post-operatively.
- It gives excellent functional and aesthetic results, if executed properly.
- It is technically less challenging as compared to extracorporeal septoplasty and prevents destabilisation of keystone area.

8.5.6.4 Disadvantages of Partial Extracorporeal Septoplasty

Moderate degree of surgical skill is required to execute this technique properly.

A thorough understanding of the deviated noses will help the budding rhinoplasty surgeon overcome the fear of this type of noses, where each case is different and beautiful in its own way.

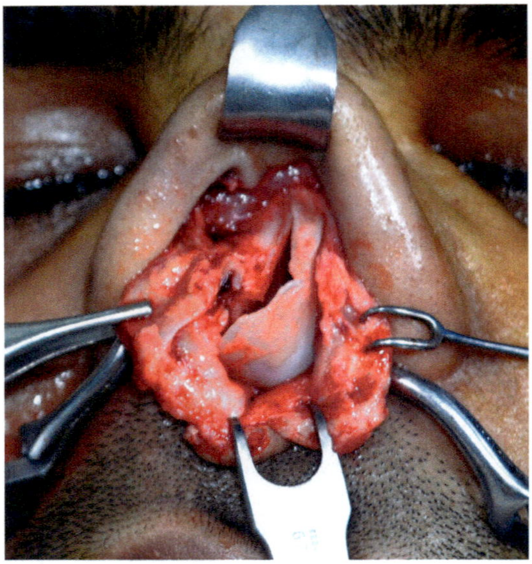

Fig. 8.79 Paramedian position of attachment of dorsal septum to keystone area

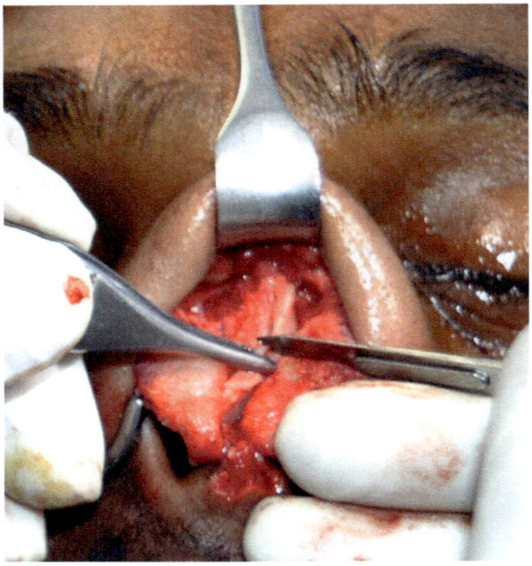

Fig. 8.80 4 mm cut made just above the point of deviation leaving straight cartilage to be used as a spreader graft attached to keystone area

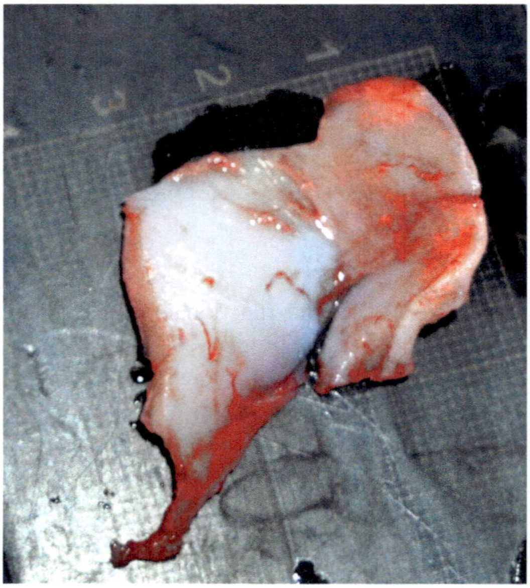

Fig. 8.81 Dimensions of original septum measured

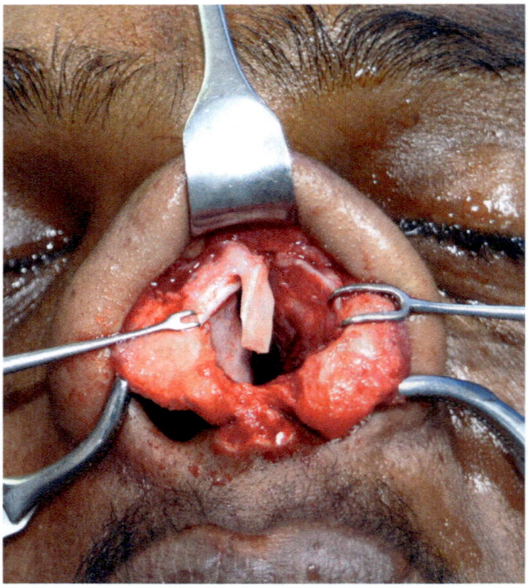

Fig. 8.82 Retained piece of cartilage at keystone area in paramedian position to be used as a spreader graft

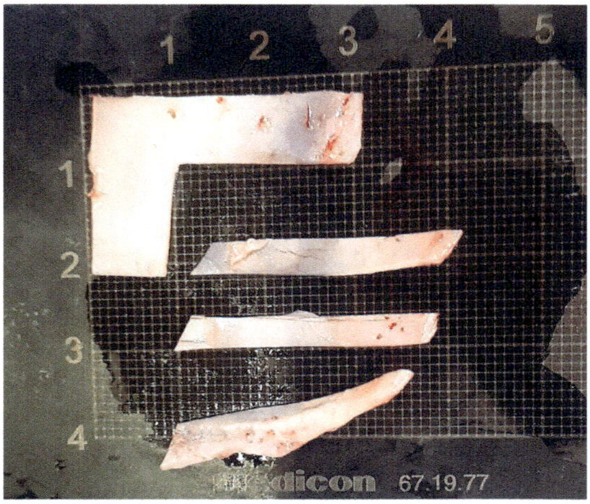

Fig. 8.83 L strut and spreader grafts from harvested cartilage

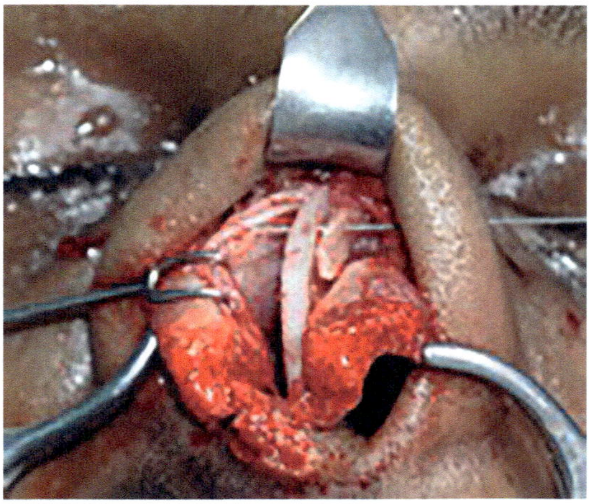

Fig. 8.84 L strut attached to medial side of retained piece of spreader graft attached to keystone area

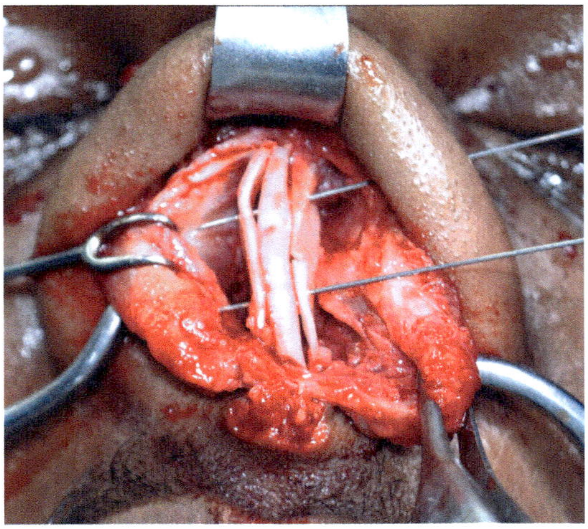

Fig. 8.85 Another spreader graft attached to lateral side of this L strut with percutaneous needles

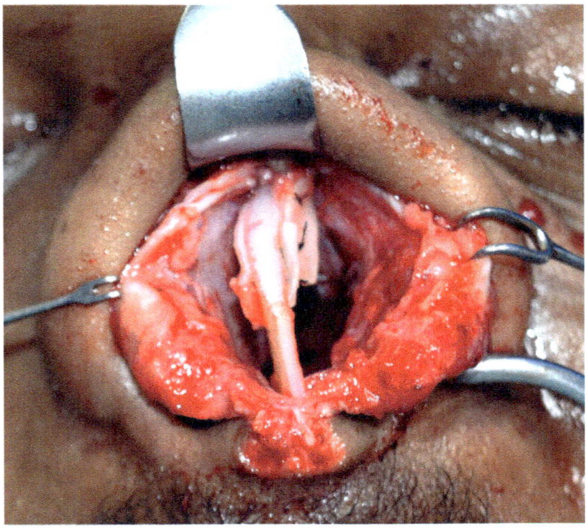

Fig. 8.86 This assembly of neo-septum secured with sutures and caudal septum sutures to ANS

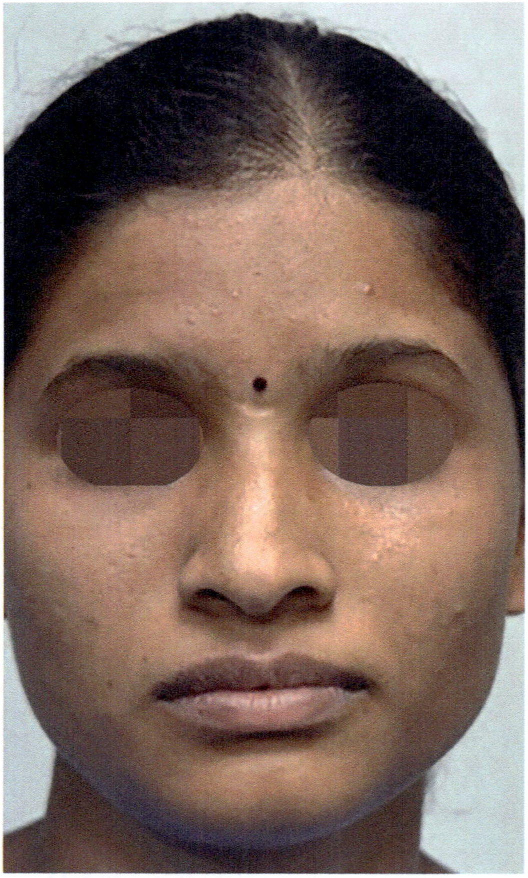

Fig. 8.87 Pre-op AP view

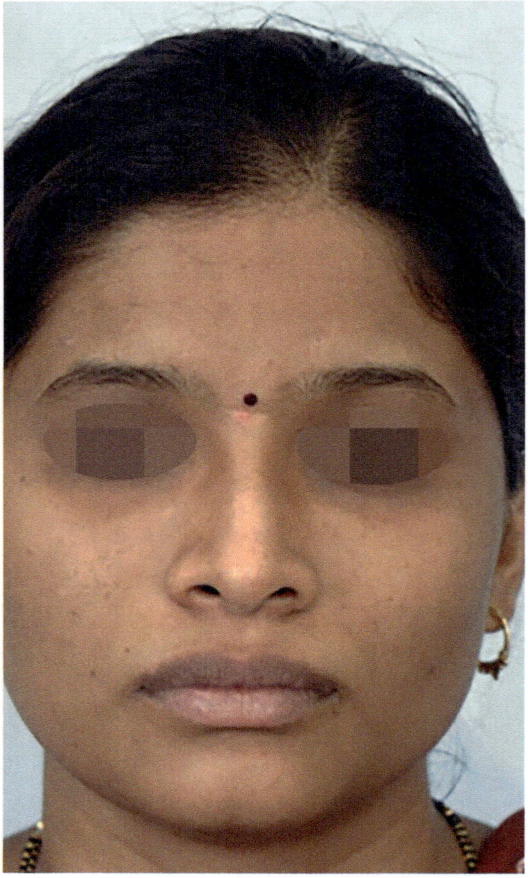

Fig. 8.88 Post-op AP view

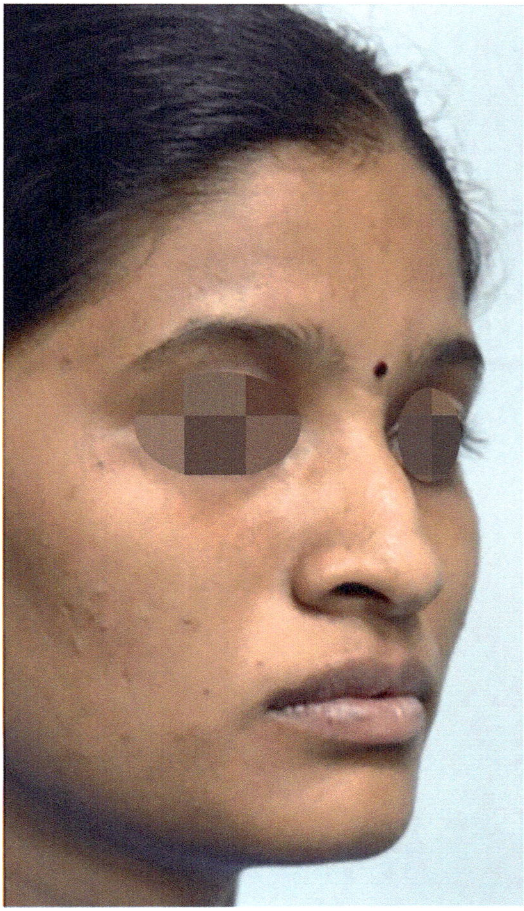

Fig. 8.89 Pre-op oblique view

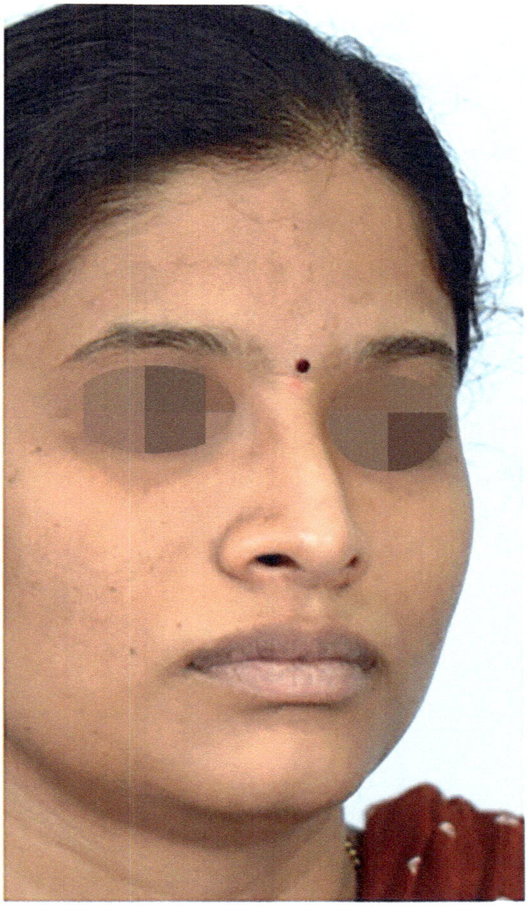

Fig. 8.90 Post-op oblique view

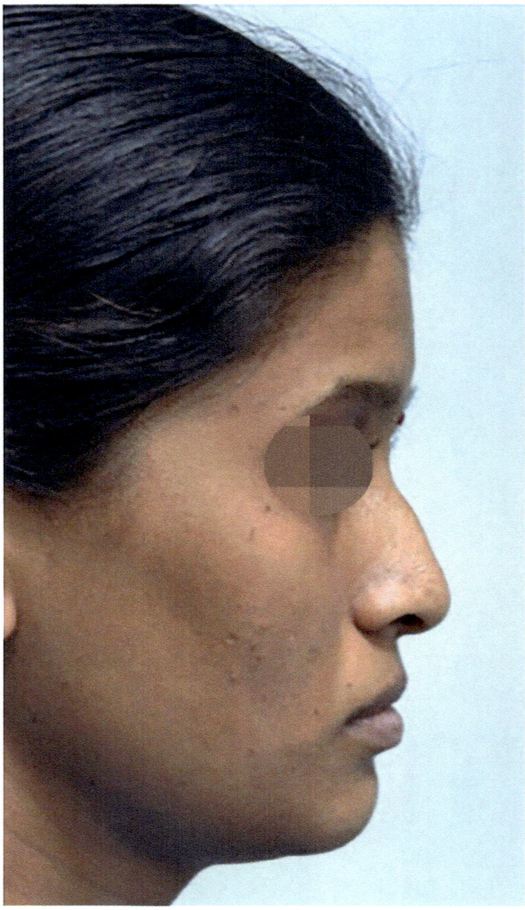

Fig. 8.91 Pre-op lateral view

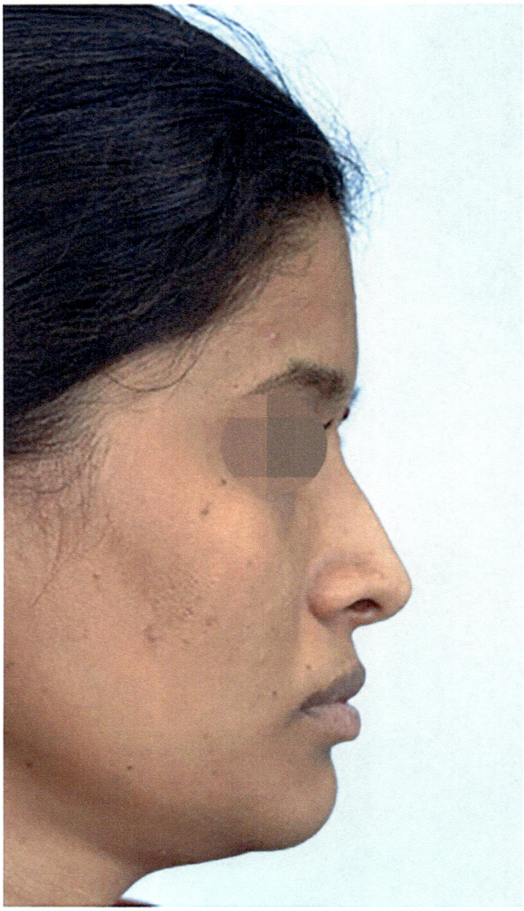

Fig. 8.92 Post-op lateral view

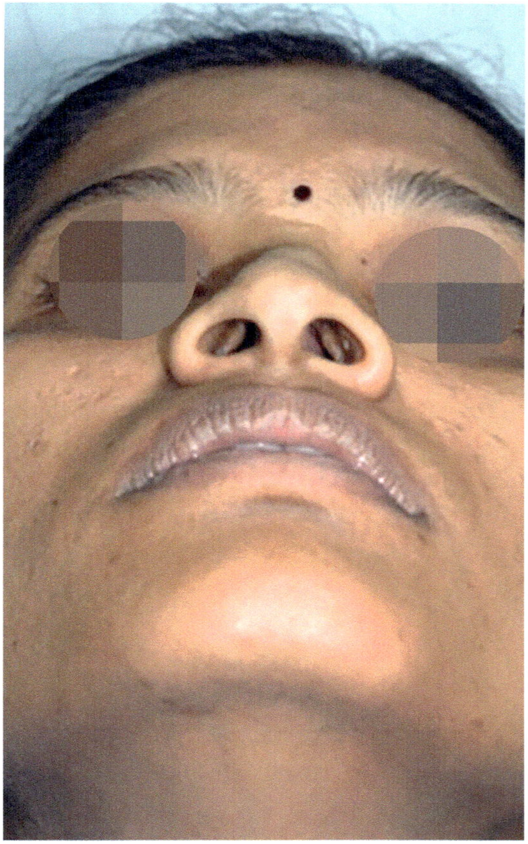

Fig. 8.93 Pre-op basal view

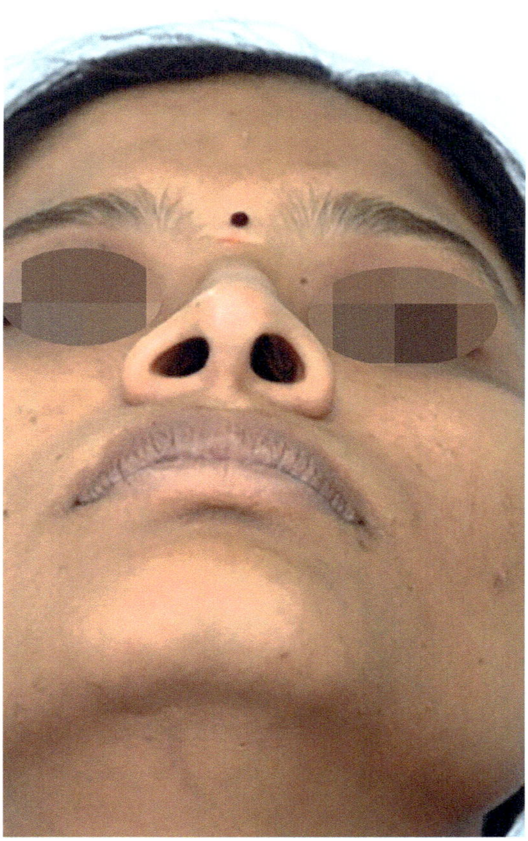

Fig. 8.94 Post-op basal view

9 Nasal Tip Deformities

Main

The nasal tip is a 3-dimensional structure of curves and angles. The anatomy of the tip determines the operative technique. The underlying alar cartilages support and configure the tip lobule. Modern *rhinoplasty* techniques allow the *tip* to be reconfigured and refined without compromising the nasal structure. Hence, understanding tip anatomy is very vital to provide aesthetic improvements to the tip.

9.1 Relevant Surgical Anatomy

Understanding the anatomy of tip, analysis, deformities and surgeries is quite complex yet very interesting as it involves very intricate details. Tip of the nose consists of two domes, interdomal connective tissues and an overlying skin with lower alar cartilage constituted by three crura, i.e. lateral, middle and medial crura (Figs. 9.1 and 9.2).

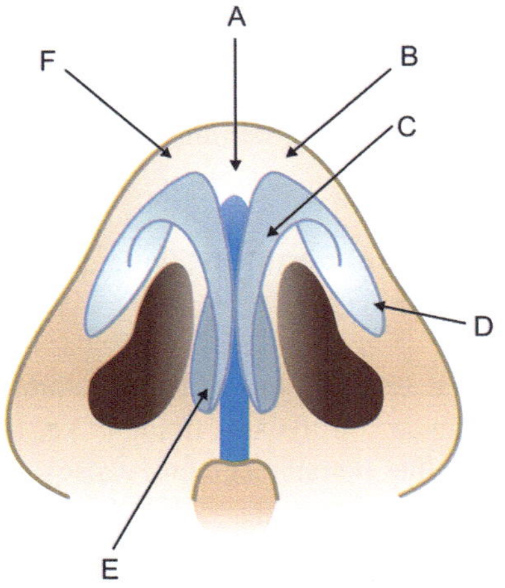

Fig. 9.1 Schematic diagram showing. (A) Interdomal area. (B/F) Dome. (C) Intermediate crus. (D) Lateral crus. (E) Medial crus

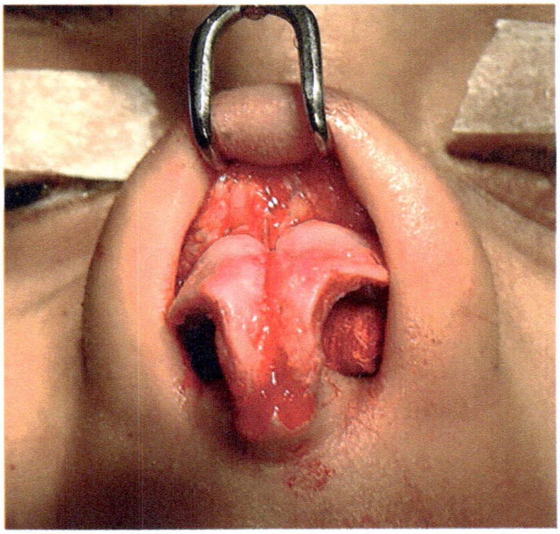

Fig. 9.2 Picture with three crura of lower alar cartilages

V. Ghaisas, *Indian Ethnic Rhinoplasty*, https://doi.org/10.1007/978-981-16-2478-0_9

The lobule of the nose is the lower third of the external nasal pyramid. It is made of two lower alar cartilages, muscle fibres, ligaments, subcutaneous connective and fatty tissues and thick skin. The lower alar cartilages are horseshoe-shaped cartilages that support the lobule structure. They determine the position and form of the tip, alae and columella and configuration of nares and vestibules.

9.1.1 Tip Support

In rhinoplasty, maintaining nasal tip support is important in order to achieve long-lasting aesthetic and functional outcomes. Anderson described the 'the nasal tripod' as a paradigm to explain the tip structure to describe tip rotation and projection which is explained in detail further.

Tardy et al. however divided the tip support into major and minor with the three major structures including the following:

Major tip mechanisms

Tip supporting elements

1. Anterior border of the septum
2. Connections between upper lateral cartilages and the lower alar cartilages (i.e. scroll region)
3. Connections between the medial crura of the lower alar cartilages to the caudal septum
4. Alar cartilage size and shape

Minor tip mechanisms

1. Interdomal soft tissue
2. Cartilaginous dorsal septum
3. Soft tissue sesamoid complex
4. Alar cartilage attachment to the skin and soft tissue
5. Anterior nasal spine
6. Membranous septum

9.2 Lateral Crura (Fig. 9.3)

The anatomy of the lower alar cartilage varies according to the ethnicity of the patient. Size, shape and orientation of the lateral crura of the lower alar cartilage greatly influence the aesthetics and function of the lower one-third of the nose. As the lateral crura extend laterally from the intermediate crura, a mild concavity typically exists.

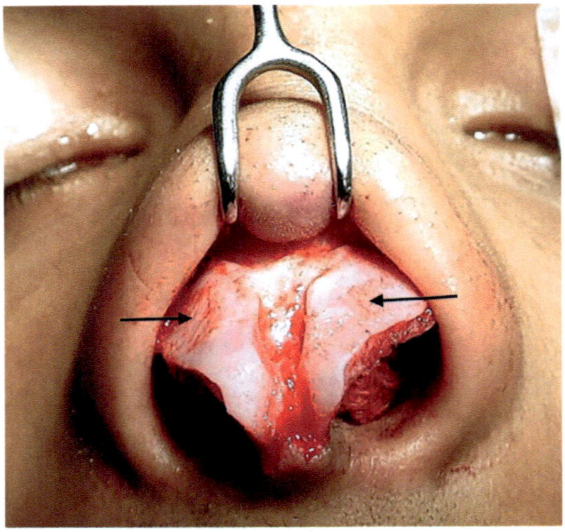

Fig. 9.3 Two black arrows showing lateral crus of LAC

9.3 Intermediate Crura (Figs. 9.4 and 9.5)

It *is* made up of domal and lobular segment. The concave edge of the crura is the domal segment. And the most anteriorly projecting part of domal segment forms the tip defining point.

9.3.1 Domal Segment (Figs. 9.6 and 9.7)

The domal segment has a distinct domal notch that influences on the soft triangle, i.e. different shape of the domal segment causes different shape of the soft triangle.

This varies in shape from concave, smooth and convex, and a varying degree of convexity of the domal segment gives more aesthetic tip.

9.3.2 Soft Triangle (Figs. 9.8 and 9.9)

It is an area of lobule between external and vestibular skin inferior to dome, devoid of cartilage, more prominent in females and is considered as a

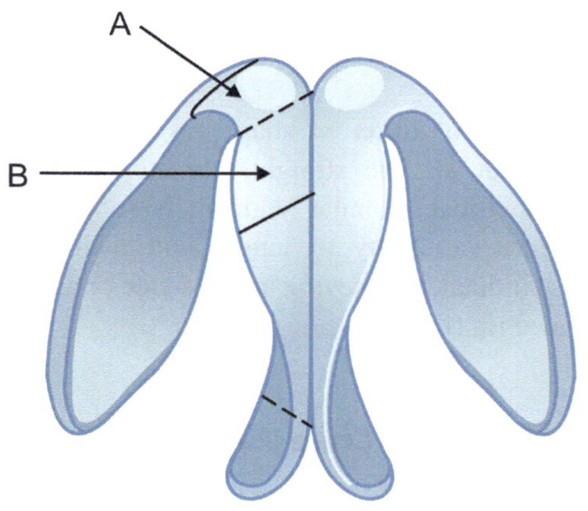

Fig. 9.4 Schematic diagram showing intermediate crura with (A) domal and (B) lobular segment

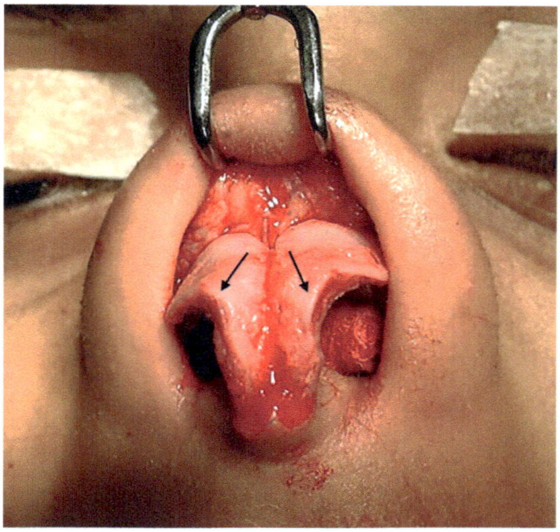

Fig. 9.5 In the picture two black arrows showing intermediate crura

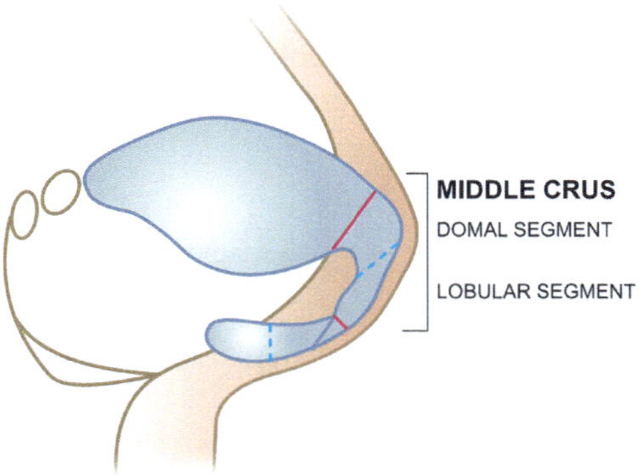

Fig. 9.6 Schematic diagram of lateral crus showing domal and lobular segment of middle crus

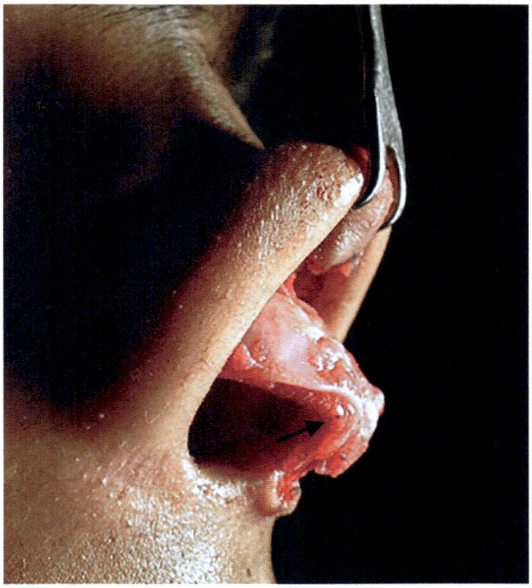

Fig. 9.7 Corresponding picture showing intermediate crus

beauty spot. And thus while closing the infracartilaginous incision, sutures in this area may lead to notching and should be avoided.

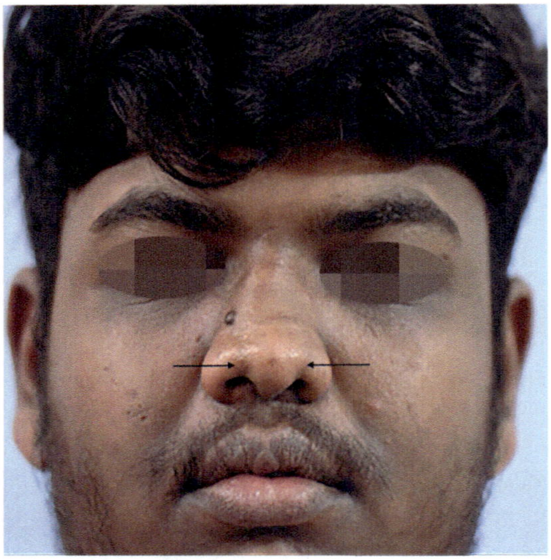

Fig. 9.8 Here is a soft triangle deformity showing a notched up domal part which is seen if the domal segment is concave. In such cases, forming the ideal convex domal segment might reduce this notching

9.3.2.1 Soft Triangle Deformity

9.3.3 Lobular Segment

It can be of different shapes as expressed by Natvig et al. like straight, curved and totally asymmetrical. Lobular segment is subjected to extreme variability in length and width. And these influence on having an uprotated or a downrotated tip (Fig. 9.10).

9.3.4 Medial Crura (Fig. 9.11)

It's the pillar of strength on which the tip rests. It has got two parts, i.e. a superior columellar and a lower footplate segment. The columellar segment influences on the length of the columella, whereas the width of the columella is influenced by three factors—the intrinsic shape of the medial crus, extrinsic influence of caudal septum and soft tissue of the membranous septum. During open rhinoplasty, the central soft tissue is raised with the columellar flap, and lack of this soft tissue laterally can lead to medial crus notching.

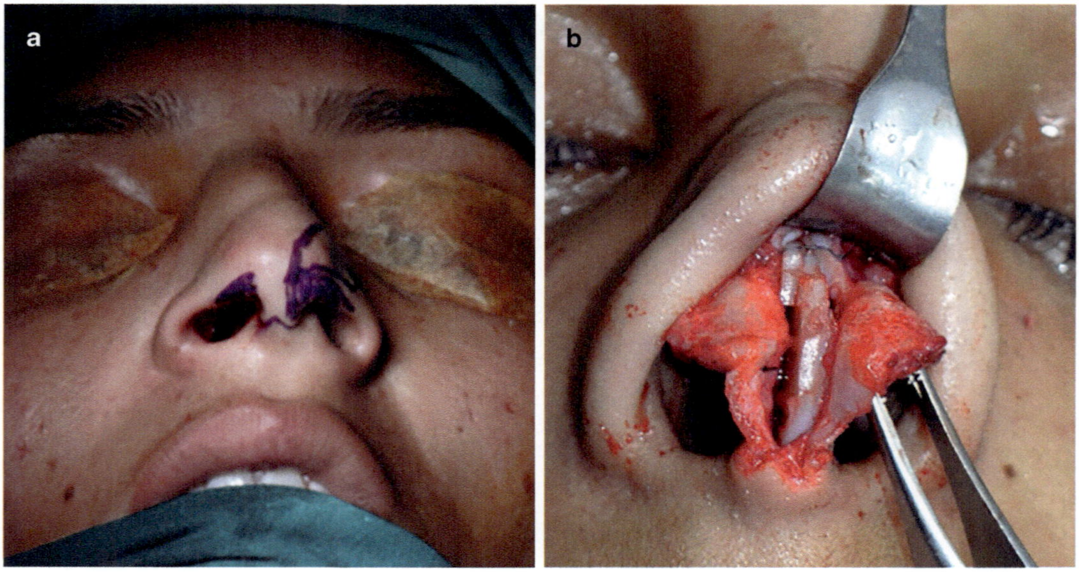

Fig. 9.9 (**a**) Shaded area with blue and the (**b**) forceps showing the soft triangle in the domal part of intermediate crus

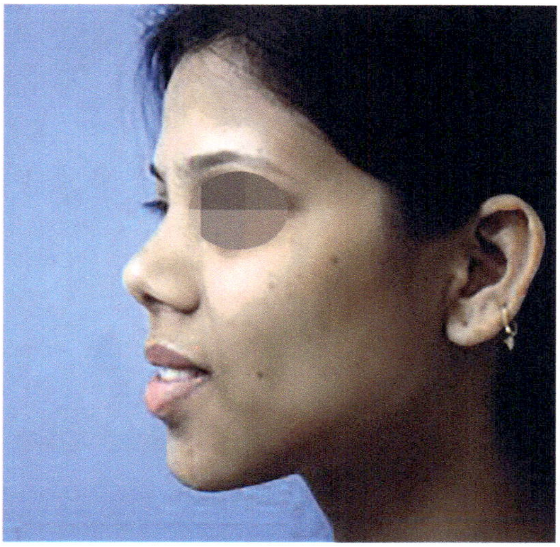

Fig. 9.10 For example, short lobular segment causes a snubbed tip

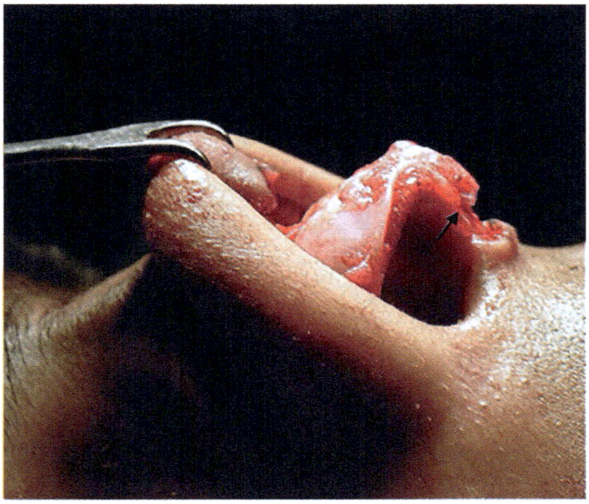

Fig. 9.11 Lateral view of the nose opened showing medial crus of LAC

9.4 Footplate Deformities

If Exists

We need to cut the soft tissue in between and suture the footplate. At the same time, one should avoid cutting of footplate to avoid loss of support.

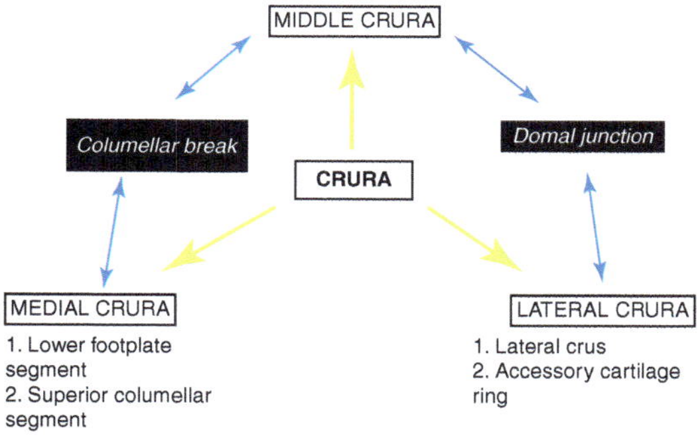

9.4.1 Interdomal Ligament (Figs. 9.12 and 9.13)

This is the ligament that runs between the two middle crura in a more posterior and cephalic direction. It is easily found in all noses and is often quite rigid. During open rhinoplasty this ligament is cut, and routinely an interdomal suture is inserted to narrow the interdomal distance.

Pitanguy's midline ligament is a dermodomal ligament (Fig. 9.14) where it's origin is from the midline SMAS layer. Pitanguy's midline ligament divides into a 'superficial portion', which passes above the interdomal ligament and becomes continuous with the superficial orbicularis oris nasalis muscle, and a 'deep portion', which passes below the interdomal ligament and becomes continuous with the depressor septi nasi muscle.

Surgically, division and repair of Pitanguy's midline ligament has become an important method, thus reducing the supratip dead space and potentially stabilising the tip.

However, it must be emphasised that it is the deep portion that is repaired, whereas the superficial portion is usually irreparably disrupted during exposure.

AESTHETIC ANATOMY of the nose comprises intrinsic and extrinsic factors.

INTRINSIC FACTORS are defined by:

1. *Tip definition* which is the adjacent relationship between domal segment and lateral crura with the skin above.

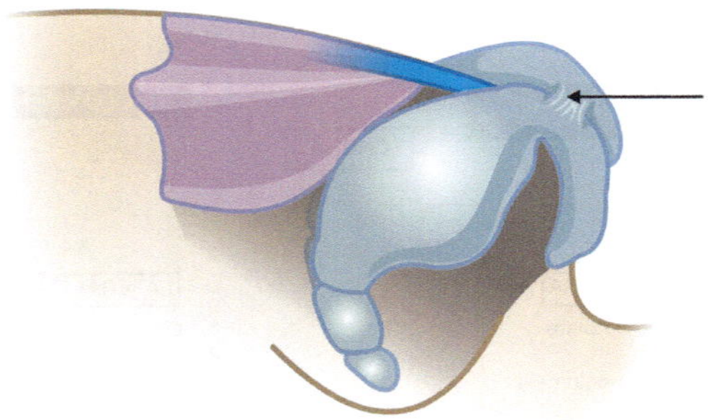

Fig. 9.12 Schematic diagram showing interdomal ligament

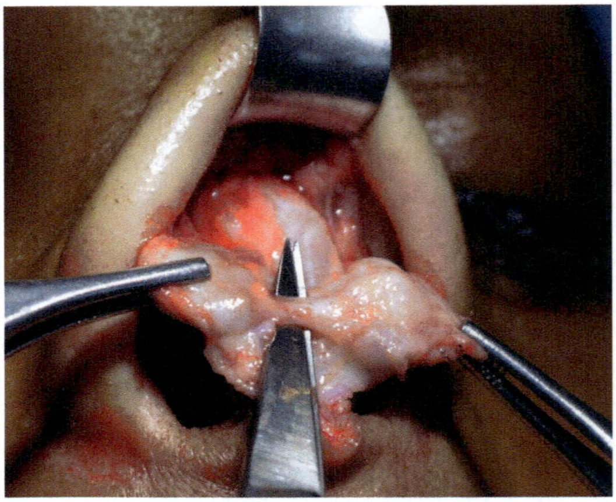

Fig. 9.13 Corresponding picture showing interdomal ligament

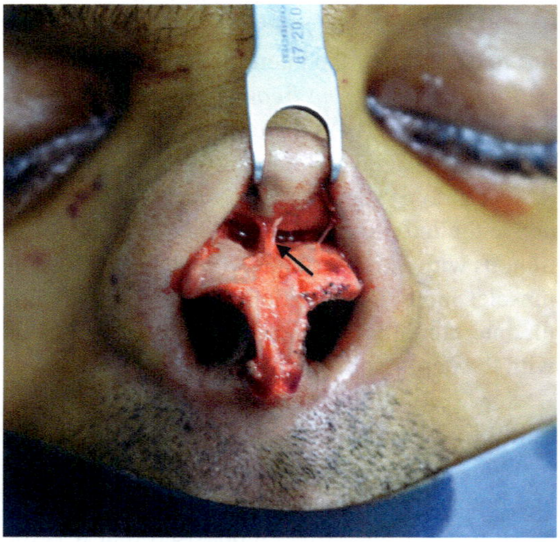

Fig. 9.14 Dermodomal ligament—Pitanguy's ligament

There are three kinds—smooth convex, acutely convex and concave in which smooth convex domal and concave lateral crura provide an acceptable aesthetic kind (Figs. 9.15 and 9.16).

2. *Tip width* is the interdomal distance.

It is an ideal distance which correlates with dorsal lines and philtral columns (Figs. 9.17 and 9.18).

3. *Tip volume is* formed solely by the lateral crura of both sides (Figs. 9.19 and 9.20):
   (a) To reduce the tip volume—a lateral crural sliding technique (for overprojected and downrotated tip) or excision is done which reduces the tip volume where the tip rotates upwards, deprojects and becomes smaller (Figs. 9.21, 9.22, 9.23, and 9.24).
   (b) If the cartilage is weak, then to strengthen it, a lateral crural underlay or infolding is done (Fig. 9.25).

(c) A lateral crural strut graft is placed for lateral crural collapse (Figs. 9.26, 9.27 and 9.28).

EXTRINSIC FACTORS

1. *PROJECTION* (Figs. 9.29, 9.30 and 9.31)
   It is defined as the distance from a vertical facial plane passing through the alar crease to the nasal tip.

IDEAL TIP PROJECTION is considered to be two-thirds the ideal dorsal length.

If there is a long tip, that means that there are long alar cartilages and a large cartilaginous vault.

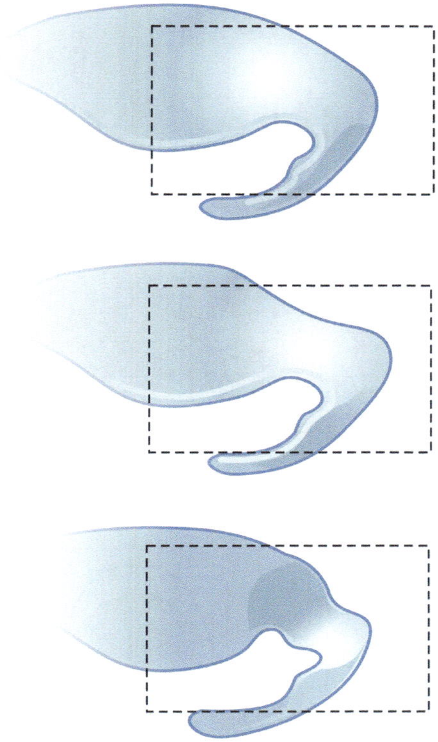

Fig. 9.15 Smooth, concave and convex type of domes

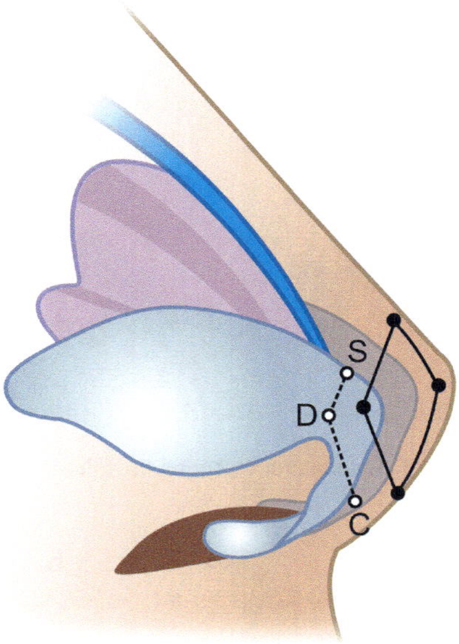

Fig. 9.16 Schematic diagram showing an anatomical (D), surgical (S) and clinical (C) domes

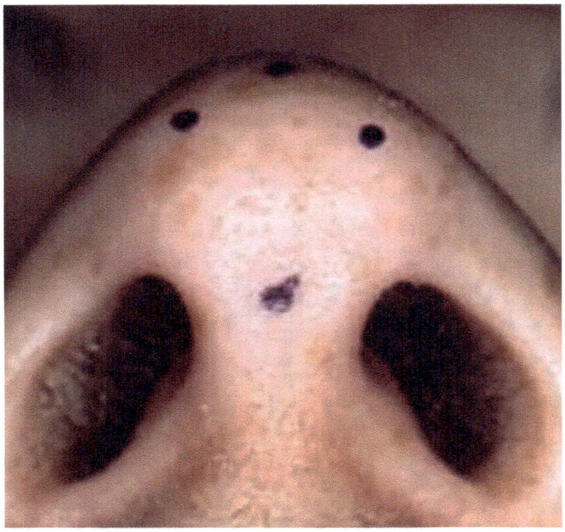

Fig. 9.17 Tip-defining points

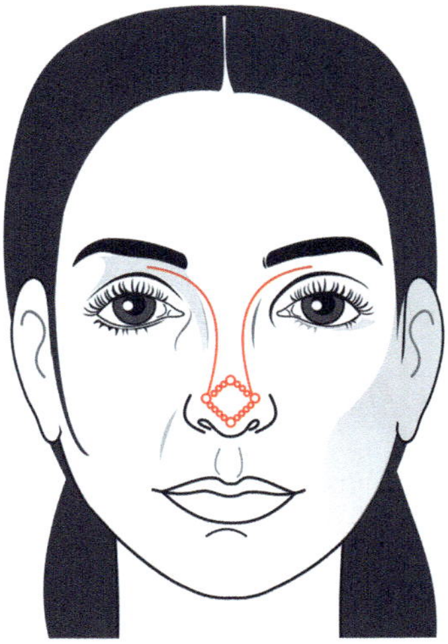

Fig. 9.18 Dorsal aesthetic lines

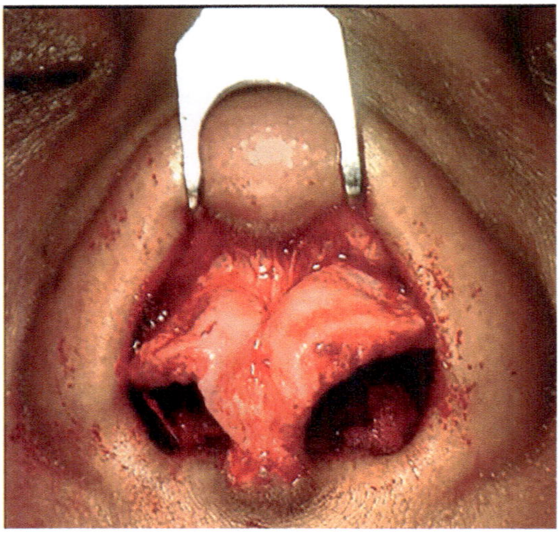

Fig. 9.19 Lateral crura forming tip volume

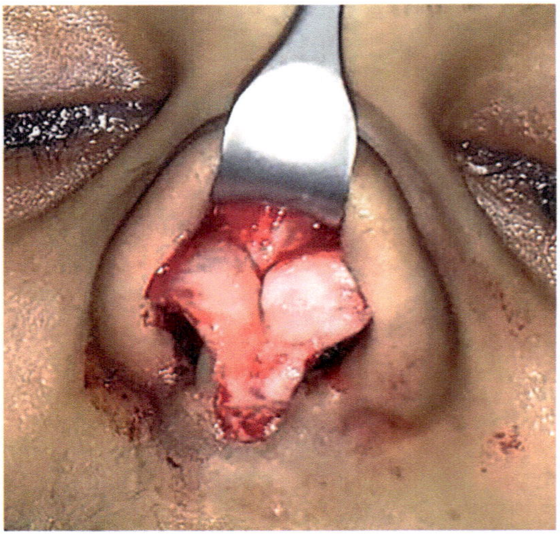

Fig. 9.20 Tip volume formed by lateral crura

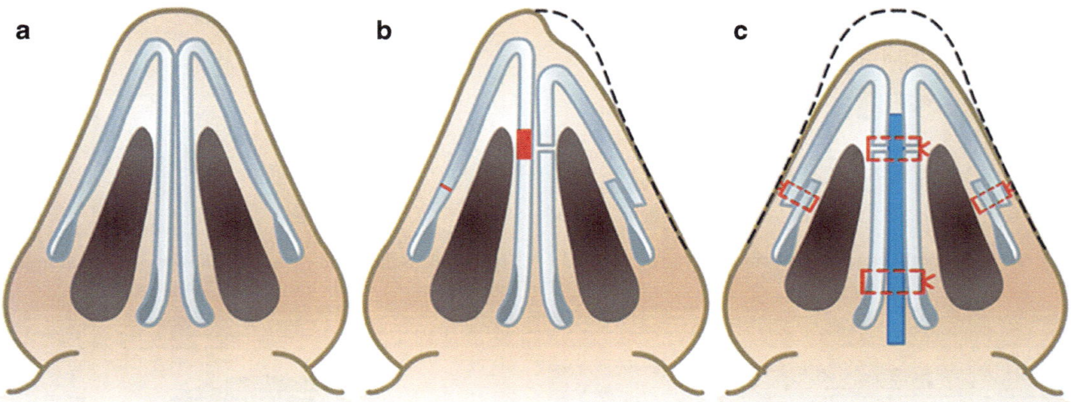

Fig. 9.21 (**a**) Overprojected tip. (**b**) Medial crus resected and lateral crus resected and repositioned. (**c**) Resected crura with columellar strut in between sutured and shortening of the nose achieved

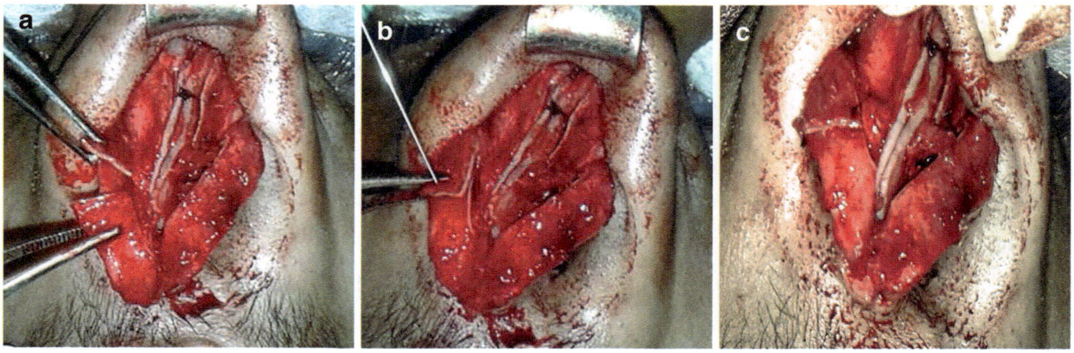

Fig. 9.22 (**a**) Cutting of right lateral crura. (**b**) Sliding over another. (**c**) Sutured with 5-0 PDS

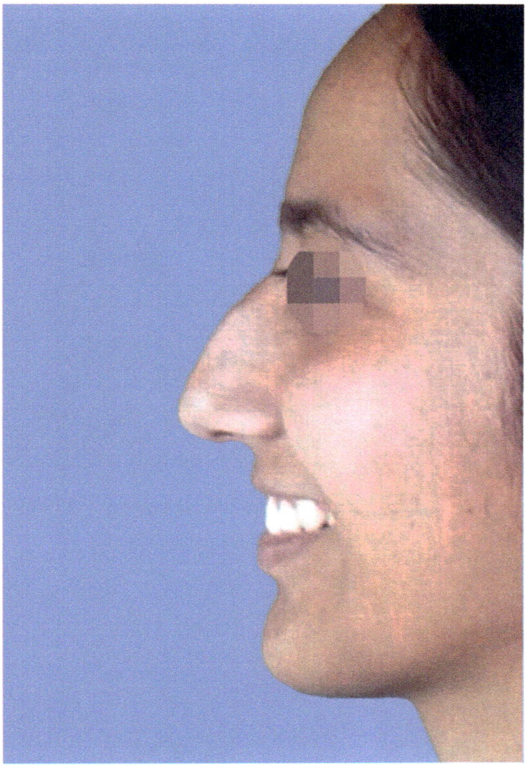

Fig. 9.23 Pre-op hump nose—drooping tip

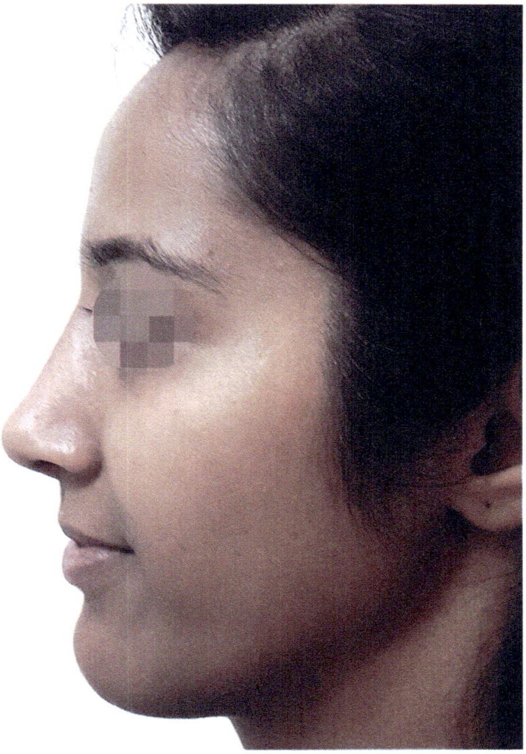

Fig. 9.24 Post-op picture showing an improvement in the tip rotation and projection

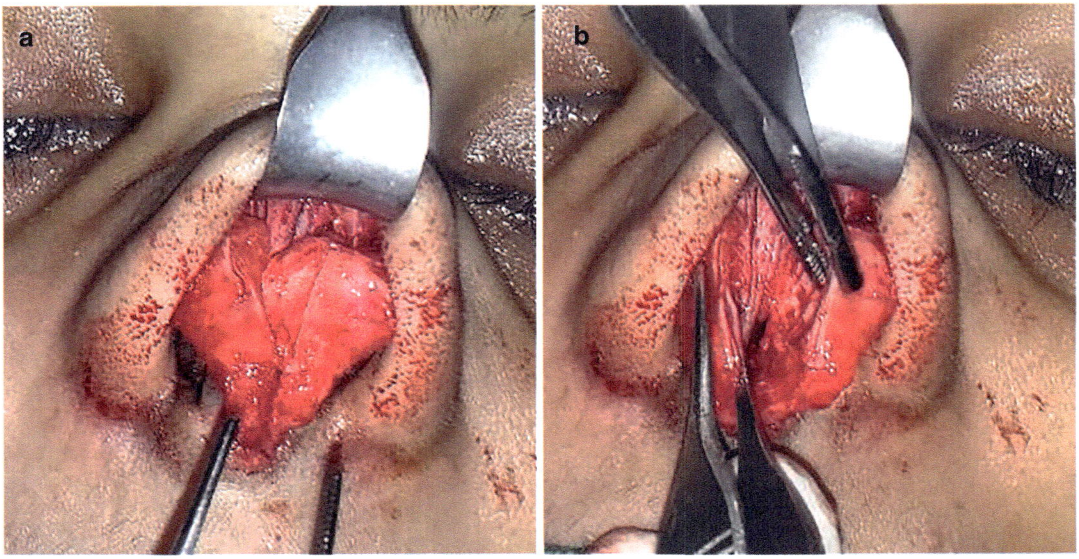

Fig. 9.25 (**a**, **b**) Pictures showing lateral crural underlay or infolding

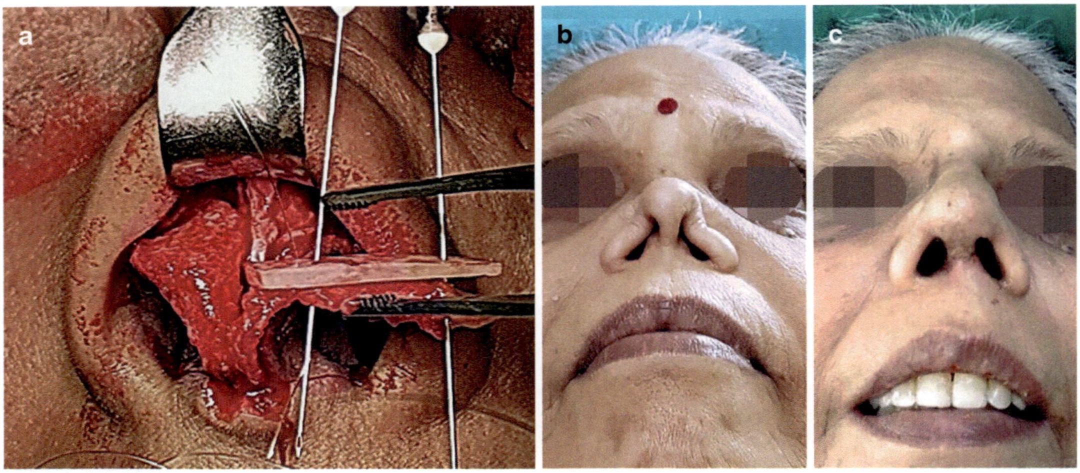

Fig. 9.26 (**a**) Lateral crural strut graft for collapse of lateral crus. (**b**) Pre-operative lateral crural collapse. (**c**) Post-operative lateral crural strut graft

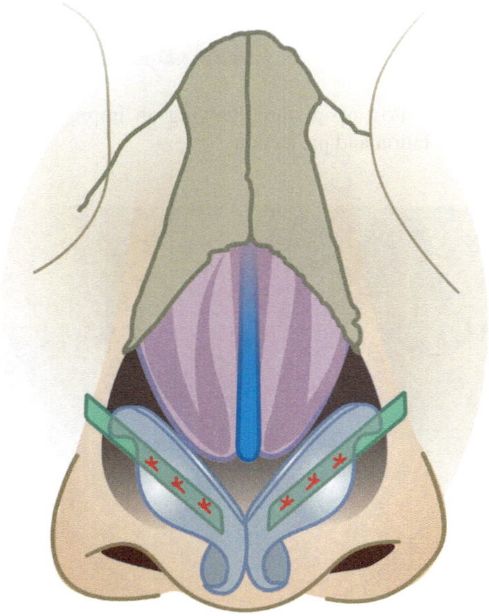

Fig. 9.27 Frontal view of lateral crural overlay or lateral crural strut graft

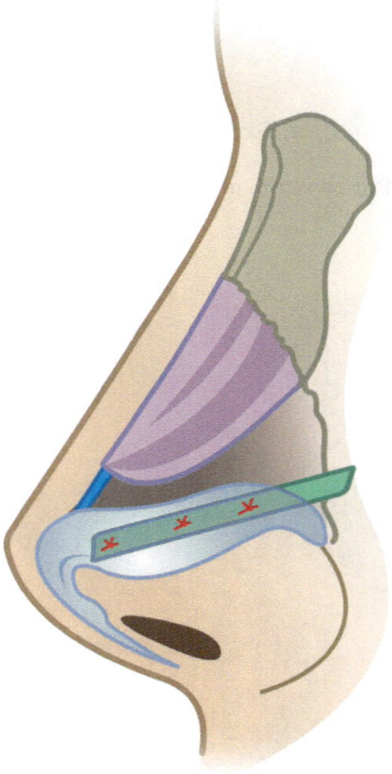

Fig. 9.28 Frontal view of lateral crural overlay or lateral crural strut graft

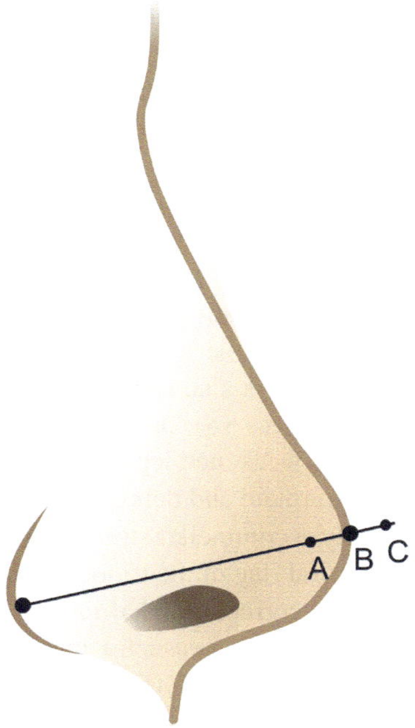

Fig. 9.29 Tip projection points. (A) Underprojected tip. (B) Ideal tip. (C) Overprojected tip

2. *ROTATION* (Figs. 9.32, 9.33, 9.34 and 9.35)

   It is defined as the *tip angle.*
   IDEAL NASOLABIAL ANGLE

- *In females—110*
- *In males—90*

An acute or obtuse nasolabial angle is produced due to problems in either of the three crura, caudal septum or anterior nasal spine.

For example, the *downrotated tip or drooping tip* could be because of large crura or long caudal septum or both (Figs. 9.36, 9.37 and 9.38).

For example, the *upwardly rotated tip* could be because of severely concave lateral crura or short lobular segment of middle crus or both (Figs. 9.39 and 9.40).

3. *TIP POSITION* (Fig. 9.41)

- Tip position refers to the location of the tip along the dorsal line. This is important in deciding the formation of a new tip while shortening a long nose.

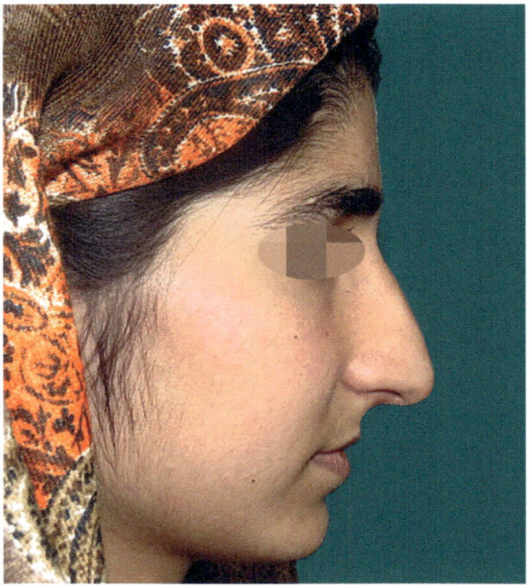

Fig. 9.30 An overprojected tip

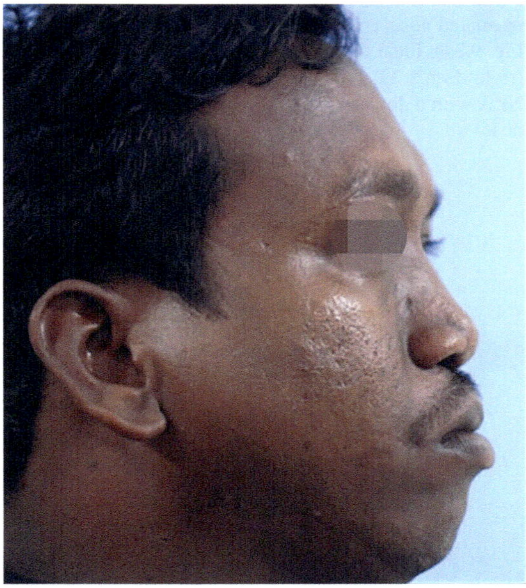

Fig. 9.31 An underprojected tip

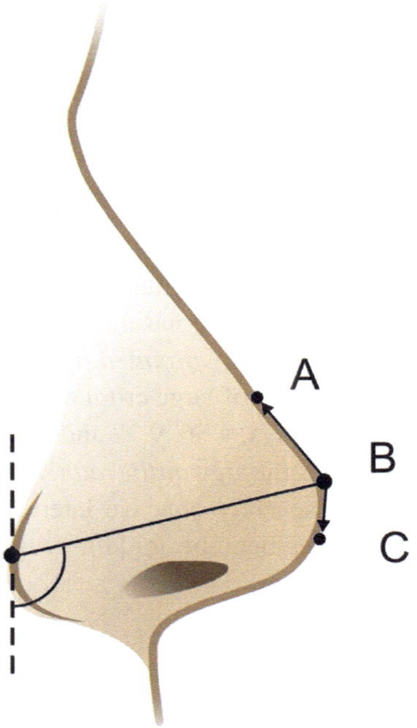

Fig. 9.32 Tip rotation. (A) Uprotated tip. (B) Ideal tip. (C) Downrotated tip. With nasolabial angle indicated at the base of the nose

9.5 Anderson Tip Tripod Concept (Figs. 9.42 and 9.43)

When considering the effect of surgical techniques on the nose, one may think of the tip as a tripod, with each lateral crus composing one leg of the tripod, and the paired medial crura composing the third leg. Shortening the two 'lateral crural' legs will cause the tripod to fall in that direction, thereby 'rotating and deprojecting' the tripod. Weakening these two legs (as with cephalic resection) is also said to have the same effect (although less so), as the healing forces applied to these weakened legs of the tripod will cause the tip to rotate and deproject slightly over time. Similarly, a columellar strut will strengthen the 'medial crural' leg of the tripod. Use of a columellar strut to correct buckled medial or intermediate crura may increase tip projection and rotation. Even though the tripod concept oversimplifies the dynamics of the nasal tip, it provides those with little experience in rhinoplasty with a method of predicting the effects of specific techniques.

Figs. 9.33–9.35 (left: Fig. 9.33): Obtuse NLA with an uprotated nose; (middle: Fig. 9.34): Ideal tip nose; (right: Fig. 3.23): Acute NLA with a downrotated nose

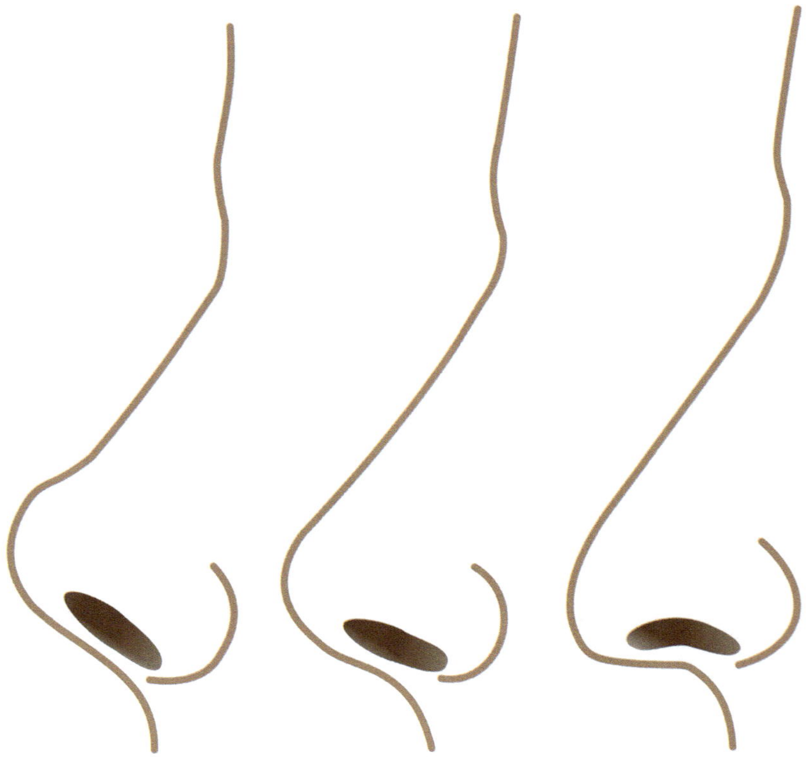

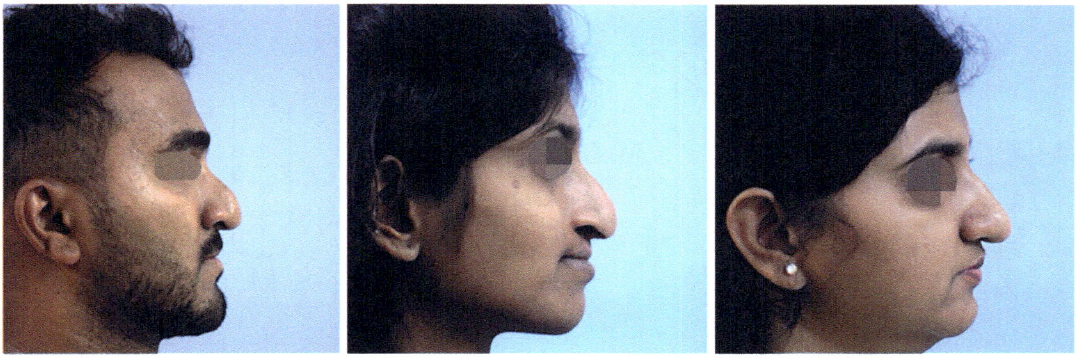

Figs. 9.36–9.38 (left: Fig. 9.36): Downrotated tip; (middle: Fig. 9.37): Downrotated tip; (right: Fig. 9.38): Downrotated tip

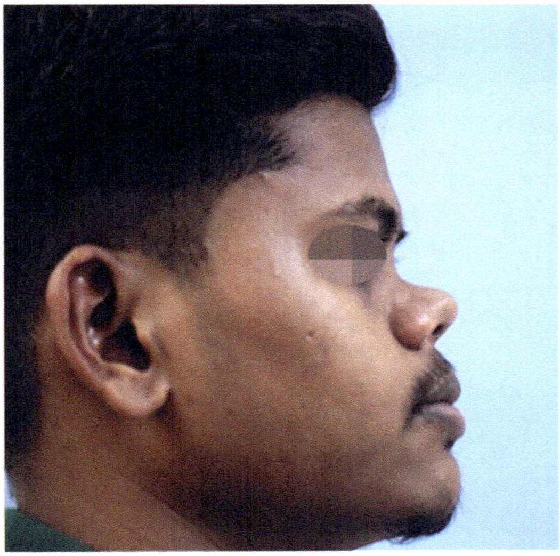

Fig. 9.39 Upwardly rotated tip

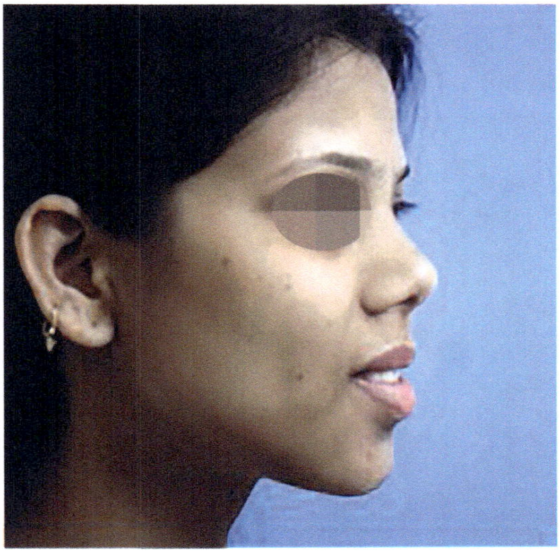

Fig. 9.40 Upwardly rotated tip

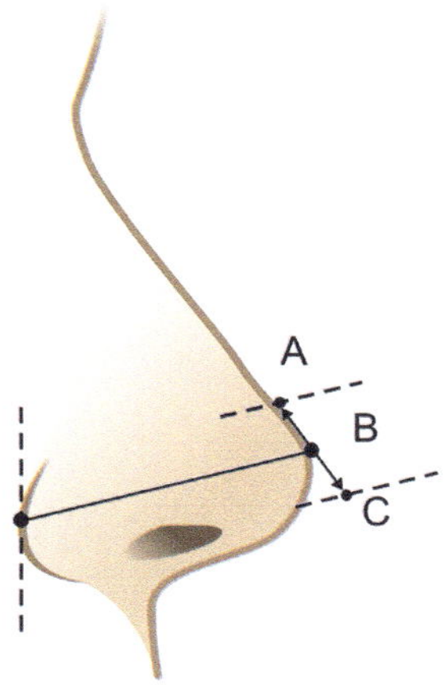

Fig. 9.41 Tip position. (A) Short tip. (B) Ideal tip. (C) Long tip

9.5.1 Other Deformities of Tip

1. *Broad and bulbous tip* (Figs. 9.44, 9.45, 9.46 and 9.47)

Domes and lateral crura in a broad bulbous tip are continuous without any tip definition (Figs. 9.48 and 9.49).

2. *Boxy tip* (Figs. 9.50 and 9.51)

In a boxy tip, the lateral crura convexity (LAC) defines tip width.

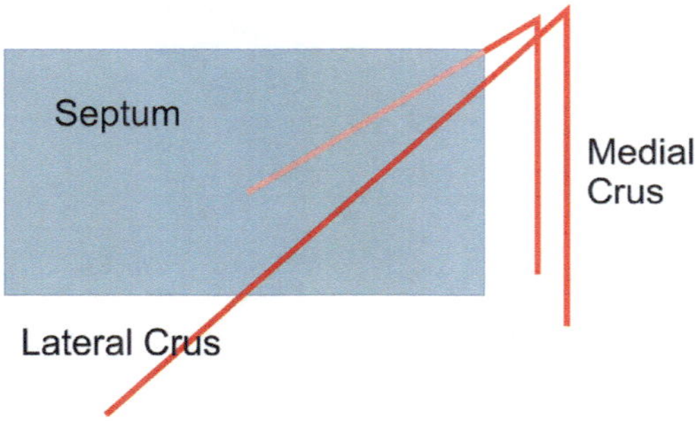

Fig. 9.42 Schematic diagram of medial and lateral crus

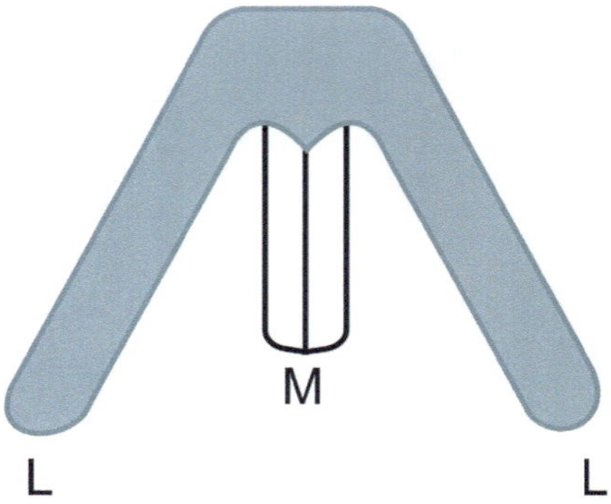

Fig. 9.43 Schematic diagram comparing the three limbs of crura to a tripod

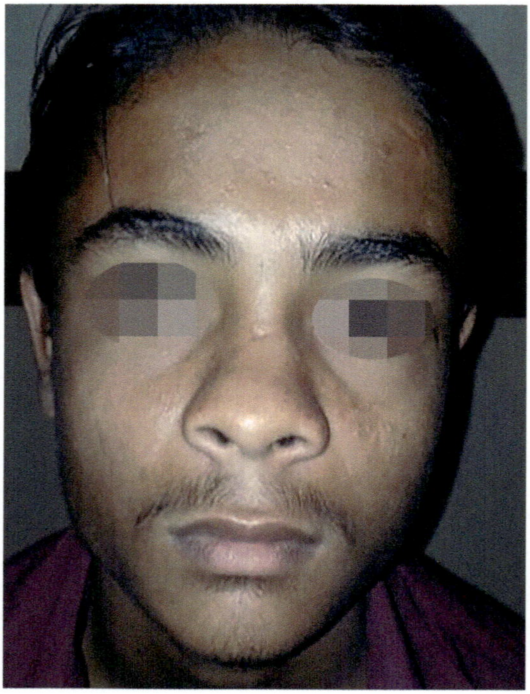

Fig. 9.44 Frontal view of a broad tip nose

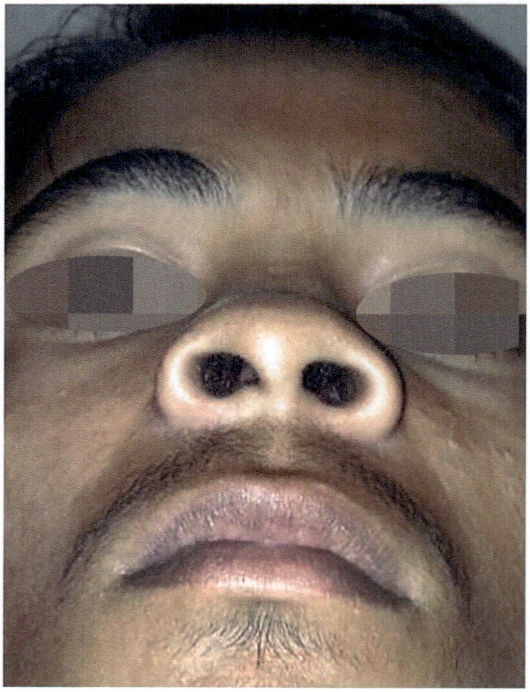

Fig. 9.45 Basal view of a broad tip nose

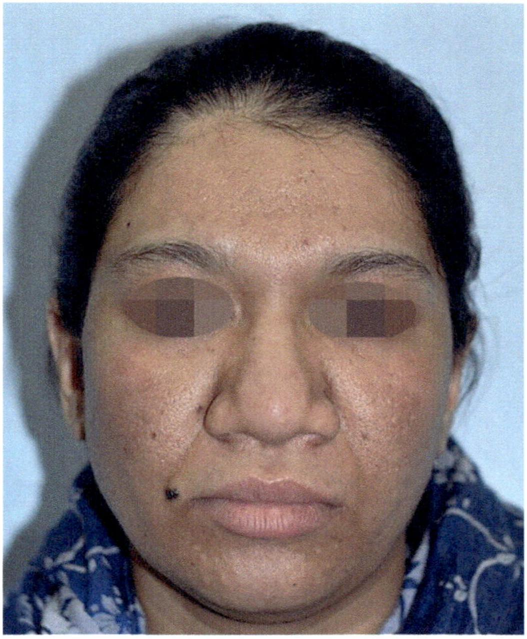

Fig. 9.46 Frontal view of a bulbous tip nose

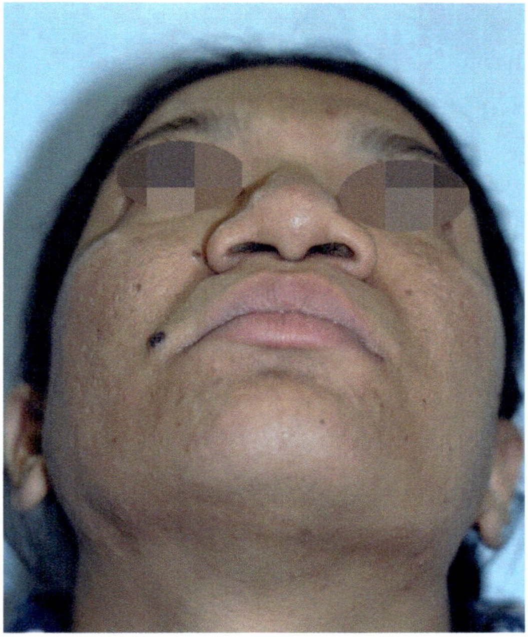

Fig. 9.47 Basal view of a bulbous tip nose

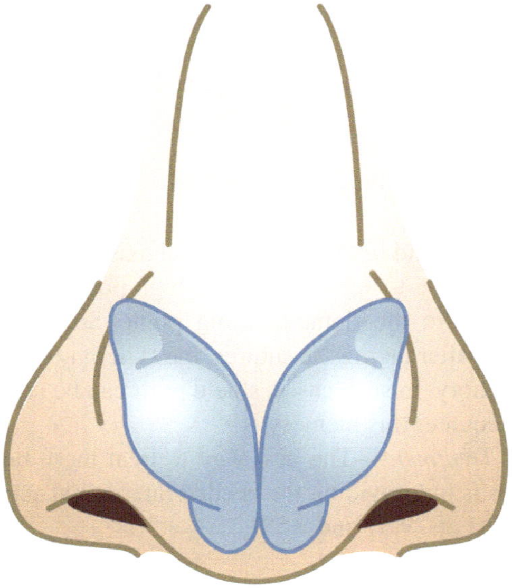

Fig. 9.48 Schematic diagram (two blue arrows) showing convex dome and lateral crura being continuous

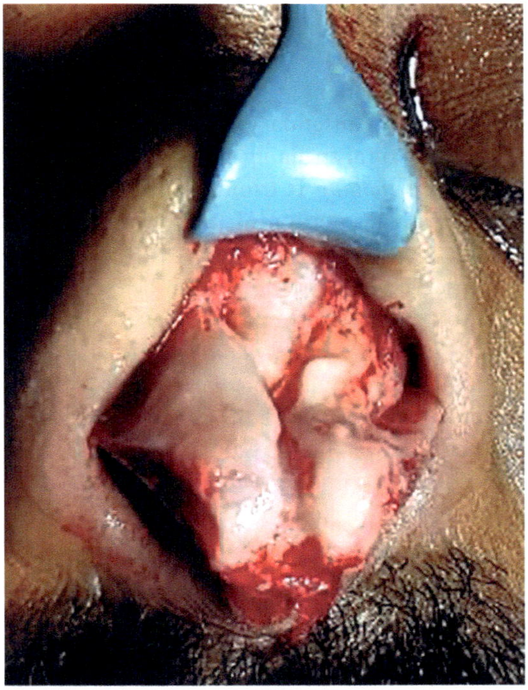

Fig. 9.49 Picture of convex dome and lateral crura being continuous

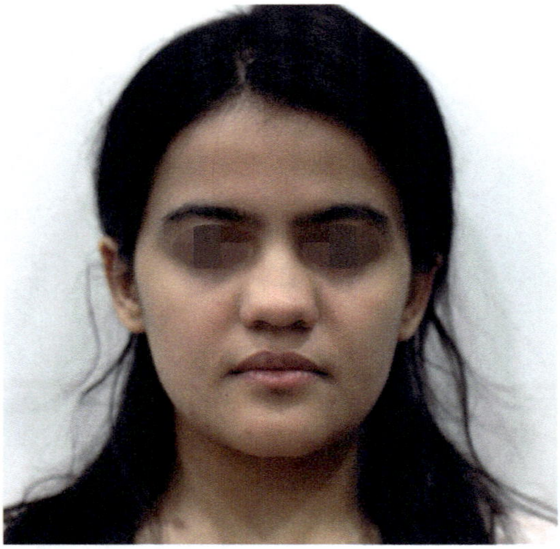

Fig. 9.50 Boxy tip frontal view

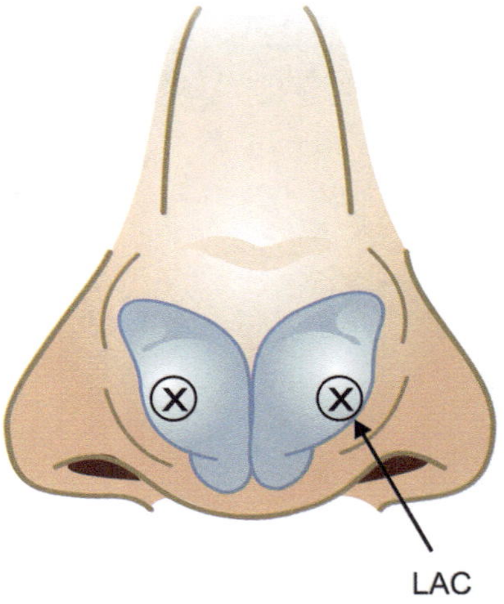

Fig. 9.51 Schematic diagram of lateral crural convexity defining the tip in frontal view

The most common sequences of treating a broad, bulbous and boxy tip are by (Fig. 9.52a–d):

(a) Placing a columellar strut and cephalic trimming
(b) Domal creation
(c) Domal equalisation
(d)Lateral crural spanning sutures

Cephalic trimming is trimming or infolding of the cephalic portion of the lower alar cartilage where at least 7 mm of the cartilage is preserved and the rest can be shaved or infolded.

A classic lateral crural spanning suture is passed through a portion of one lateral crus and then through a portion of the other lateral crura, and tied over the dorsal septum. The suture then passes through the dorsal septum and the knot is tied just over the septum.

Columellar Strut (Fig. 9.53)
Create a pocket in the membranous septum in between the medial crura (cross-check with you sir). Touch the anterior nasal spine just below the dome.

Stitch properly with 5-0 PDS. This provides a good tip support.

If it is placed too deep, then sublabial palpation of the graft is done.

Domal Creation (Fig. 9.54)
The most aesthetic configuration of the tip is convex domal segment adjacent to concave lateral crura.

This configuration is gained with *DOMAL SUTURES*.

3. *Bifid tip* (Figs. 9.55 and 9.56)

In a bifid tip, the lateral crural axis shifts from transverse to vertical, and the high point (HP) is lateral to the dome-defining point. Sometimes even after taking the sutures, the skin may have a memory. In such cases, shield graft can be added to counter this memory.

Treatment—The best way to treat these bifid tips is by providing the needed interdomal suturing (Figs. 9.57 and 9.58).

9.6 Grafts

TIP ONLAY GRAFT—Either one or multiple can be placed (Fig. 9.59).

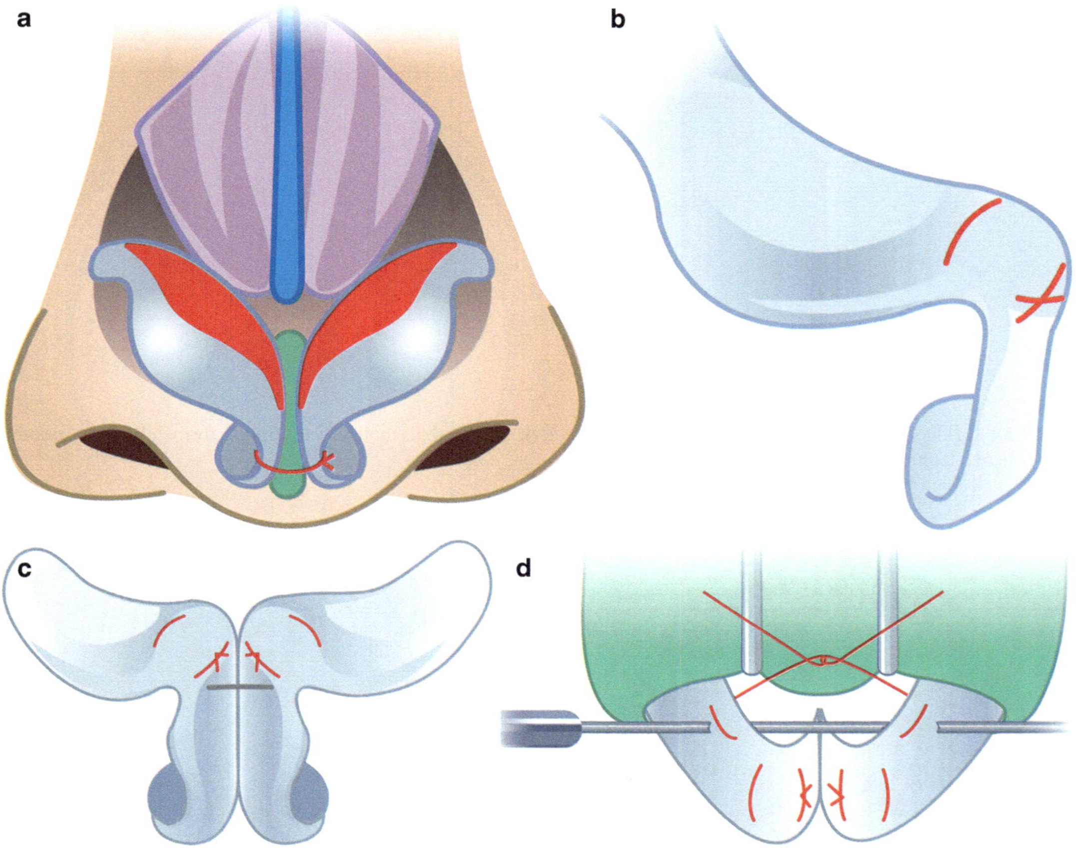

Fig. 9.52 (**a**) Columellar strut with cephalic trimming. (**b**) Domal creation. (**c**) Domal equalisation. (**d**) Lateral spanning suture

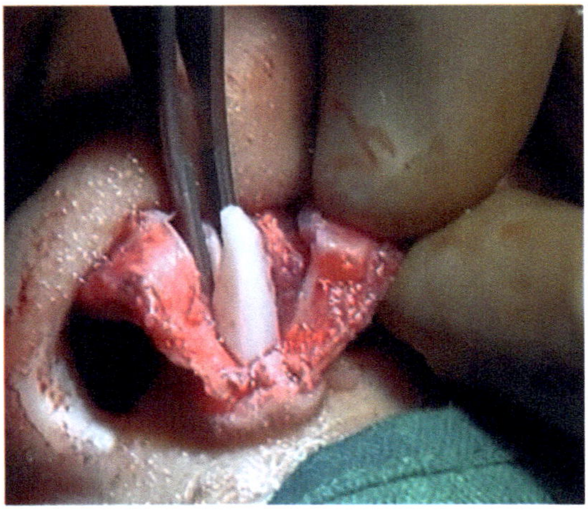

Fig. 9.53 Columellar strut

The size has to be thick and two grafts have to be placed if more tip projection is required.

The preferred cartilage for this is septal cartilage. Tip onlay graft is preferred if there is good columellar show and shield graft if there is no columellar show.

9.6.1 Infratip Lobular or Shield Graft

This grafting is done by creating a pocket which should not be wider than the medial crural breadth, and the superior aspect of the length of the graft is maintained about 3–4 mm above more than dome (Figs 9.60 and 9.61).

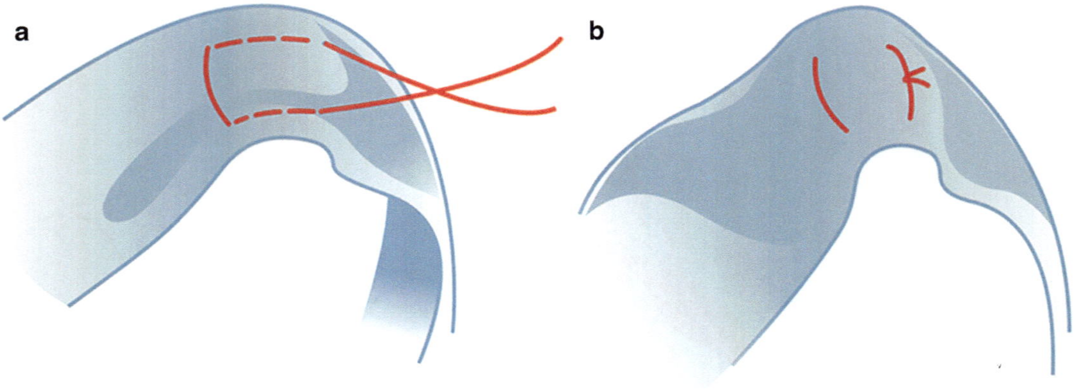

Fig. 9.54 (**a**) Domal sutures placed on the domal segment. (**b**) An ideal aesthetic configuration formed by convex dome and concave lateral segment

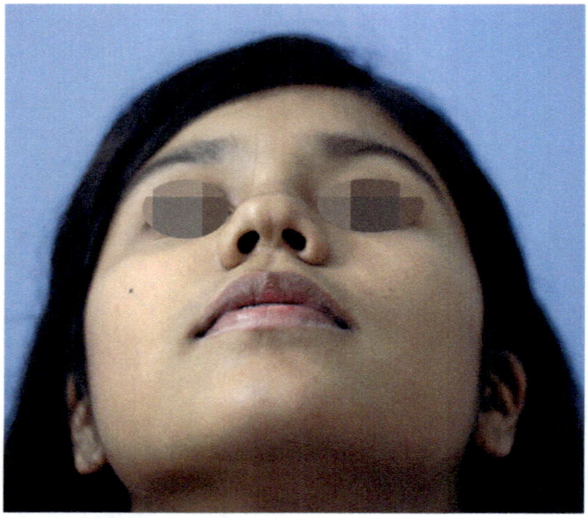

Fig. 9.55 Bifid tip basal view

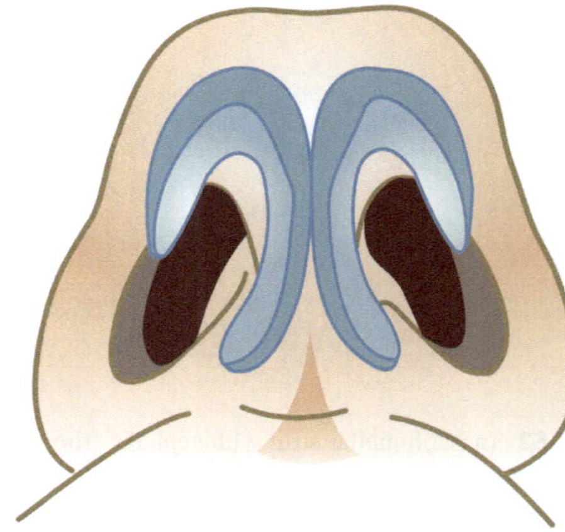

Fig. 9.56 Schematic diagram showing bifid tip by shift of lateral crural axis

9.6.1.1 Rim Graft

The *alar rim graft* is a technique that provides support to the external valve and improves *alar rim* contour. The alar *rim graft* is placed in a tunnel created directly along the alar margin. Preferred cartilage here is septal cartilage. A 2–3 mm pocket in breadth is done laterally from dome (Figs. 9.62, 9.63 and 9.64).

9.6.1.2 Articulated Rim Grafts

The 'articulated' alar rim graft is a modification of the conventional rim graft that improves treatment of secondary alar rim deformities, including postsurgical alar retraction. Unlike the conventional alar rim graft, the articulated rim grafts are sutured to the underlying tip complex to provide direct stationary support to the alar margin, thereby enhancing the graft efficacy (Figs. 9.65, 9.66, 9.67, 9.68, 9.69 and 9.70).

9.6.2 Alar Base Deformity

Alar flare is a common feature that contributes to the width of the lower third of the nose. Alar flare reduction can improve nasal harmony and facial aesthetic balance; however, it is also difficult to

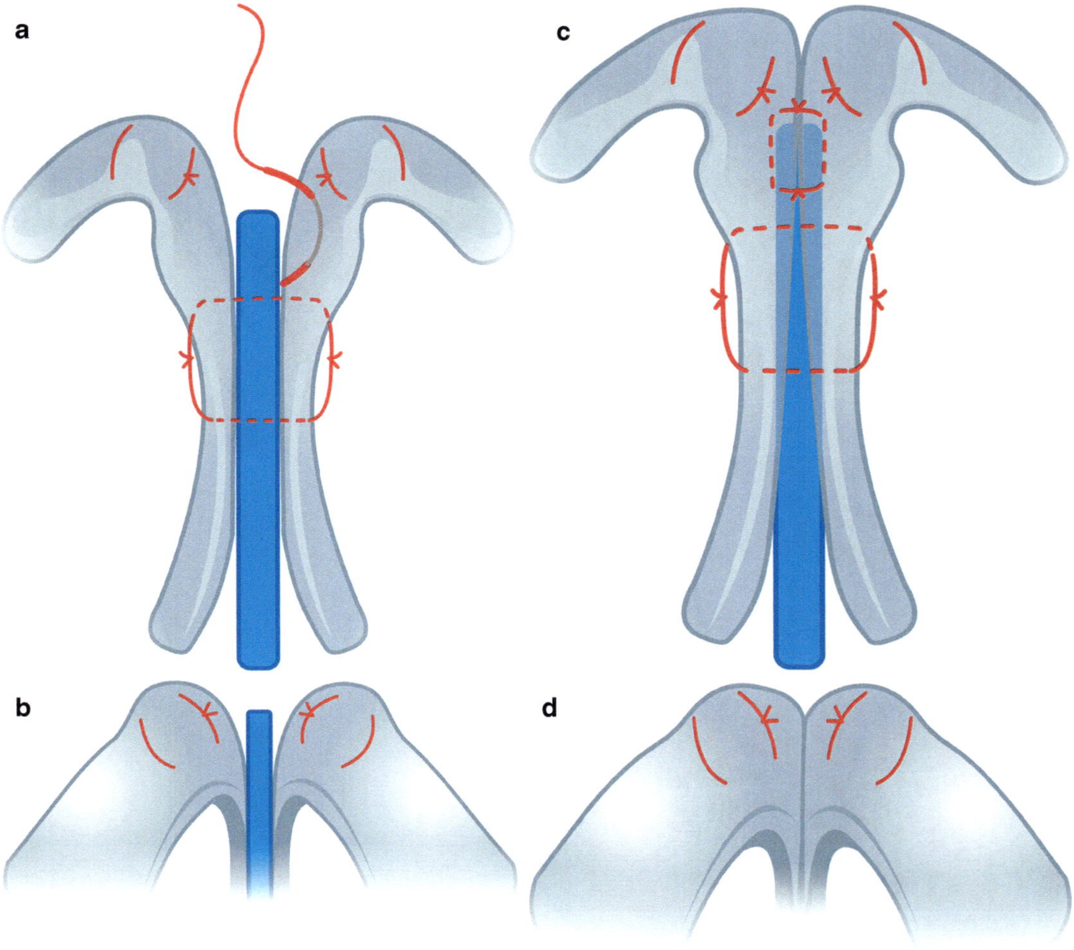

Fig. 9.57 Schematic diagram showing (**a**, **b**) intradomal suturing of both sides with columellar strut graft placed between two crura. (**c**, **d**) Interdomal suturing done with a columellar strut buried in between

correct if performed inappropriately or overzealously (Figs. 9.71, 9.72, 9.73 and 9.74).

- *Wedge.* Wedge excisions reduce nasal flaring by removing wedges of ala, or the fleshy curved lower part of the nose that attaches to the cheek.
- *Sill.* Sill excisions are used to narrow the base of the ala, or where it attaches to the cheek which helps to reduce the nostril width.
- *Weir or hockey stick* excision is a combination of both.

Alaplasty—Alar base reduction is done using sill excision (Fig. 9.75).

9.6.3 Hanging Columella (Figs. 9.76)

Hanging columella is when a person's *columella* is placed such that more than 4 mm of the nostril is visible on his/her profile view and usually mentioned as a columellar show.

Tongue-in-groove operation is done for treating the hanging columella.

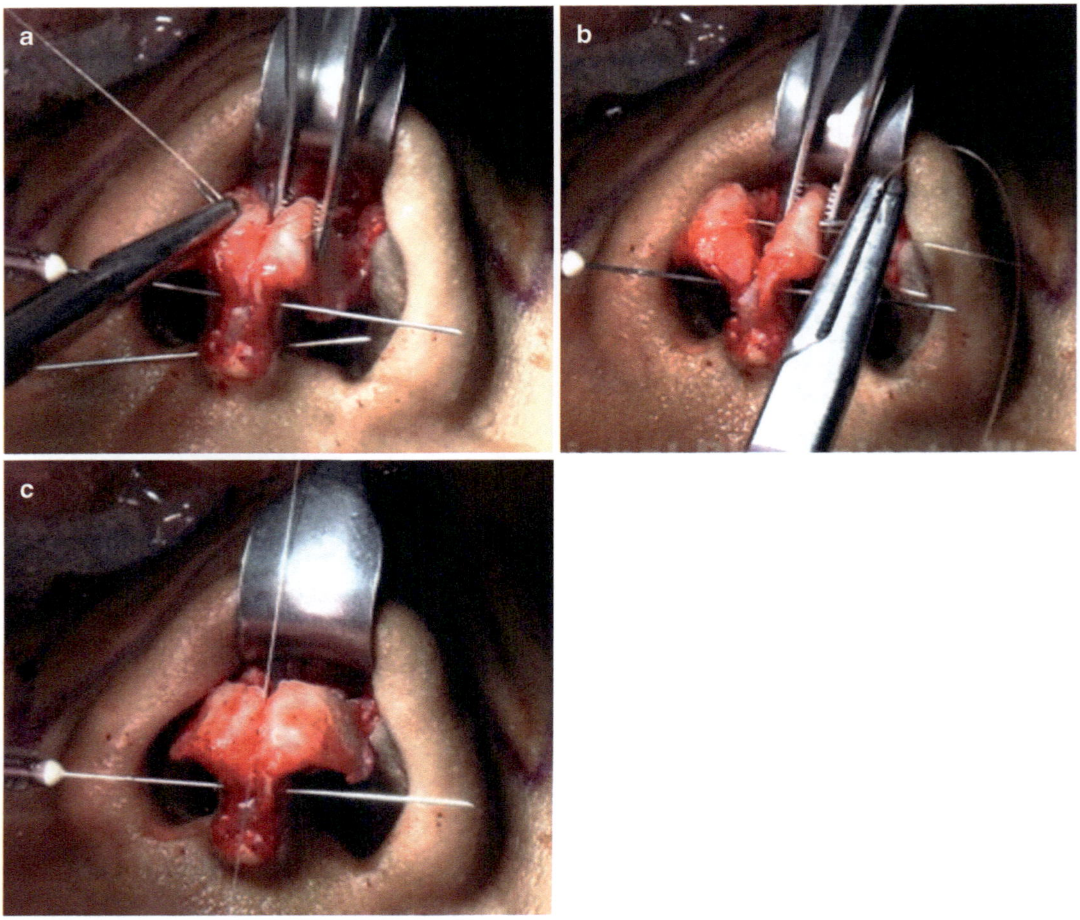

Fig. 9.58 (**a**) Domal creation. (**b**) Domal equalisation. (**c**) Domal stabilisation with suturing by 5-0 PDS

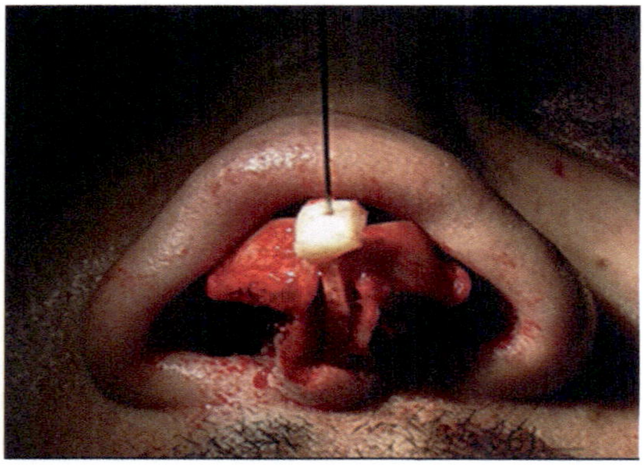

Fig. 9.59 Tip onlay graft

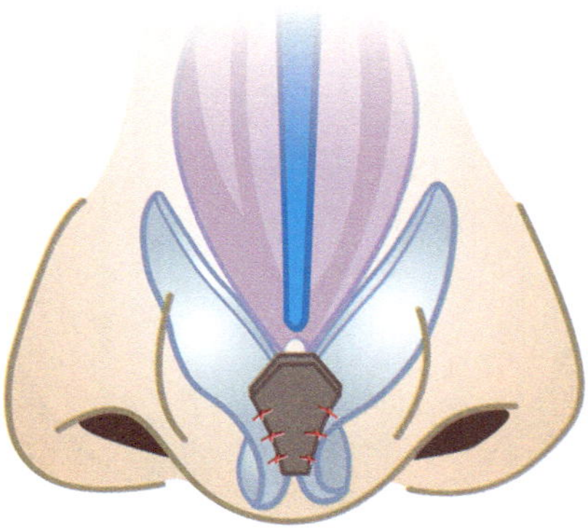

Fig. 9.60 Shield graft

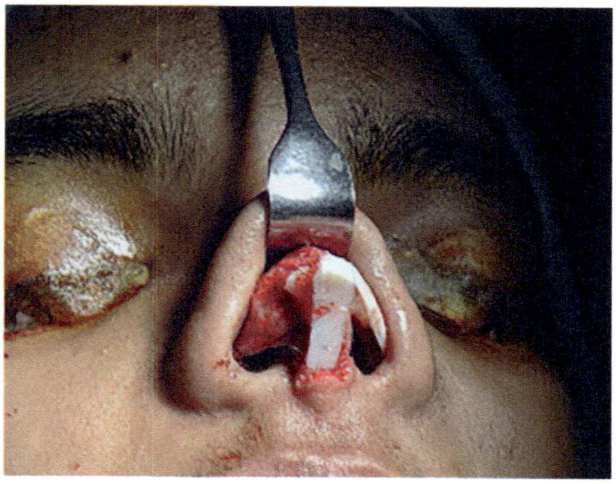

Fig. 9.61 Shield graft with additional left alar overlay graft

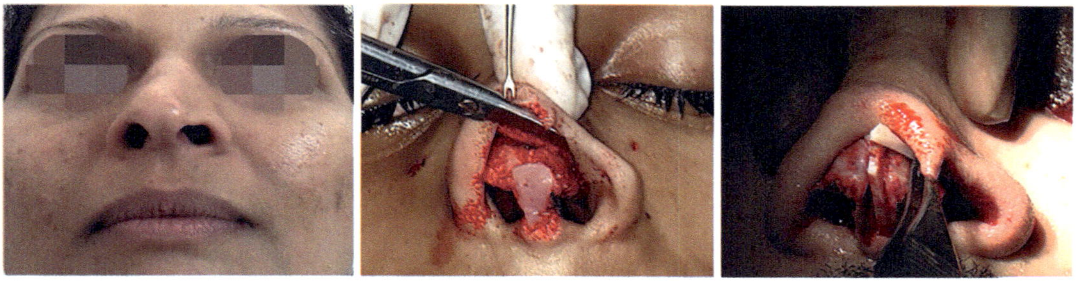

Figs. 9.62–9.64 (left: Fig. 9.62): Asymmetrical shape of the ala with left alar deformity; (middle: Fig. 9.63): A 2–3 mm pocket in breadth is made laterally from dome; (right: Fig. 9.64): Placing of a rim graft on the left side of ala

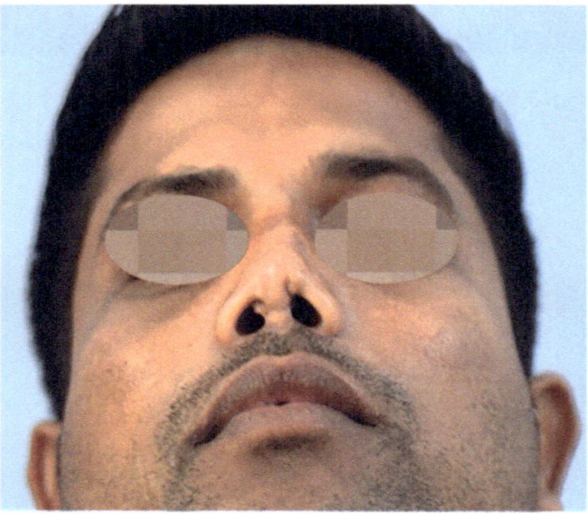

Fig. 9.65 Picture showing postsurgical alar retraction

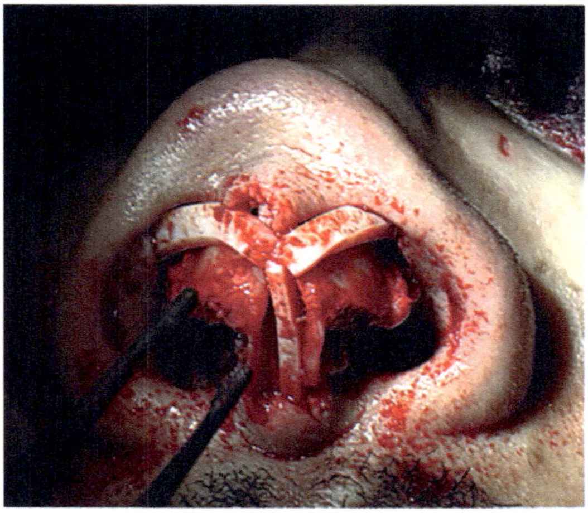

Fig. 9.66 Correction with bilateral articulated rim grafts

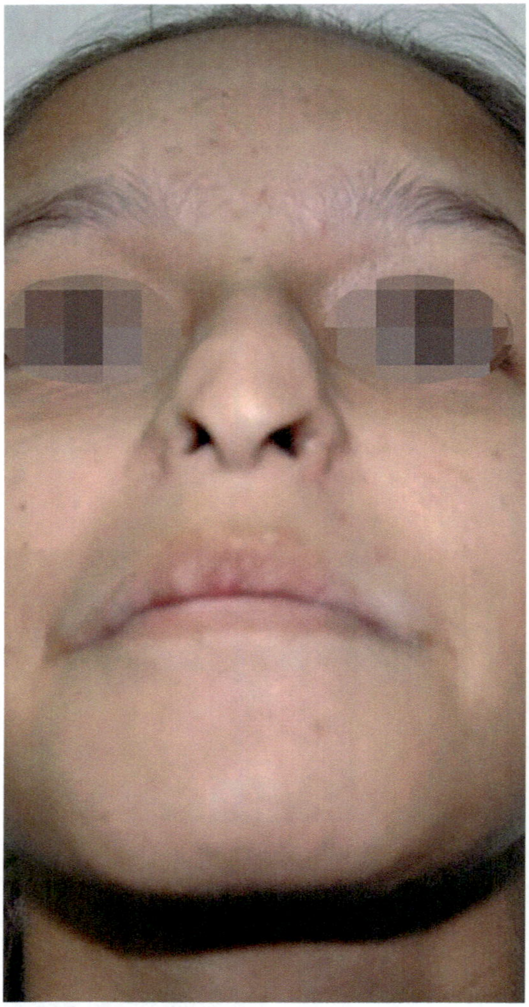

Fig. 9.67 Bilateral alar retraction

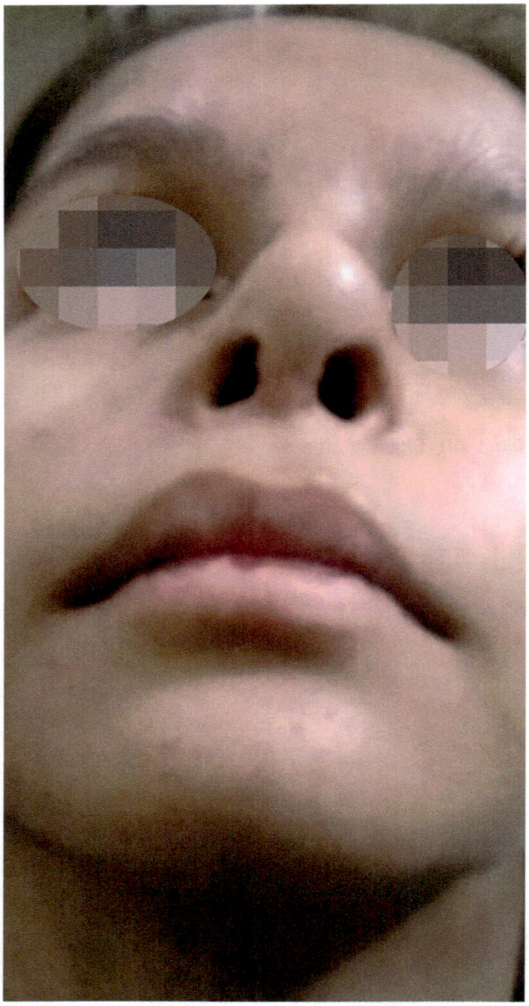

Fig. 9.68 Post-op articulated rim grafts

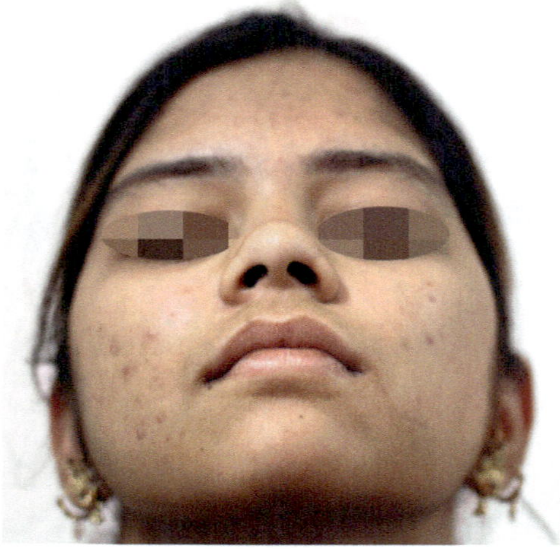

Fig. 9.69 Pre-op alar asymmetry

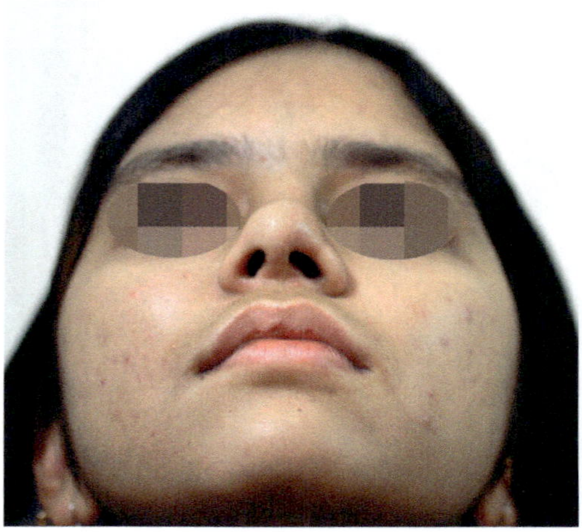

Fig. 9.70 Asymmetry treated with articulated rim grafts

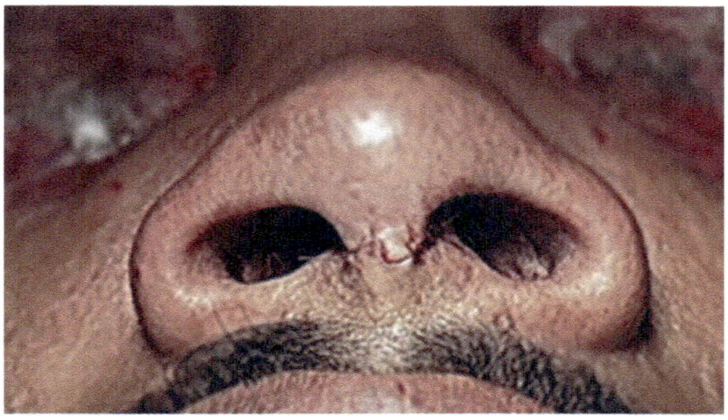

Fig. 9.71 Broad and wide ala

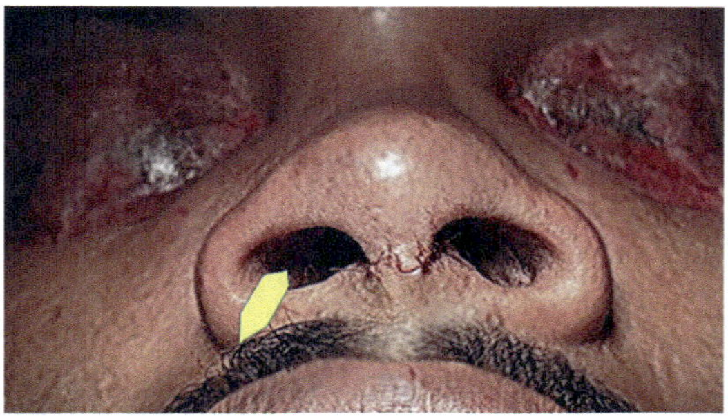

Fig. 9.72 Sill excision depicted by yellow mark

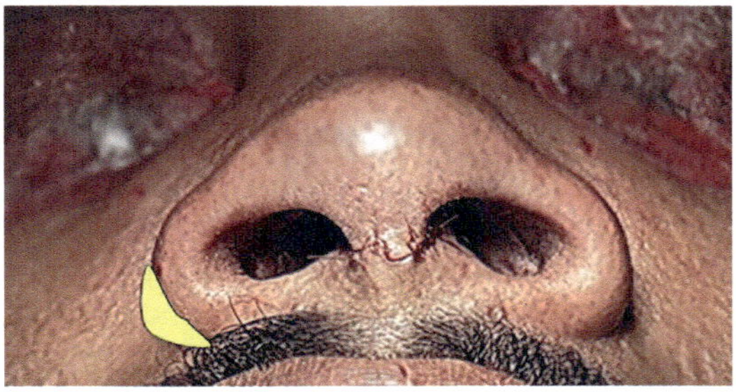

Fig. 9.73 Wedge excision

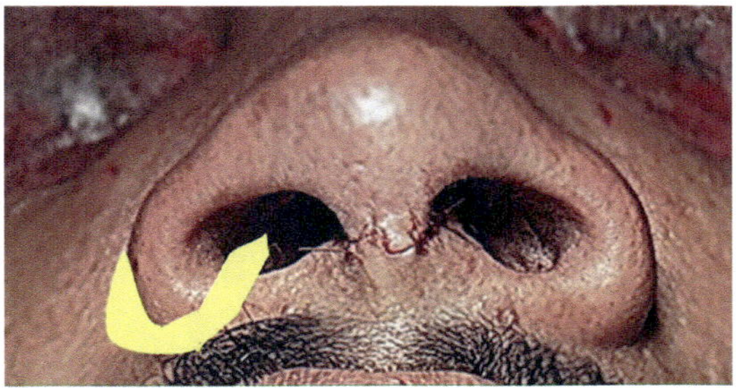

Fig. 9.74 Hockey stick excision

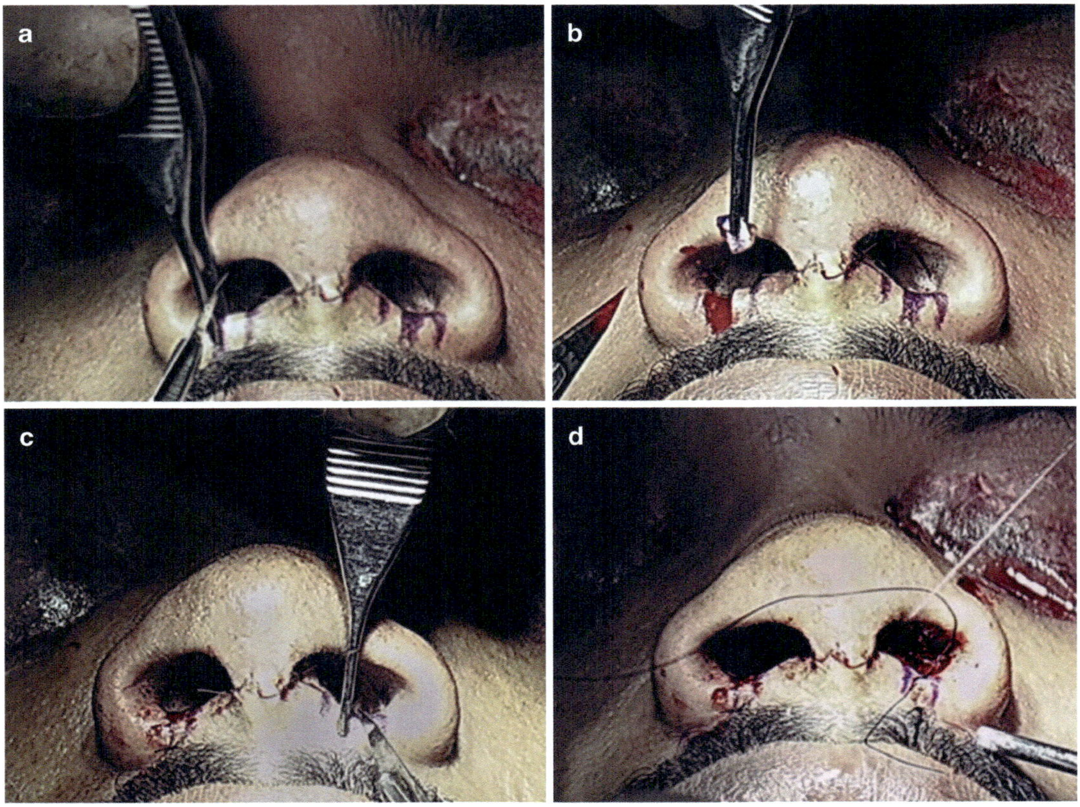

Fig. 9.75 (**a**) Alar base incision. (**b**) Sill excision. (**c**) Sill excision on both sides. (**d**) Suture using 5-0 Ethilon

The specific steps are as follows:

1. Correction of any caudal septal deviation through bilateral full-transfixion incisions

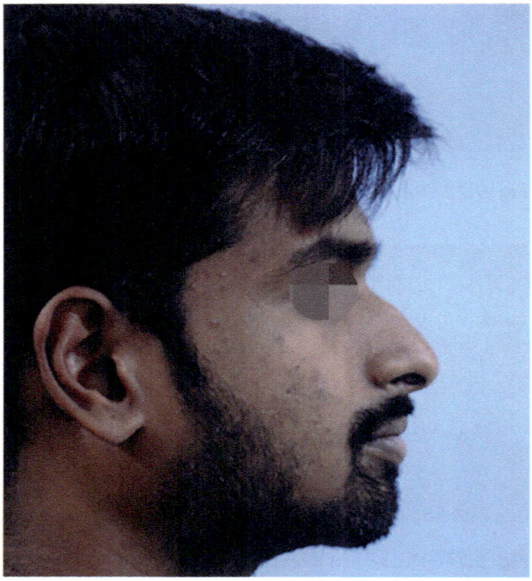

Fig. 9.76 Hanging columella

2. Retrograde dissection between medial crura with optional soft tissue excision
3. Telescoping of the columellar tissue onto the caudal septum
4. Fixation with 5-0 PDS sutures
5. Bilateral membranous septum excision

The most common errors include the following:

1. Underresection of the anterior nasal spine
2. Persistent deviation of the caudal septum
3. Excessive upward tip rotation

9.6.4 Columellar Retraction

A retracted columella is referred to as an aesthetic condition wherein the nose tip projection appears as retracted or pulled in when viewed from the front or in profile view (Figs. 9.77 and 9.78).

Septal extension grafting is used for treating columellar retraction.

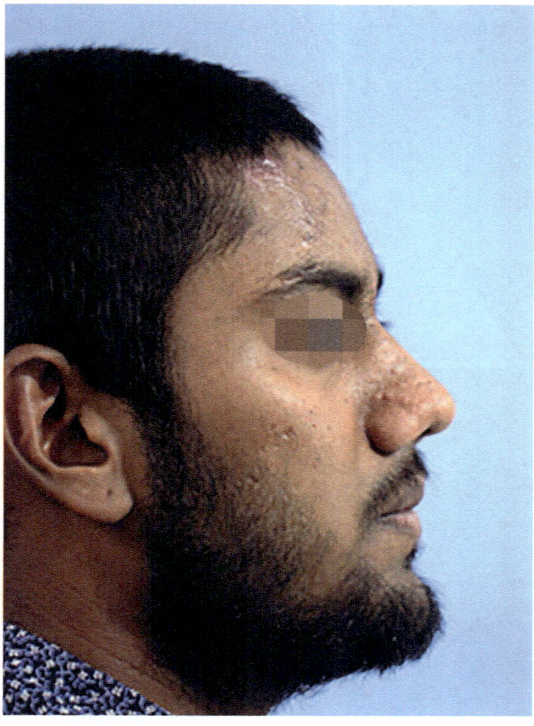

Fig. 9.77 Columellar retraction

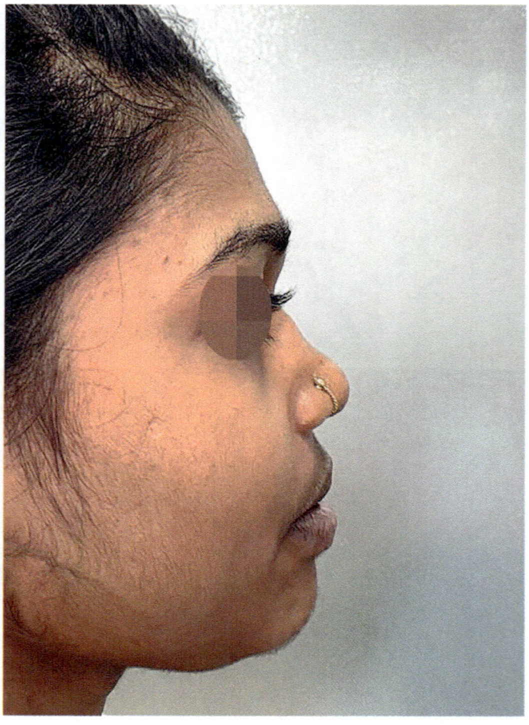

Fig. 9.78 Columellar retraction

9.6.5 Septal Extension Graft (Fig. 9.79)

The septal extension graft is a very useful method of controlling nasal lengthening and tip projection, rotation and shape by fixing a graft to the septum, which leads to a strong supporting structure. It gives a good size and shape to the tip, causes reinforcement of the tip and gives a good tip support.

The graft is placed from the caudal border of the septum till medial crura. And if more lengthening is required, then extend it along with extended spreader grafts.

Following this, side-to-side suturing is done or end-to-end suturing is done.

Three-point fixation to be done:

- Ala, septum and extended spreader grafts.
- Grafts used are the rib and septum.
- It causes an excellent control of support and tip rotation.

Disadvantages:

- Causes thickening of septum and hardens the tip

9.6.6 Anthropological Variations of Tip and Surgical Solution

SOUTH INDIA—Tip is bulbous with weak cartilage, and therefore an underlay or overlay graft needs to be placed for the alar cartilages. Also repositioning of lateral crura is very important during lengthening.

NORTH-EAST—Short noses with tip being bifid mostly also with weak cartilage. Here therefore lengthening of the nose with septal extension graft and articulated rim grafts will be what has to be focused upon.

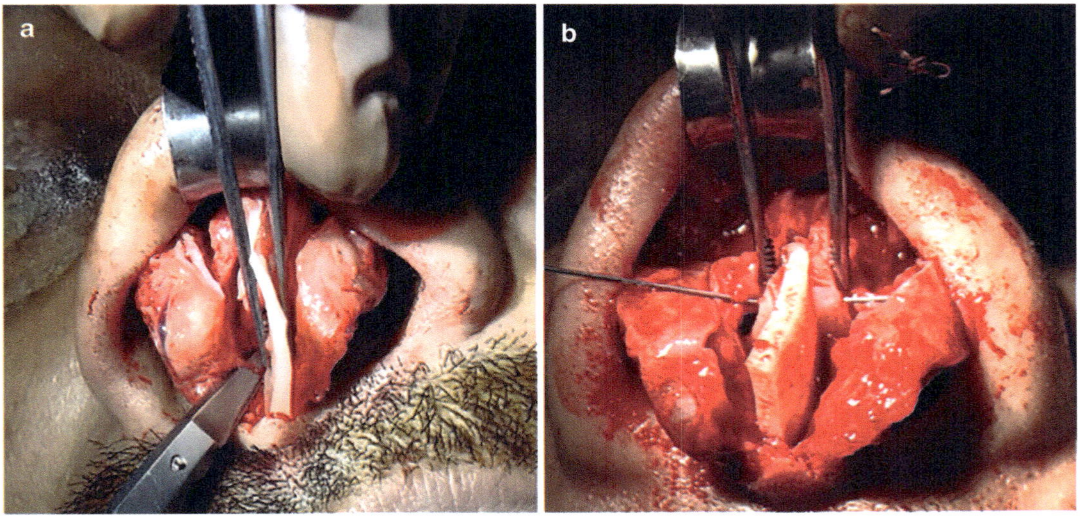

Fig. 9.79 (**a**) Septal extension graft is placed and sutured to the side caudal aspect of the septum. (**b**) SEG is sutured to the extended spreader grafts

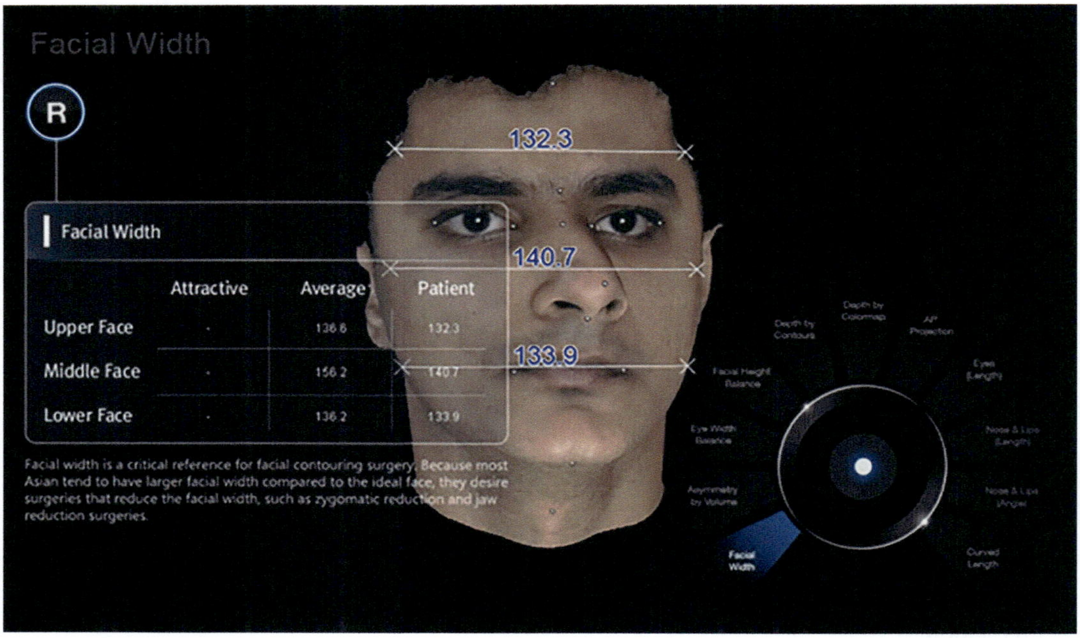

Fig. 9.80 3D scanning with facial proportions analysed

NORTH Indians have long noses with drooping tip mostly however associated with strong cartilages, and these require good reduction of tip.

CUTTING EDGE IN ANALYSIS OF TIP IN RHINOPLASTY is 3D scanning where the tip is analysed with facial proportions (Fig. 9.80).

Complications of Rhinoplasty 10

Main

A surgeon should be critical of his own results to enable improvement and be aware of the complications associated with surgeries for avoidance of problems in the future. A mind-set of continuous learning needs to be developed by a rhinoplasty surgeon when confronted with complications in practice. Unfortunately, sometimes the patient chooses to go to another centre when complications occur, and the primary surgeon is unable to assess his failures.

There is an extensive literature on revision rhinoplasty. However, assessment of rhinoplasty complications needs to be considered in more detail. Lessons for the future, a crucial step in gaining expertise, lie in the assessment of complications.

Rhinoplasty surgery has an inherent risk of complications due to the unpredictable healing of the various different types of tissues involved, which include the skin, fascia, nerves, muscle, bone and cartilage. Also, these healing patterns tend to change over a period of time, adding to the complexity of the matter.

Rhinoplasty is one of the most challenging facial surgeries and demands a thorough understanding of art and science. Complications occur in this surgery just as any other surgery. However, a few of them can cause hazardous long-term effect on the patient. The post-operative complications in rhinoplasty surgery are different because even a minor complication is seen and appreciated on the most prominent part of the face by everyone and thus becomes a major concern.

10.1 Classification of Complications of Rhinoplasty

(a) Intraoperative
(b) Immediate and early post-operative
(c) Late post-operative

10.2 Intraoperative Complications

10.2.1 Excessive Bleeding

Prevention

- It is important to rule out pre-operatively acquired coagulopathy, the commonest culprit being aspirin.
- Pre-operative BP to be controlled in hypertensive patients.
- At the time of induction, either inj tranexamic acid or inj botropase or Tab. ethamsylate with sips of water should be considered.
- Head end elevation to about 30 degrees.
- Good and sufficient local infiltration before scrubbing and draping.
- Maintain the proper plane of dissection to avoid the superficial muscular aponeurotic system (SMAS).

V. Ghaisas, *Indian Ethnic Rhinoplasty*, https://doi.org/10.1007/978-981-16-2478-0_10

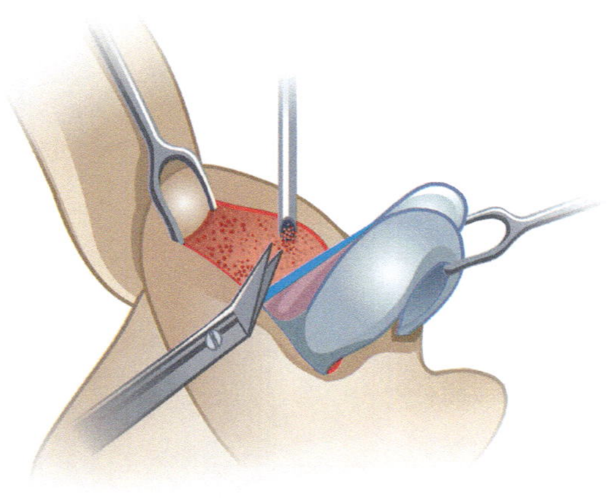

Fig. 10.1 Schematic diagram of the plane of dissection, in subperichondial and subperiosteal plane and debulking of fatty tissue from deep fatty layer

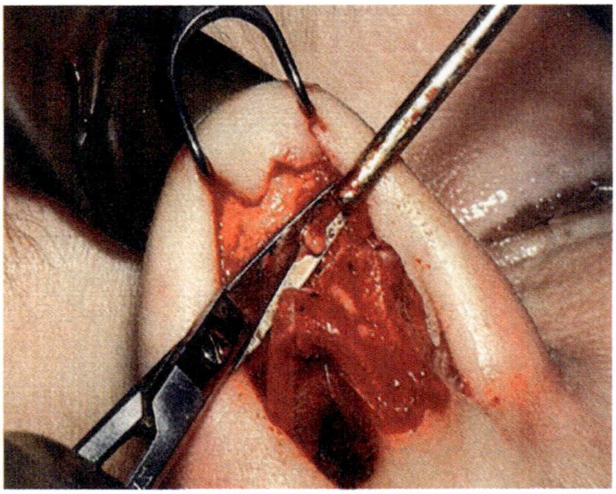

Fig. 10.2 Corresponding picture of plane of dissection and debulking of fatty tissue from deep fatty layer

10.2.1.1 Layers of SSTE

These include the skin, superficial fatty layer and deep fibromuscular layer. A rhinoplasty surgeon must be careful to not damage these layers. In an open rhinoplasty, the plane of dissection is in the subperichondrial/subperiosteal layer (Figs. 10.1 and 10.2) to prevent bleeding. And the deep fatty layer needs to be debulked for better draping of the soft tissues.

10.2.2 Button Holing of the Skin (Figs. 10.3 and 10.4)

This usually occurs during undermining of the skin during dissection and can lead to scarring. It is commonly seen:

(a) In individuals with pre-existing scars, which are bone deep
(b) In the ones undergoing revision rhinoplasty
(c) In thin-skinned individuals than thick-skinned ones

Prevention

- To give careful attention to the technique.
- Accurate non-tension suturing is done to avoid it.

10.2.3 Cautery Burns

This is usually a result of excess charring, which can lead to scarring.

Prevention

- To exercise appropriate caution when using cautery
- Bipolar cautery to be used and not monopolar
- Minimal amount of bleeding not to be cauterised

10.2.4 Tears of Mucoperichondrial Flaps

This can happen during septoplasty or during spurectomy. It can be either on one side or both sides.

- Unilateral tears
  - We should not forget to align the edges together after the entire procedure and then insert a medicated Merocel pack.

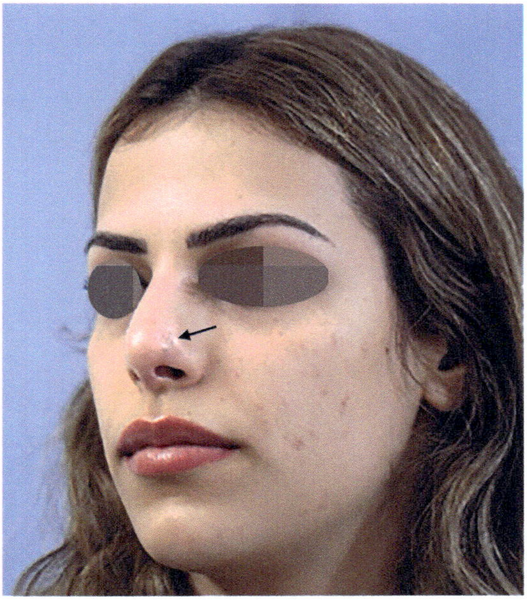

Fig. 10.3 Frontal view (*with an arrow showing a button holing of the skin*)

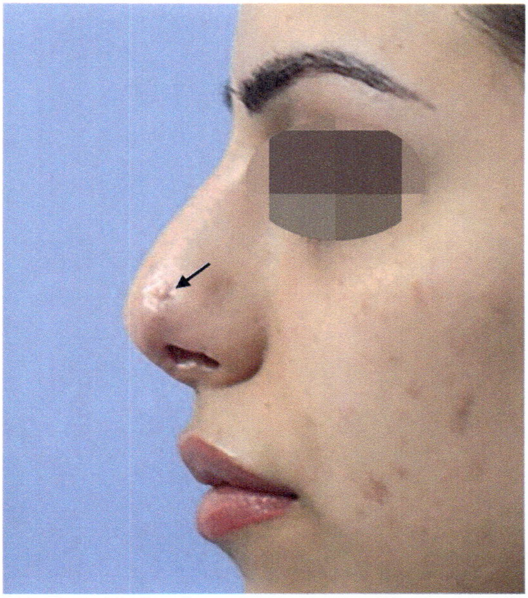

Fig. 10.4 Profile view (*with an arrow showing a button holing of the skin*)

  - Tears in the anterior aspect can be sutured using 3-0 Vicryl.
- Bilateral tears
  - If the tears are present on both sides and on the same position, then septal perforation is an anticipated complication, and this can be avoided by suturing bilateral tears by placing an intervening cartilage.

10.2.5 Disarticulation of the Upper Lateral Cartilages

Most of the time, in open rhinoplasty, both the upper lateral cartilages are cut using 11 No. blade and are approximated in the end of the procedure either by placing spreader grafts or by creating spreader flaps depending upon the deformity. But in situations where only a bony hump is present, where there is no need to cut the ULC, one has to very carefully and meticulously rasp the nasal bones and avoid incising the ULC during nasal bone periosteal elevation. If there is injury to both sides of ULC, it causes loss of length, tension and projection and leads to midvault weakness, which will lead to an inverted 'V' deformity in the frontal view. This results from medial and posterior relocation of the upper lateral cartilages and loss of a smooth continuous contour with the bony pyriform aperture. This can be prevented by avoiding excess hump removal.

Steps to ensure the prevention of excess hump removal (Figs. 10.5 and 10.6):

- *Marking to be done from the tip to NFA*: Defines the extent of removal
- *Preserve*: The underlining mucosa and the rhinion projection by not excising in a straight line.
- *Nasal bones*: As the caudal part of nasal bones is thin and overresection is avoided. On the contrary, cephalic part is generally thicker, and there is a possibility of underresection and this should not be overlooked.

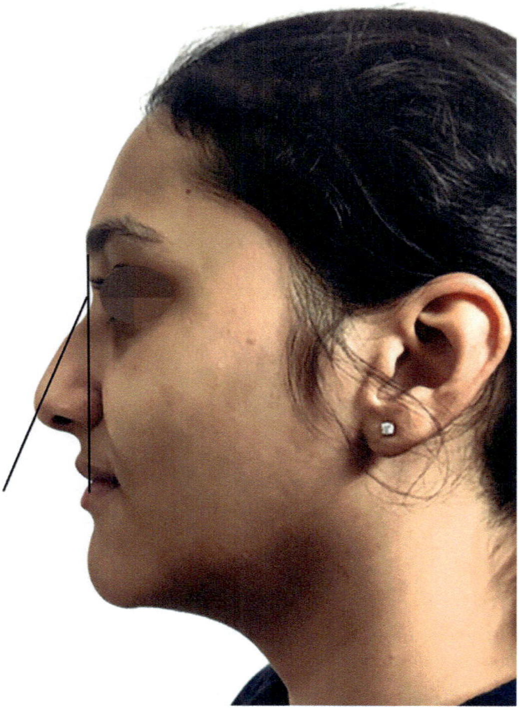

Fig. 10.5 Lateral view of bony and cartilaginous hump nose and resection is planned above the line drawn on the nose

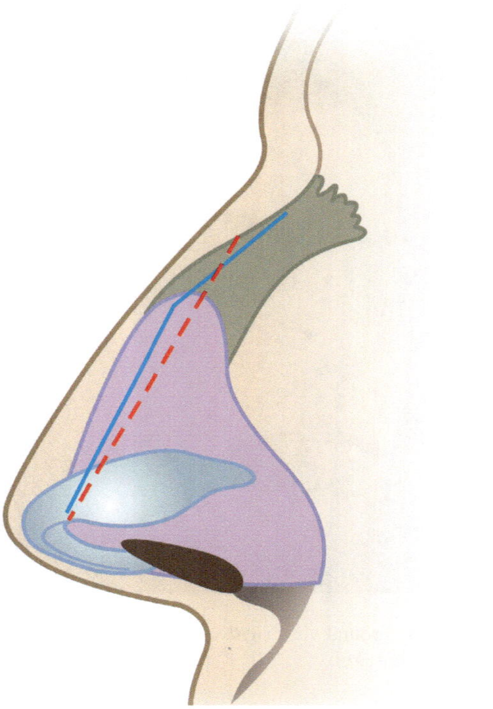

Fig. 10.6 Hump reduction. Blue line—ideal line for hump reduction. Red dotted line—to be avoided

10.2.6 Disarticulation of Septum from Keystone Area

It is one of the most dreadful intraoperative complications and happens to every rhinoplasty surgeon some or the other time in his career. Generally, it happens due to injury to this region during medial osteotomy. It can be prevented by doing paramedian osteotomy gently, preferably with a Lindemann's burr or piezoelectric device. Care should be taken that the osteotomy is complete. In case of disarticulation, the septum has to be fixed to nasal bones and upper lateral cartilages the way it is fixed in extracorporeal septoplasty.

DIFFERENT METHODS BY WHICH HUMP REDUCTION IS DONE (Figs. 10.7, 10.8, 10.9 and 10.10) (Explained in Detail in Chap. 7)

Small humps

10.2.7 Complications Due to Osteotomy

1. Injury to surrounding structures

During lateral osteotomy there is a likely possibility of injury to nasolacrimal system and angular vein which causes epiphora and bleeding,

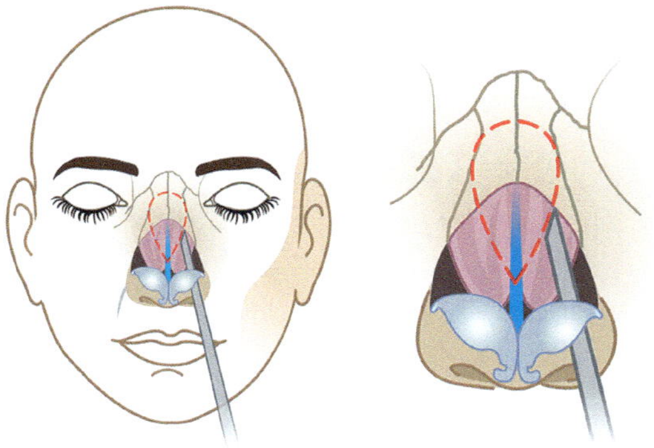

Fig. 10.7 Big cartilaginous humps are resected with 11 No. blade or scissors

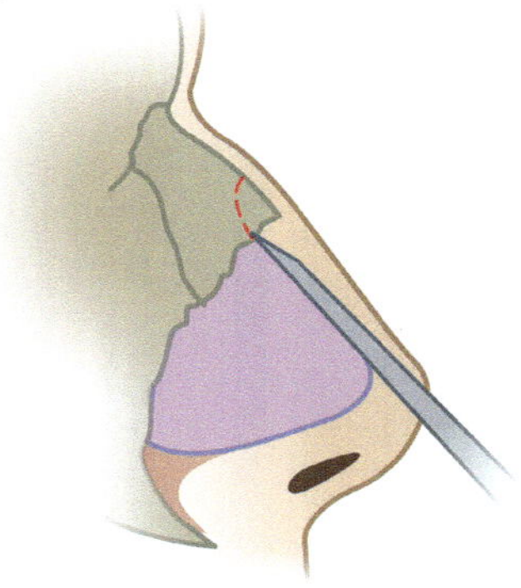

Fig. 10.8 Big bony humps are excised using chisel and hammer; however, even this can be dealt by drilling with a diamond burr or piezoelectric device

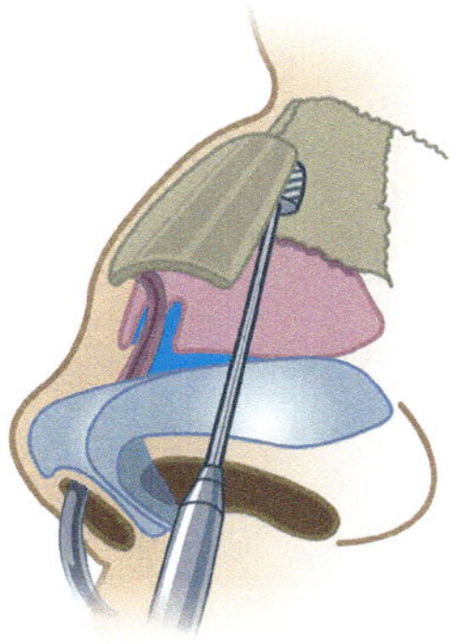

Fig. 10.9 These are reduced by drilling with coarse diamond burr

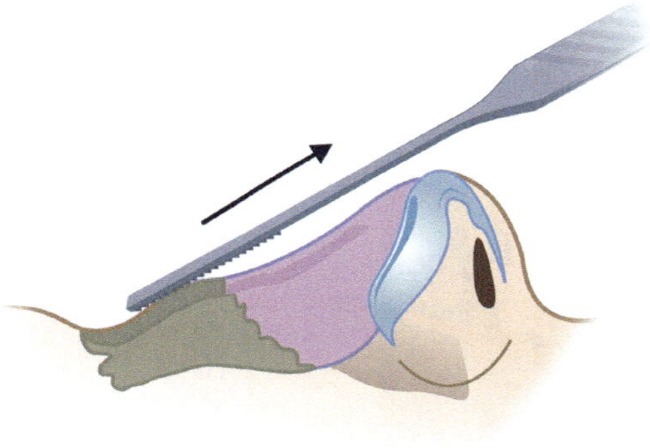

Fig. 10.10 By rasping the nasal bones

respectively, if the medial canthus is not respected. This injury can be prevented by dissecting the subperiosteal tissue with the sharp end of osteotome which will keep the angular vein and nasolacrimal system away from the osteotomy site. However, if there is bleeding, it can be prevented by applying ice packs.

2. Aesthetic deformities due to osteotomies
   (a) STEP DEFORMITY (Figs. 10.11 and 10.12)

If lateral osteotomy is performed too far medial to nasofacial groove, then a visible ridge is seen on the side of the nose on medialisation which can be prevented by performing osteotomy in the nasofacial groove.

(b) ROCKER DEFORMITY (Figs. 10.13 and 10.14)

If a straight lateral osteotomy is performed too far cephalically in the frontal process of nasal

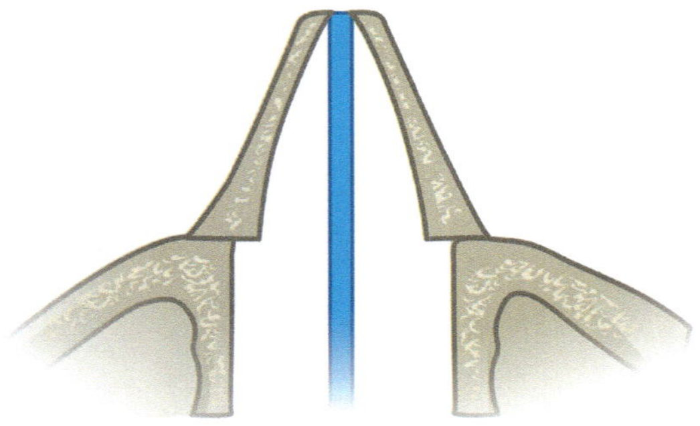

Fig. 10.11 Sketch diagram showing correct dissection in the nasofacial groove

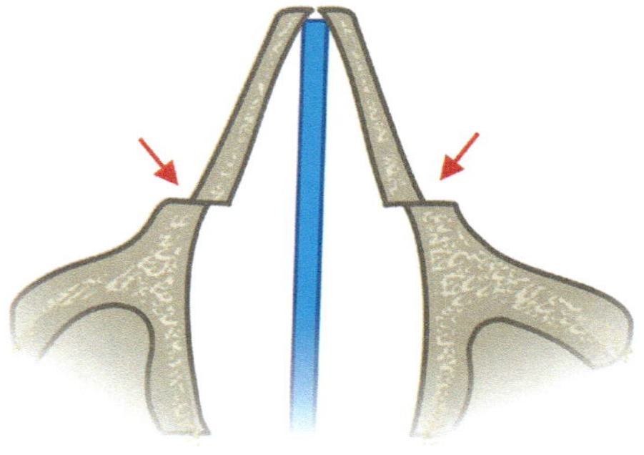

Fig. 10.12 When it is done too far medial to nasofacial groove

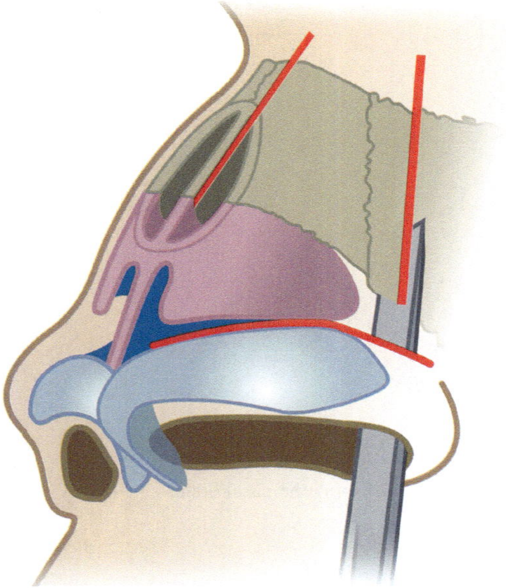

Fig. 10.13 Rocker deformity

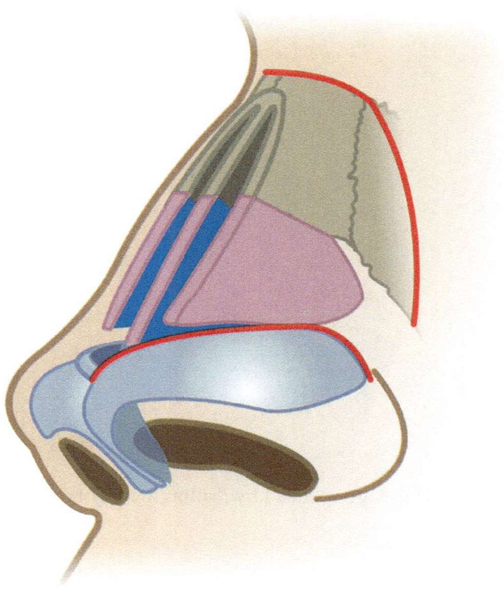

Fig. 10.14 Prevention of rocker deformity

bones, during medialisation the superior segment narrows in, while the caudal segment moves out laterally causing visible and persistent widening.

This can be prevented by not exceeding the osteotomy above the intercanthal line and curving the lateral osteotomy line at the medial canthal level to join the transverse osteotomy site.

(c) OPEN ROOF DEFORMITY (Figs. 10.15, 10.16, 10.17 and 10.18)

This is caused when the lateral segments fail to align with dorsal septum after osteotomies, with a resultant gap. Intranasal mucous membrane can adhere to the overlying soft tissue and create a depression.

Causes

1. Excessive tight nasal packing post procedure
2. High DNS
3. Incomplete osteotomy

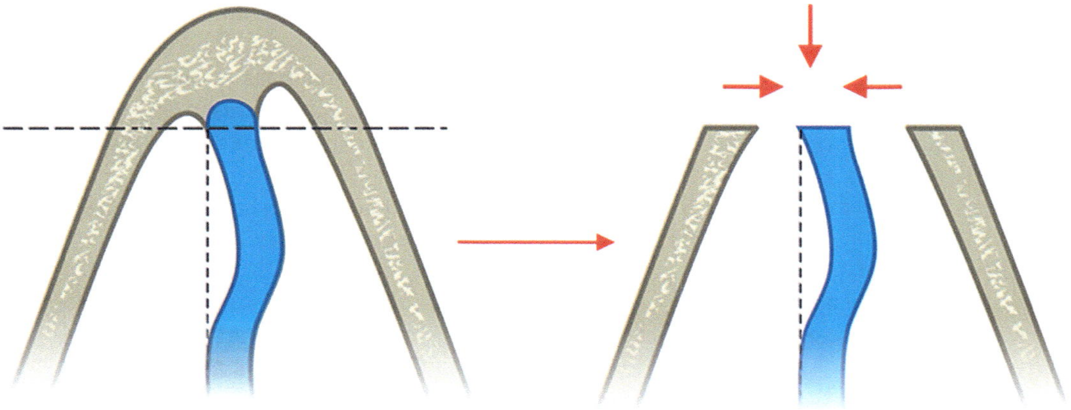

Fig. 10.15 High DNS following osteotomy leading to open-roof defomity

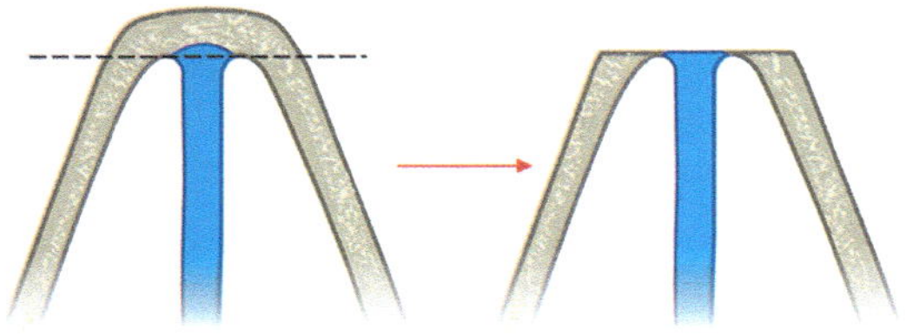

Fig. 10.16 Incomplete osteotomy causes open roof deformity

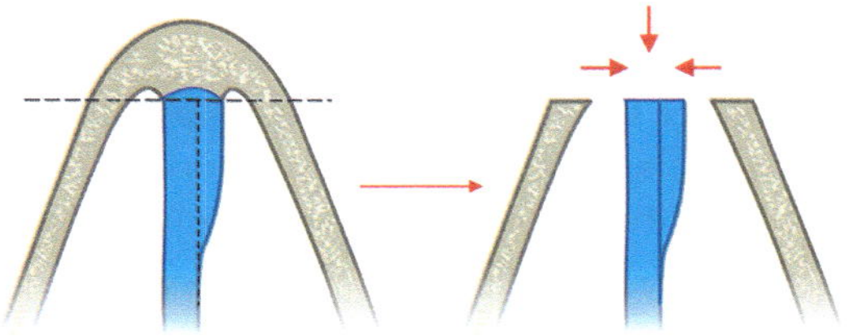

Fig. 10.17 Dorsally thick septum and osteotomy causing open roof deformity

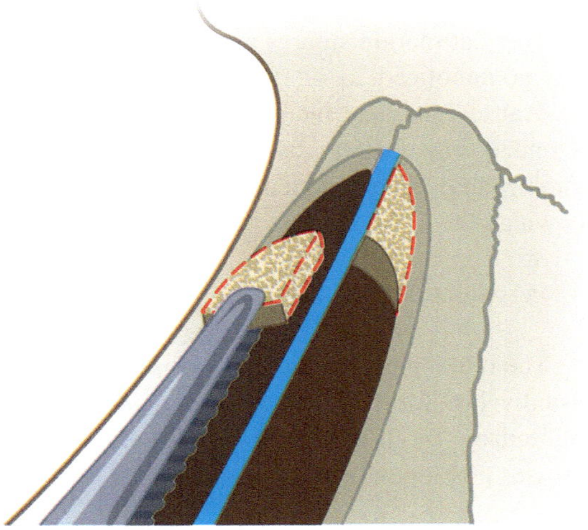

Fig. 10.18 Bone rongeurs used to remove the bony wedges formed due to incomplete medial osteotomy

4. Dorsally thick septum
5. Formation of bony wedges formed by incomplete medial or lateral osteotomy which are removed by bony rongeur before narrowing of the dorsum

Prevention of osteotomy complications by using:

1. Sharp instruments
2. Wooden or silicon hammer
3. Piezoelectric device or Lindemann's burr

FEW SALIENT FEATURES OF OSTEOTOMY TO PREVENT UNDUE COMPLICATIONS (Fig. 10.19)

- **Osteotomy is performed under supervision until mastered.**
- **Surface markings of the osteotomy site**
- **To ensure that the lateral osteotomy is done in the nasofacial groove and avoid osteotomy above intercanthal level.**

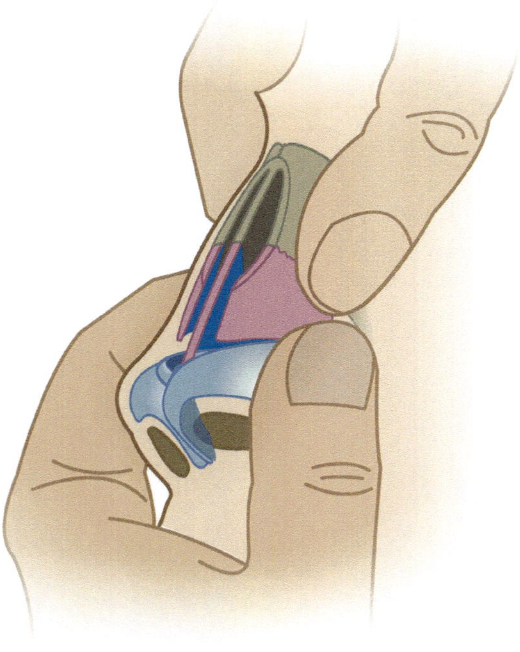

Fig. 10.19 Ideal narrowing of the nose pattern is demonstrated in this picture

- **Sequences of osteotomies** are paramedian, lateral and transverse.
- **Lateral and transverse osteotome** is performed using a 2 mm chisel
- **Paramedian osteotome** is done using a 5 mm chisel.
- **Sharp osteotomes to be used and preferably a silicon or a wooden hammer.**

10.3 Immediate Post-Operative Complications and Early Post-Operative Complications

1. Haemorrhage

This happens mostly due to improper packing ad dressing which can be managed by nasal repacking and pressure over the osteotomy site.

2. Septal haematoma

Collection of blood on either side of the septum and is managed by immediate I&D, along with antibiotics to prevent abscess formation.

3. Dehiscence of incisions

The alar margin sutures are gaped which usually go unnoticed.

Transcolumellar incision gaping must be attended immediately by resuturing. To avoid gaping, advise the patient not to pull the upper lip down and to avoid shaving of moustache.

4. Persistent oedema

The initial periorbital ecchymosis and oedema usually last for 10 days. However, this can be minimised by head elevation and cold compresses post-operatively.

5. Persistent numbness

Appreciated over the tip of the nose and the upper lip—*external nasal nerve* injury during osteotomy, which usually recovers over a period of 6 months.

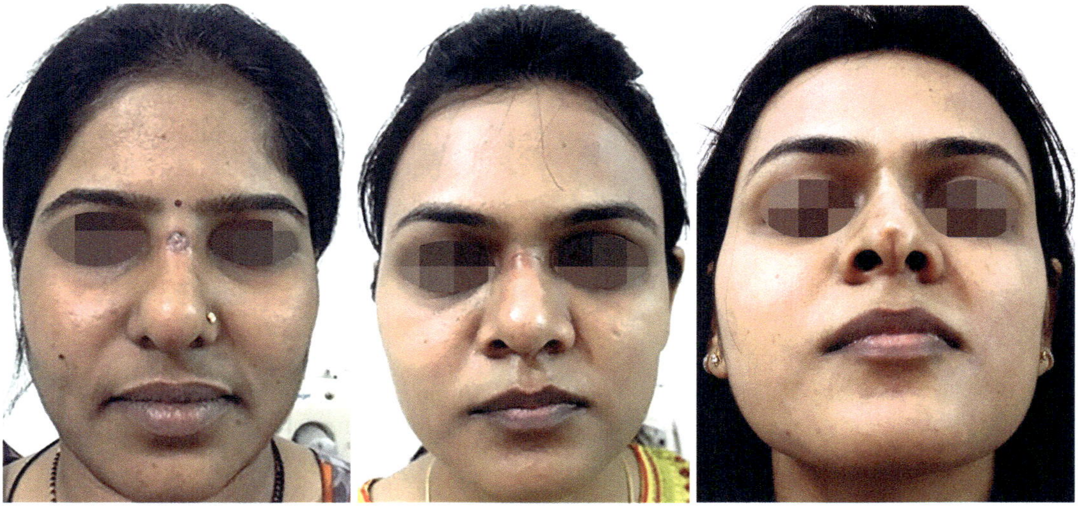

Figs. 10.20–10.21 (left and middle: Fig. 10.20): (**a**, **b**) Infection at the bridge; (right: Fig. 10.21): Infection at the tip and columella

6. Transient epiphora

Usually lasts 1–2 weeks, being secondary to soft tissue oedema blocking nasolacrimal pathway. But if a lacrimal pathway, injury due to lateral osteotomy with subperiosteal dissection takes a longer time to recover.

7. Infection (Figs. 10.20 and 10.21)

The post-operative wound infection is reported to be 2%. Localised cellulitis and small abscesses respond usually to post-operative antibiotics.

8. Acute or chronic sinusitis
   This occurs due to osteomeatal dysfunction which may require FESS if it fails to medical treatment.
9. Scarring (Fig. 10.22)

The skin of a few individuals may heal with depressed scars. We should always assess the quality of the skin and their tendency for scarring prior to surgery.

Common causes are:

(a) Occurs when there is no underlying cartilage support.

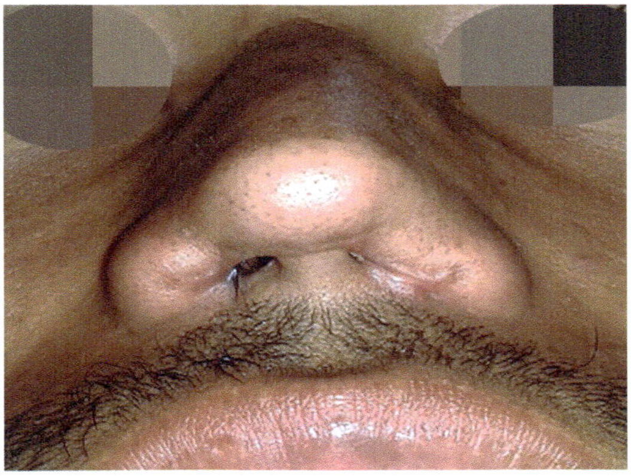

Fig. 10.22 Picture showing vestibular after scarring with total obstruction left and severe stenosis right side

Avoided by columellar strut, suturing medial crura and shield graft.

(b) Due to straight transcolumellar incision.

Avoided by inverted V transcolumellar incision.

(c) Marginal incision in the soft triangle region.

Avoided by meticulous incision and suturing.

10. Skin atrophy and discolouration
    (a) Vascular supply and lymphatics to the skin and soft tissue envelope are located in the subcutaneous layer of tissue superficial to nasal musculature.
    (b) Dissection should be in supraperichondrial plane in lower 2/3rd with transition to subperiosteal plane at nasal bone.
    (c) Dissection superficially in subcutaneous layer disrupts vascular supply causing atrophic skin and increases the visibility of cutaneous vessels.

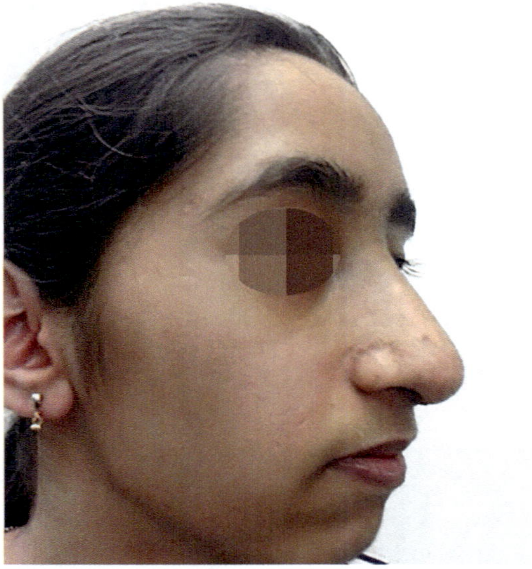

Fig. 10.23 Hard pollybeak deformity

10.4 Late Post-Operative Complications

A. Hump nose
   Due to insufficient dorsal hump reduction.
B. Pollybeak nasal deformity
   This is characterised by absence of a supratip dip created.

- *Hard pollybeak* (Fig. 10.23)
  This is due to undercorrection of cartilaginous dorsum and superior septal angle region.
- *Soft pollybeak* (Fig. 10.24)
  This is due to loss of tip support and excessive accumulation of soft tissue scarring.

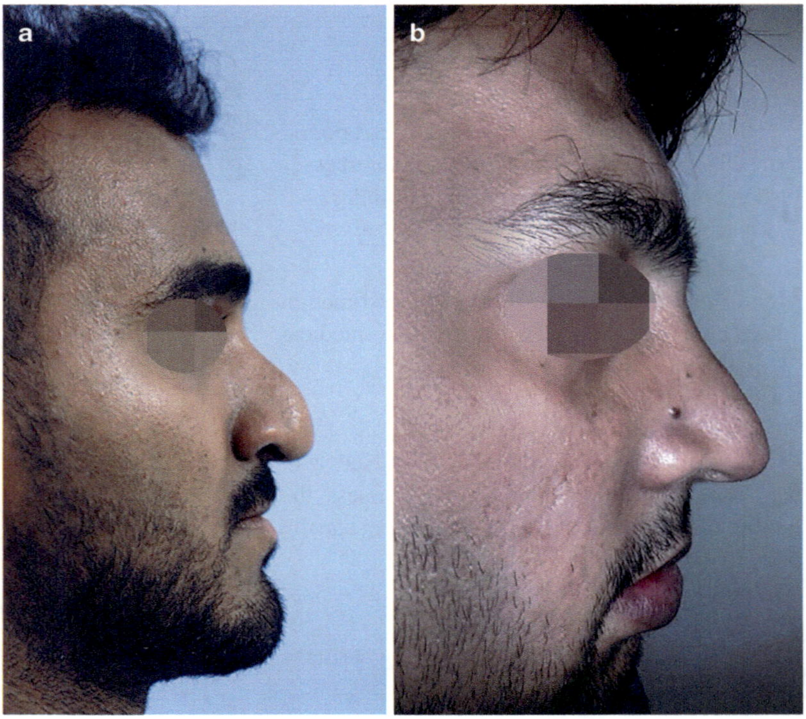

Fig. 10.24 (**a**, **b**) Soft pollybeak deformity

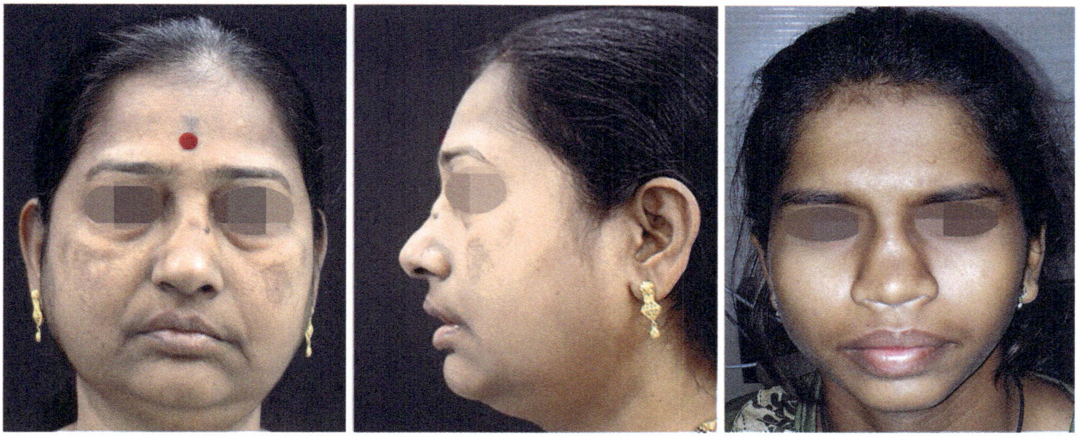

Figs. 10.25–10.26 (left and middle: Fig. 10.25): (**a**) Frontal view of inverted V deformity. (**b**) Lateral view of inverted V deformity; (right: Fig. 10.26): Frontal view of inverted V deformity

In South Indian noses, if a soft tissue polly-beak is formed, it is usually due to excess accumulation of soft tissue in the supratip area in the subdermis (thick skin). In such cases inj triamcinolone after 3 weeks after surgery with insulin syringe has to be given.

C. Pinocchio nose

It is seen in a big nose with no lateral and medial sliding technique executed to reduce the lower alar cartilages.

D. Inverted V deformity (explained earlier) (Figs. 10.25 and 10.26)

INVERTED V DEFORMITY

Inverted V deformity can be prevented by placing spreader grafts to prevent the loss of stability at the 'K' area and to retain the smooth contour of the pyriform aperture.

E. Saddle nose

Saddle noses are all mainly due to graft deformities.

There are two types of graft complications:

(a) *Autogenous graft complications*
(b) *Allograft graft complications*

AUTOGRAFT

These are the most acceptable and reliable type of grafts. These can be placed directly under the skin with no fear of infection. However, they are known to have a few complications like resorption, displacement and extrusion which are quite rare.

Donor site complications are also seen like:

1. Post septal cartilage harvest, there is a fear of saddling of the nose (Fig. 10.27).

POST-SEPTOPLASTY DEFORMITY

Picture showing a post-septoplasty deformity where the dorsal support is lost with underprojected tip and colummelar retraction.

2. Conchal site causes a crumpled look of the pinna.
3. Costal cartilage site causes relatively more pain and sometimes pneumothorax.

This is explained in detail in Chap. 6.

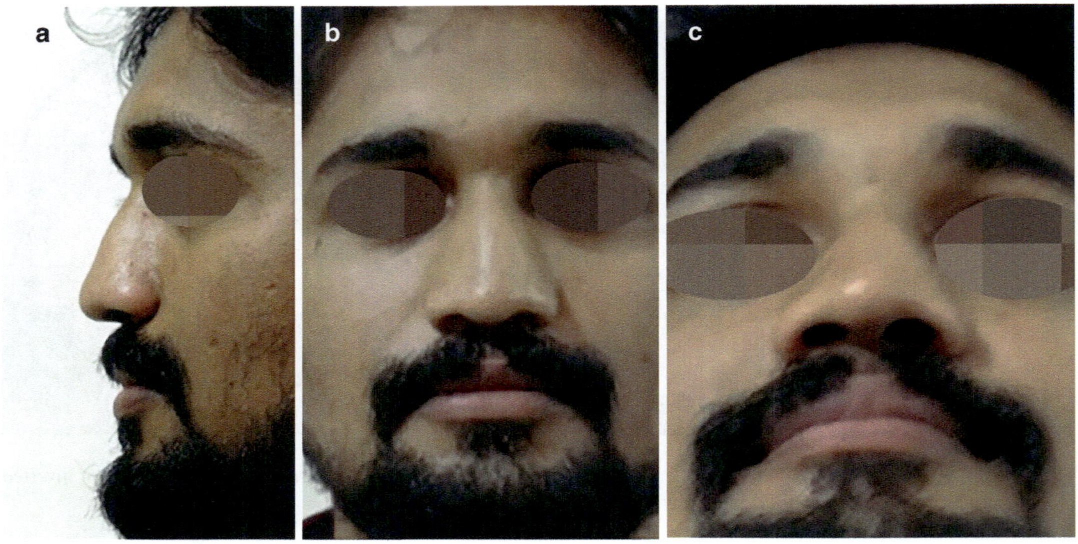

Fig. 10.27 (**a**) Lateral view; (**b**) frontal view; (**c**) basal view

ALLOGRAFT

I do not generally use allograft cartilage/bone materials. However, few surgeons prefer to use irradiated allograft cartilages.

These are known to cause more complications which are explained under:

1. *Immediate*
   (a) Infection
   (b) Extrusion
   (c) Dislocation
   (d) Resorption
   (e) Calcification of the graft
2. *Long term*
   (a) Extrusion
   (b) Dislocation
   (c) Bending

Some common complications are considered in brief here:

1. *Infection*

Common causes are:

(a) Narrow transplant bed
(b) Accumulation of blood in the pocket created
(c) Ischaemia of overlying mucosa/skin

They usually present with:

(a) Fever
(b) Pain on site of the graft/over the dressing

Treatments

(a) Partially open incision to drain the pus
(b) Pus to be sent for culture and sensitivity
(c) Start IV antibiotics
(d) Daily inspection and cleaning of the incision site
(e) Antibiotics considered to be changed if necessary, according to culture and sensitivity report
(f) Not to be neglected as can lead to graft extrusion, if untreated

2. *Extrusion of graft* (Fig. 10.28)

Causes are:

(a) Uncontrolled infection
(b) Trauma
(c) Extruded through necrosis of the skin or mucosa especially on the dorsum and lobule

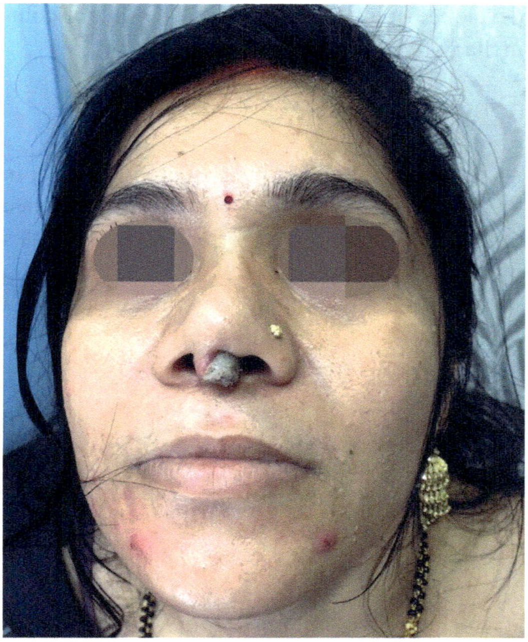

Fig. 10.28 Extrusion of the graft

3. *Dislocation*

Causes are due to graft malposition or improper fixation.

4. *Bending/warping of cartilage* (Fig. 10.29)

Warping of cartilage is harvested cartilage which is twisted out of shape by being bent.

It is usually seen in freeze-dried costal cartilage, which has a high tendency of warping.

5. *Resorption*

This is seen in cartilage used for augmentation for either support or reconstruction.

Septal Complications

1. *Septal haematoma*
   (a) Post-operatively seen commonly located posteriorly

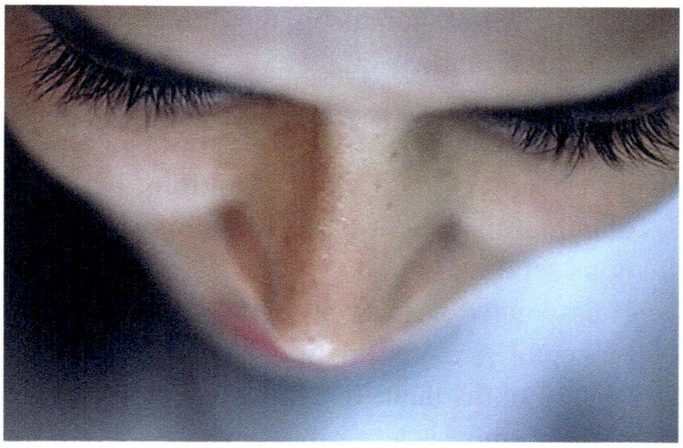

Fig. 10.29 Warping of the cartilage on the nasal dorsum

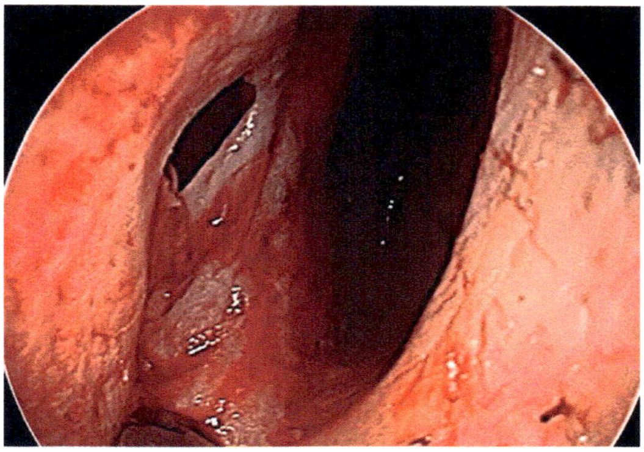

Fig. 10.30 Septal perforation

   (b) Diagnosed on examination of the nose after nasal decongestion and spraying local anaesthesia by palpation with a blunt instrument
   (c) Treatment: Incision and drain
   (d) Awareness important as untreated can lead to abscess and septal perforation

2. *Septal abscess*

   (a) Untreated haematoma can lead to septal abscess.
   (b) It usually presents with fever and pain.

Treatment: I&D with IV antibiotics

3. *Septal perforation* (Fig. 10.30)

This is seen if there is bilateral mucoperichondrial flap tear at the same area:

- Location and size are important to be noted.
- The height of the defect should not be larger than half the height of the remaining cartilaginous septum.
- If associated with external deformities, repair of septal perforation first is performed, and 9–12 months later, revision surgery for external deformity is advisable.

GENERAL DEFORMITY is due to other complications (Figs. 10.31, 10.32, 10.33, 10.34, 10.35, 10.36 and 10.37):

1. External nasal valve collapse where pinching of the nose is seen.

   It is caused commonly by:

   (a) Aggressive cephalic trimming; hence, a minimum of 8 mm shouldbe preserved. And it can be managed by alar batten graft.

2. Pug nose deformity

Surgery went on for 7 hours in the learning phase and the DCF got infected. Patient also developed columellar necrosis. The skin of columella got necrosed and was sutured.

3. Bossa formation

These are protuberances that may arise in the region of nasal tip which has an incidence of 2% and caused by uncorrected irregularities of LLC.

It is usually seen in a nose with a triad of thin skin, strong cartilage and bifidity which indicate patient is prone for bossae.

Specific surgical causes are:

(a) Domal separation
(b) Improper tip grafts
(c) Asymmetric domal sutures
(d) Improper vertical dome division

Therefore, by minimising the cartilage excision, reinforcing areas of weakness, avoiding asymmetry and irregularity and maintaining alar integrity, bossa formation can be reduced.

4. Synechia formation
   (a) May or may not be symptomatic
   (b) Endoscopic excision and subsequent stenting

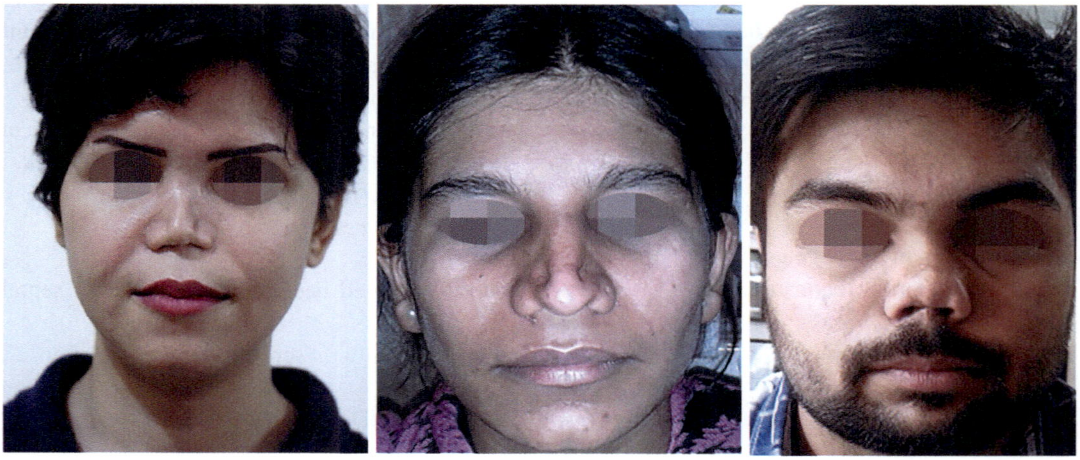

Figs. 10.31–10.33 (left: Fig. 10.31): Nasal valve pinching due to aggressive cephalic trimming and weakening or overresection of the lateral crura; (middle: Fig. 10.32): Excessive trimming results in retraction of the alae, pinching results from insufficient support by the lateral cruara; (right: Fig. 10.33): Pug nose deformity—upturned nose secondary to infection

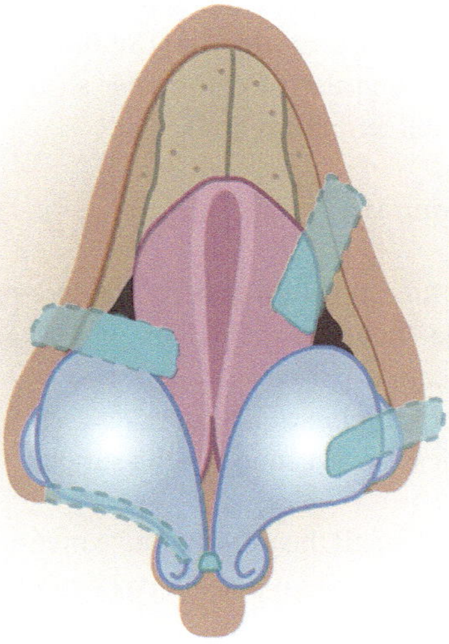

Fig. 10.34 Diagram showing areas of weakness being reinforced to avoid bossa formation

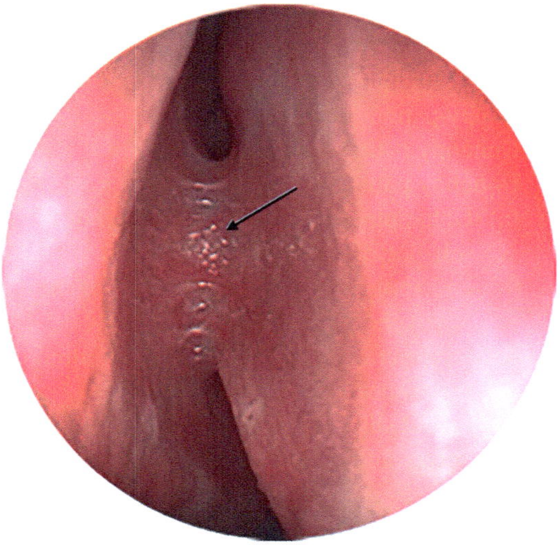

Fig. 10.35 Synechiae between inferior turbinate and septum

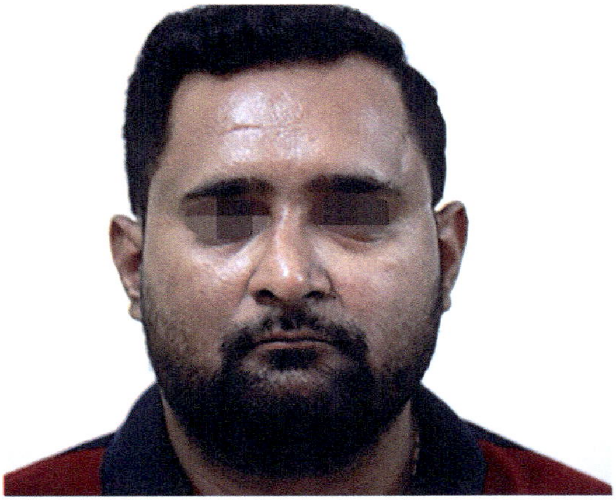

Fig. 10.36 A crooked nose with a dorsal deviation

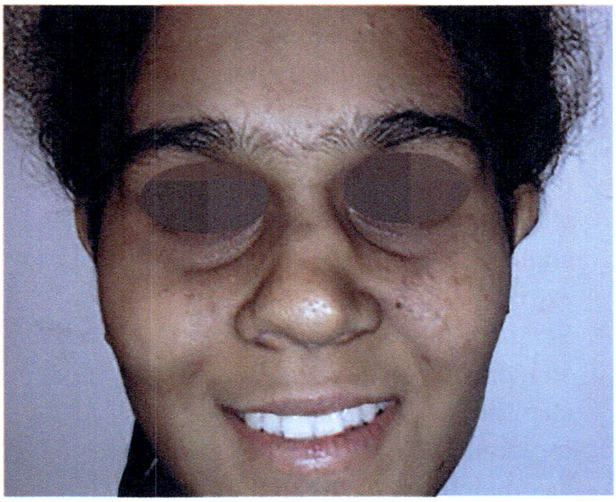

Fig. 10.37 Saddling and deviation in the middle 1/3rd of the nose

5. Mucosal cyst

Although rare, this is seen if the nasal mucosa is displaced into the subcutaneous tissue. It usually presents with gustatory rhinorrhoea:

(a) Parasympathetic and sympathetic cross-excitation as a result of misdirected regeneration of nerve fibres subsequent to the trauma of surgery may cause rhinorrhoea during eating.
(b) Antihistaminics may help, but definitive treatment is excision of the cyst.

6. Persistent deformity (Figs. 10.36 and 10.37)

Despite good surgical procedure, few end up with persistent deformity.

THERE ARE USUALLY FOUR OUTCOMES IN A SURGEON-PATIENT RELATIONSHIP.

Four outcomes:

1. Happy patient, happy surgeon
2. Happy patient, unhappy surgeon
3. Unhappy patient, happy surgeon
4. Unhappy patient, unhappy surgeon
    (a) Unhappiness of surgeon—relates to self-perfection.
    (b) Unhappiness of patient—can be genuine or psychological.
    (c) Pre-operative psychological evaluation recommended.
    (d) Establishing a good rapport between the doctor and patient can help.

In our country, I have always explained about the diversity of the noses seen. Revision also has the same outlook:

1. We usually find hump noses in the northern part of our country, where hump reduction with spreader grafts or spreader flaps is used and there is a possible complication of inverted V deformity which needs to be corrected.
2. North eastern and the southern part of country the most likely complication we would face would be graft-related issues, which either could be graft absorbed, dislocated or extruded.
3. Southern part of noses usually have wide ala and mostly incomplete alaplasty or undone alaplasty is seen in such cases.
4. In addition to the above regional variations, incomplete septoplasty and incomplete osteotomy should be always looked for no matter what the pre-existing deformity is.

10.5 Revision Rhinoplasty

Complication of a previous case can or will become a revision case in a year's time.

Why is a revision required for patients in the first place has to be looked into:

1. If it was due to incomplete pre-op evaluation of the patient in the first surgery
2. Due to improper techniques used
3. Due to loss of tip support due to incorrect graft—e.g. use of columellar strut in place of a septal extension graft

It requires:

- Careful estimation of deformity pre-operatively
- Understanding the techniques available for correction
- Proposed plan of action
- Meticulous execution of the surgical technique

Inspite of all the pre-operative measures taken, the following two types of errors can occur:

- *Errors of omission:*

Certain surgical manoeuvres were not performed in the primary procedure that would have enabled achievement of the desired refinement.

- *Errors of commission:*

When too much surgery was done—for instance, if a patient has a dorsal hump and excessive removal of the hump results in a saddle nose deformity.

Also, whether the complication from the previous surgery is because of surgeon's misjudgement or there is an undue unfortunate real complication despite all the good work has to be assessed.

In cases of body dysmorphic syndrome—surgeons would have done a good job, but the patient and his perception about his body will be a problem no matter how well the surgery has been done.

ALWAYS AND ALWAYS TO evaluate and go back to AND ASSESS the pre-existing deformity is important:

- To know if the case previously treated was a hump, a saddle or a deviated nose.
- To know the type of graft used also becomes very important:

For example, if warping seen—to know if rib cartilage was used or not

- And if there has been use of diced cartilage with or without fascia and if or not stacked cartilage is used.

ONCE DECIDED TO BE REOPENED, A REVISION CASE SHOULD BE DONE ONLY AFTER 1 YEAR.

In revision cases:

- Tissue fibrosis is usually seen, so careful dissection is necessary to avoid tears.

If an ENT surgeon has operated the the septum availalbility becomes doubtful whilst a plastic surgeon will retain the septum in most cases.

In North Indian noses—Ample amount of septum would be found, so rib harvest may not be required.

Southern and North-eastern—If the grafts used are not infected, the same can be reused or rib grafting becomes essential:

- If incomplete septoplasty—septum to be harvested or extracorporeal septoplasty to be done.
- In deviated noses, nasal bones are asymmetrical—assessing if they are concave or convex would be ideal. If incomplete osteotomy, complete it. To complete an incomplete osteotomy, piezoelectric device is very helpful here.
- Anterior nasal spine, which in most cases will be neglected, to be addressed in deviated nose.
- Have to focus on tip for aesthetic nose—Improper evaluation would have caused loss of tip support/supratip depression.
- An incomplete alaplasty to be completed.
- Scar of alaplasty itself can cause a problem.

If severe vestibular stenosis is seen, it is usually due to an overdone alaplasty.

The aim is to give a final wrap-up on these patients with a neat aesthetic outcome. A good septal support with a septal extension graft, completing the osteotomy and drilling the nasal bones if uneven has to be done.

And of course our free diced cartilage, to camouflage and cover up minor deformities,should be used.

An awareness of the complications, their prevention and treatment is a part of the learning process and should not intimidate the rhinoplasty surgeon. Accepting, treating and discussing with mentors and senior colleagues are important steps of the process of learning rhinoplasty surgery.

11 Special Cases: Advanced Reconstructive Rhinoplasty—Cleft Nose Deformity and Binder's Syndrome

Main
Unilateral cleft lip and Binder's syndrome are common indications requiring reconstructive aesthetic rhinoplasty. The well-defined and relatively consistent pattern of deformities in these cases is mainly a result of midface asymmetry, the lack of continuity of perilabial musculature, anomalous position and underdeveloped underlying osseous structures (i.e. premaxilla and pyriform aperture).

11.1 Cleft Lip Nose Deformity

Our country has an incidence rate of 1.10 per 1000 live births for craniofacial anomalies (cleft lip+ cleft palate and cleft palate alone). The aetiology for clefts can be genetic as well as environmental (maternal exposure to radiation/illness in first trimester/intoxication/teratogenic medication).

The ideal approach for the management of children born with clefts requires a combined multidisciplinary approach by various specialities including orthodontist, maxillofacial surgeon, plastic surgeon, ENT surgeon and speech therapist. These children require intervention from day 1 of their lives. Early rehabilitation in the form of palatal obturator/feeding appliance/lip taping is introduced for initial 0–12 weeks. This overcomes the difficulty faced during nursing. Primary repair of the lip is usually planned at around 2–3 months of age. Subsequently the palate repair should be performed at around 6–12 months of age. The role of speech therapy remains crucial in the management of clefts, which can ideally be started as early as 3–4 years. On an average, around 6 years of age, the premolars are near eruption, and orthodontic procedures for nasoalveolar moulding in the form of fixed/removable appliances can be employed around this age. A cancellous bone graft in the cleft area provides a good scaffold and helps in prevention of alveolar and hard palate collapse. In case of bilateral clefts, the bone graft helps in closing oronasal fistulas and stabilises the premaxilla. Once the lip and palate procedures are done, the focus now shifts to dentition. By the age of 14–15 years, most of the facial and maxillary development is achieved. It is advisable to perform orthognathic surgery and rhinoplasty around the teenage. The most common orthognathic surgery performed is the Le Fort 1 osteotomy to manage class 1 and 2 malocclusions. In severe cases the Le Fort 1 has to be combined with a bilateral sagittal split for the mandible along with bone grafting to fill the gaps in the maxilla following the advancement. Though children with cleft have a gross unilateral deviation of the septum, paediatric septoplasty should be deferred owing to the crucial role of the nasal septum in growth of the midface skeleton. Rhinoplasty is the last definitive surgery to be performed in cleft patients.

V. Ghaisas, *Indian Ethnic Rhinoplasty*, https://doi.org/10.1007/978-981-16-2478-0_11

11.2 Unilateral Cleft Lip Nose

Unilateral cleft lip/palate is one of the commonest craniofacial anomalies encountered.

11.2.1 Relevant Anatomy

The complexity of deformities involves all layers including the skin, mucosa, cartilaginous and bony framework.

A cleft lip forms from improper fusion of the medial and lateral nasal prominences with the maxillary prominence during embryologic development. Studies have shown that the medial nasal process remains centralised and fails to fuse with the maxillary process in cleft patients.

In complete unilateral clefts of the lip, the transverse nasal muscle lacks to attach to the anterior nasal spine and hence remains lateral to the cleft. Medially, the muscles of the non-cleft side are inserted onto the cartilaginous nasal septum and the anterior nasal spine. The unopposed forces from these muscles lead the septum to deviate to the non-cleft side causing considerate obstruction (Figs. 11.1, 11.2, 11.3, 11.4 and 11.5).

Diagrammatic representation of underlying septal and lower lateral cartilage anatomy responsible for deformity in cleft lip nose

Maxillary hypoplasia leads to posterolateral displacement of the pyriform aperture. Because of the lack of skeletal support at the pyriform aperture, the alar base insertion on the cleft side is retropositioned. The ala on the cleft side is lengthened vertically and lies below the alae on the non-cleft side. The lower lateral cartilage is depressed and spread across the cleft. The nasal tip is deviated towards the cleft side. Due to unequal opposing forces of the orbicularis oris, the columella is obliquely oriented with shortening on the cleft side. Bilateral alar bases/sills are asymmetric, with the cleft side alar base inferiorly and posteriorly displaced.

11.2.2 Evaluation

A thorough pre-operative history and examination should be performed. The history of previous surgeries and procedures should be discussed in detail with the patient to rule out surprising findings intraoperatively.

Pre-op photography with standard views should be done. A detailed discussion with patient regarding their concerns and deliverable results is a must before deciding the operative goals.

A meticulous intraoral examination should be done and the following should be noted—high-

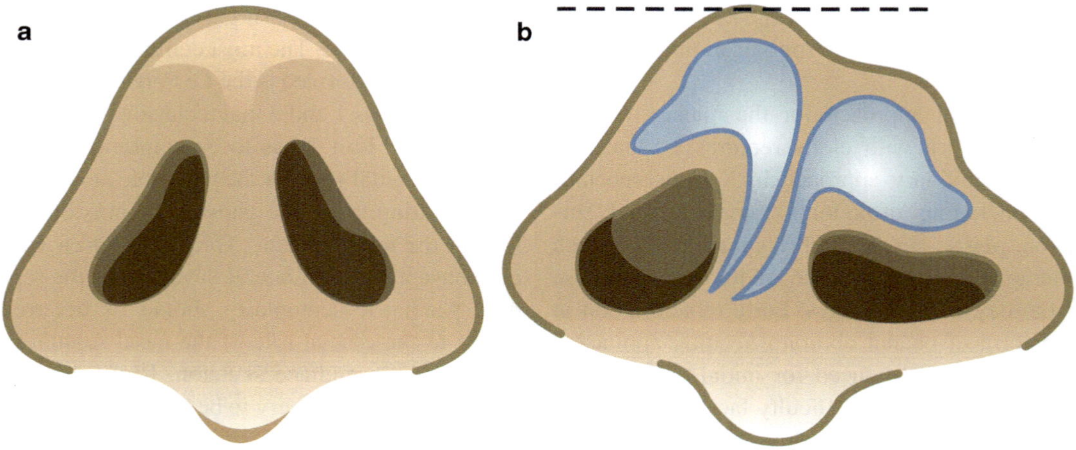

Fig. 11.1 (**a**, **b**) Tip asymmetry on basal view as compared to normal tip symmetry

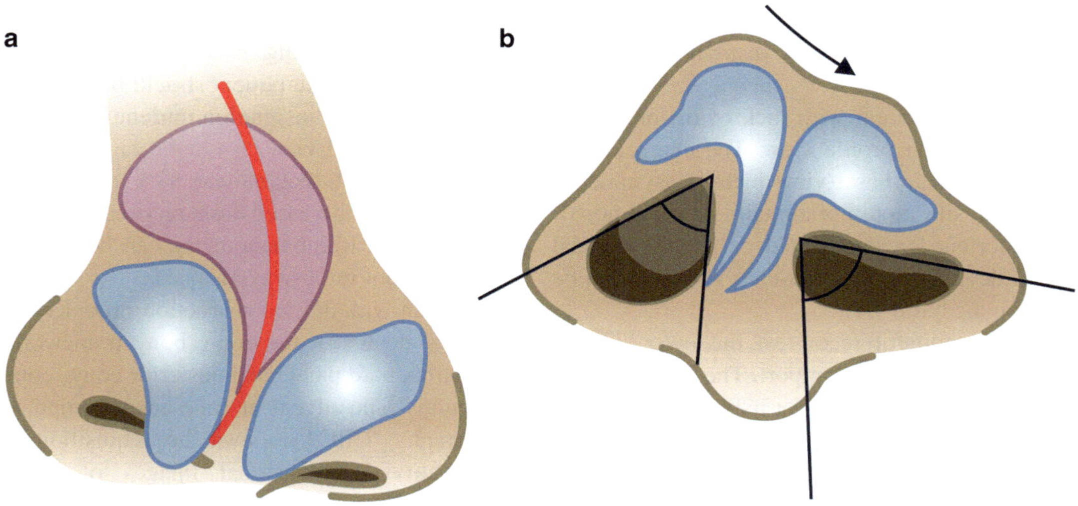

Fig. 11.2 (**a**, **b**) Deviation of septum to non-cleft side and asymmetric orientation of LLC and hence the nostril shape

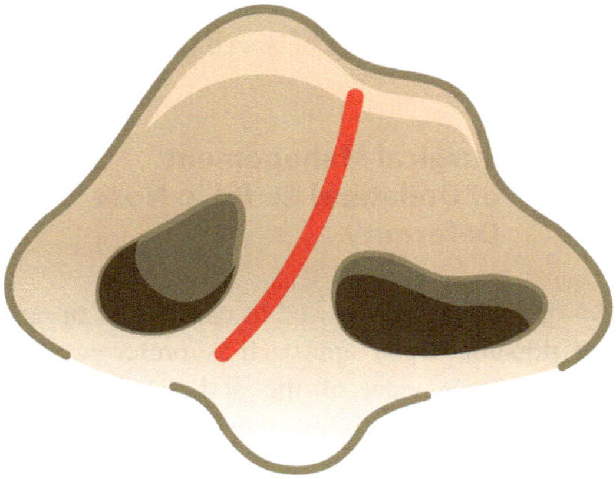

Fig. 11.3 Horizontal configuration of nostrils on cleft side

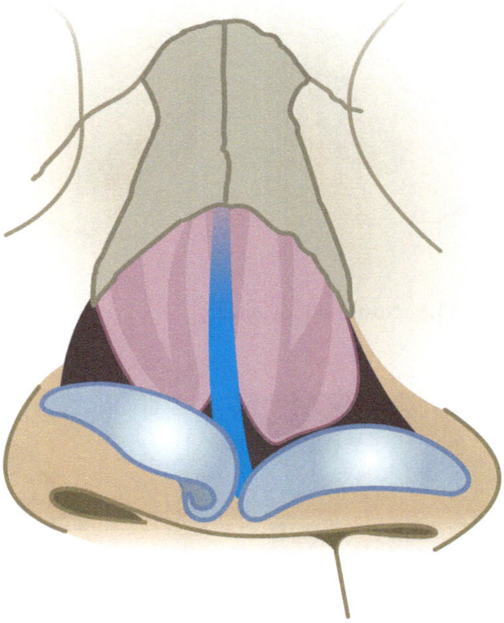

Fig. 11.4 Posterolateral displacement of pyriform aperture leading to displacement of alar base insertion laterally

arched palate, submucous cleft, soft palate function and examination of the sublabial area—to rule out oronasal fistulas.

Facial asymmetry is a consistent finding in cleft patients. The nasal root is usually deviated to the non-cleft side. The upper 1/3 is broader at the base bony width. Mid 1/3rd of the nose is relatively straighter and follows the root of the nose. The nasal tip is quite asymmetric secondary to weak and malpositioned LLC on the cleft side. The dome on the cleft side is depressed, and the ala is flattened horizontally as compared to the non-cleft side. The ala is thicker on the cleft side. Secondary to posterior and inferior rotation of the LLC, the nostrils appear hooded; also the LLC tends to protrude in the vestibule (Figs. 11.6, 11.7 and 11.8).

Mild bony hump with lack of tip projection can be seen on profile view. The characteristic features seen in basal view include asymmetric alar base, sill, more horizontally oriented nostril and shortened and deviated columella. Caudal septal deviation to the non-cleft side also can be seen on the basal view.

On palpation/tip recoil test, the lower 1/3rd of the nose lacks proper support. The anterior nasal spine should be palpated for its position.

The functional aspects can be studied via a nasal endoscopy and rhinomanometry. Deviated septum usually from the maxillary crest going towards the non-cleft side is a usual finding. Turbinate hypertrophy/sinusitis/polyposis should be ruled out and if present have to be addressed. Any mucosal webbing in the vestibular area should be noted. The patient should be asked to perform a forceful inspiration to demonstrate an external valve collapse.

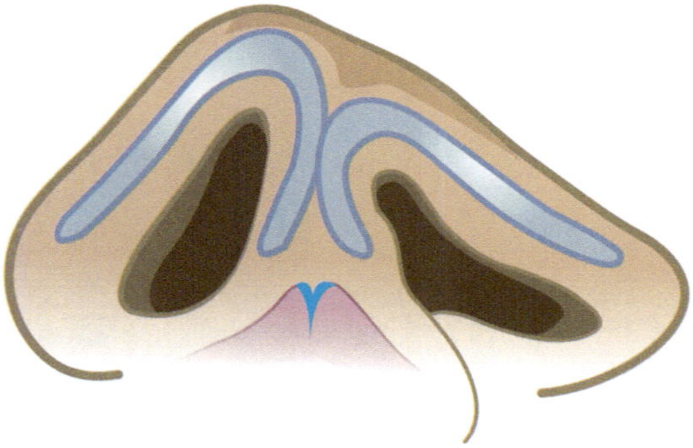

Fig. 11.5 Nostril sill asymmetry

Studies report that almost 88% of patients with cleft show increased nasal resistance on rhinomanometry. Rhinomanometry can be a good diagnostic tool for airway analysis.

CT scan with 3D reconstruction provides the structural details of the entire bony framework, premaxilla, hard palate and posterior bony septal deflections. The advent of cone-beam computed tomography (CBCT) allows the acquisition of high-quality 3-dimensional images of facial structures with reduced radiation doses compared with multisection CT (Fig. 11.9).

Cephalometric analysis can also be done. It gives additional information regarding the position of the maxilla. If orthognathic surgery is not performed previously, it can be suggested for achieving aesthetically balanced facial features.

11.2.3 Surgical Management of Unilateral Cleft Lip Nose Deformity

An open approach is used to expose the tip and the dorsum. Open approach is preferred as it allows direct view of the alar cartilages. An inverted V incision followed by marginal incision

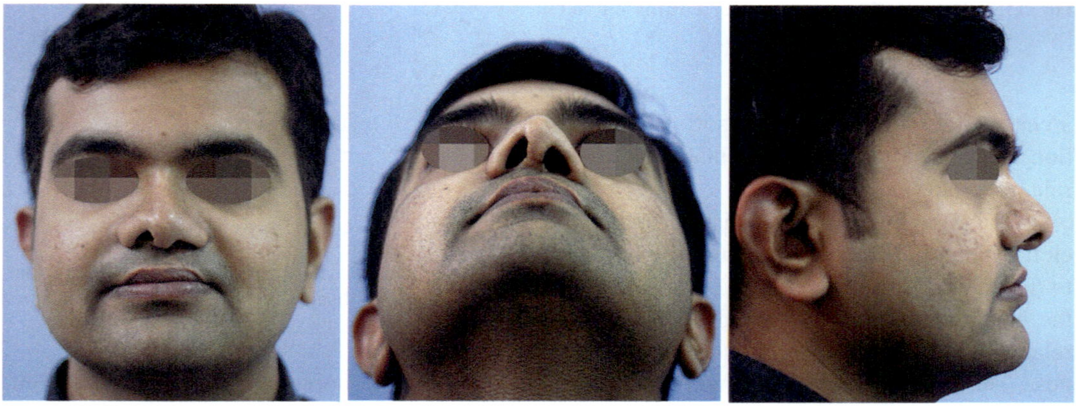

Figs. 11.6–11.8 (left: Fig. 11.6): Frontal view; (middle: Fig. 11.7): Basal view; (right: Fig. 11.8): Lateral view

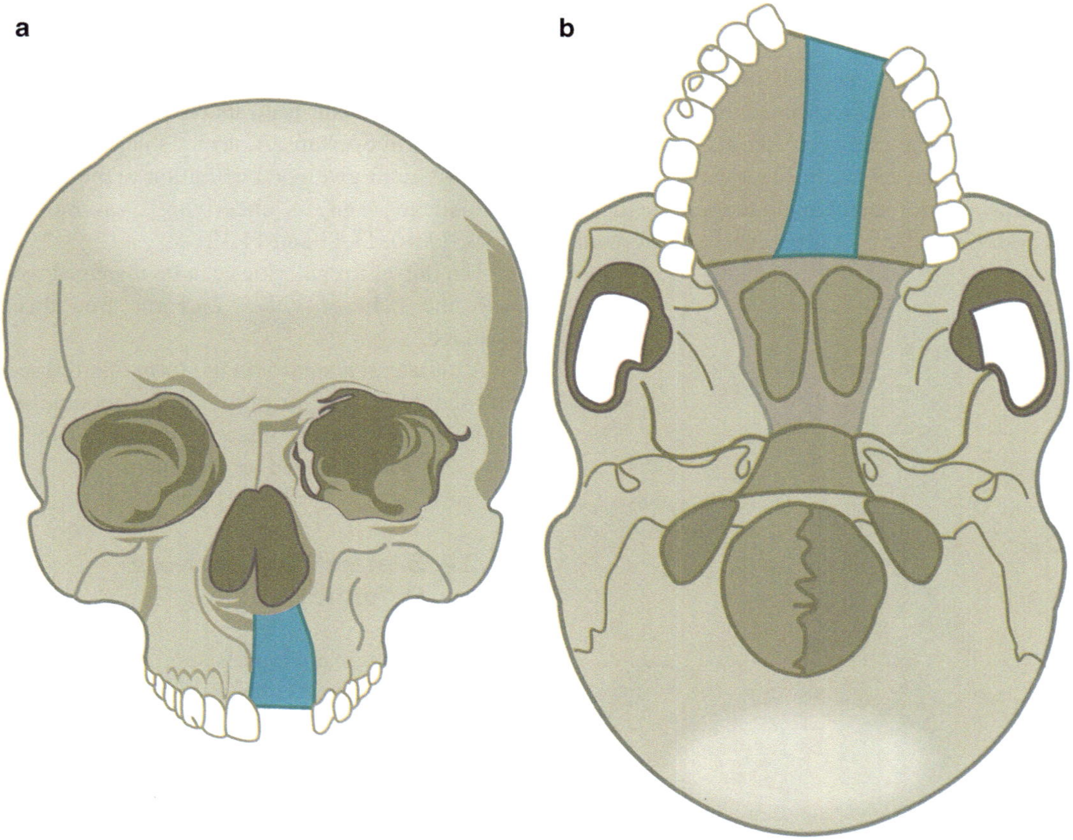

Fig. 11.9 (**a**, **b**) CT image (blue colour) suggestive of bony deformity of the premaxilla and hard palate

or a Tajima inverted U incision combined with or without the Dibbell technique to correct overhanging ala contour should be given. The tip split approach provides a bidirectional approach to the septum and also aids in creation a strong structural foundation. After opening one can reassess the operative plan and the grafts required.

The costal cartilage serves as an abundant source for carving various grafts required in the surgery. Costal cartilage can simultaneously be harvested by a colleague/team member simultaneously to save time. Harvest of the rectus fascia and both the ninth and tenth costal cartilage usually provides abundant material for the grafts.

Steps of routine rhinoplasty—septal dissection and release of septum from maxillary crest followed by septal cartilage harvest to be performed. If deviation is severe, an extracorporeal septoplasty should be planned. This should be followed by the paramedian, lateral and transverse osteotomy to straighten and narrow the bony nasal pyramid. In case of a severely deviated septum, an extracorporeal septoplasty may become necessary.

The anterior nasal spine though deviated should not be fractured. Its stability is important as it is the anchoring point for the structural grafts. Use of the piezoelectric device/diamond drill in this area can help avoid instability.

Extended spreader grafts along with a septal extension graft provide a strong structural support. These grafts should be secured with a nonabsorbable suture to the nasal bones, the anterior nasal spine and the upper lateral cartilage.

The premaxilla should be augmented using either a DCF (rectus fascial sleeve filled with diced cartilage) or solid rib cartilage graft, which is inserted through a pocket created by inserting dissecting scissors via horizontal limbs of the columellar incision.

The tip support has to be reconstructed next. Complete lateral dissection of the lateral crus of the LLC on the cleft side should be done. The LLC should be advanced (lateral crural steal) on the new anterior septal angle to increase the projection. Cephalic trimming can be performed if the LLC is found to be wide. The LLC on the cleft side is usually flaccid and concave; this can be modified by using a lateral crural onlay graft and articulated rim graft extending laterally till the pyriform aperture. A strong shield graft and tip onlay graft give good definition to the tip and camouflage any underlying asymmetry (Figs. 11.10, 11.11 and 11.12).

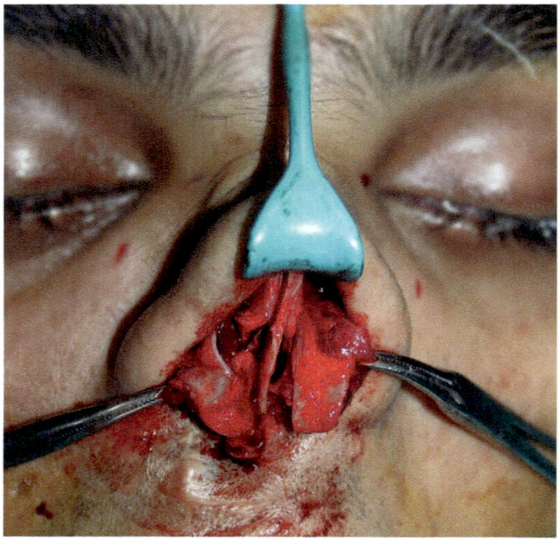

Fig. 11.10 Release of right LLC from the underlying vestibular skin

The dorsal irregularities can be managed well with the help of either DCF or free diced cartilage.

A unilateral alaplasty in the form of sill resection should be performed to achieve good nostril symmetry. However, finer refinements can be done as a part of staged procedures.

11.2.4 Bilateral Cleft Lip Nose Deformity

The underlying pathology is similar to unilateral cleft, but this group of patients shows much better facial symmetry. The septum is usually in midline. The soft tissue between the nasal tip and vermillion border in the lip is significantly less in bilateral cleft lip patients leading to shortening of columella. These cases require a timely intervention for the nasoalveolar moulding via orthodon-

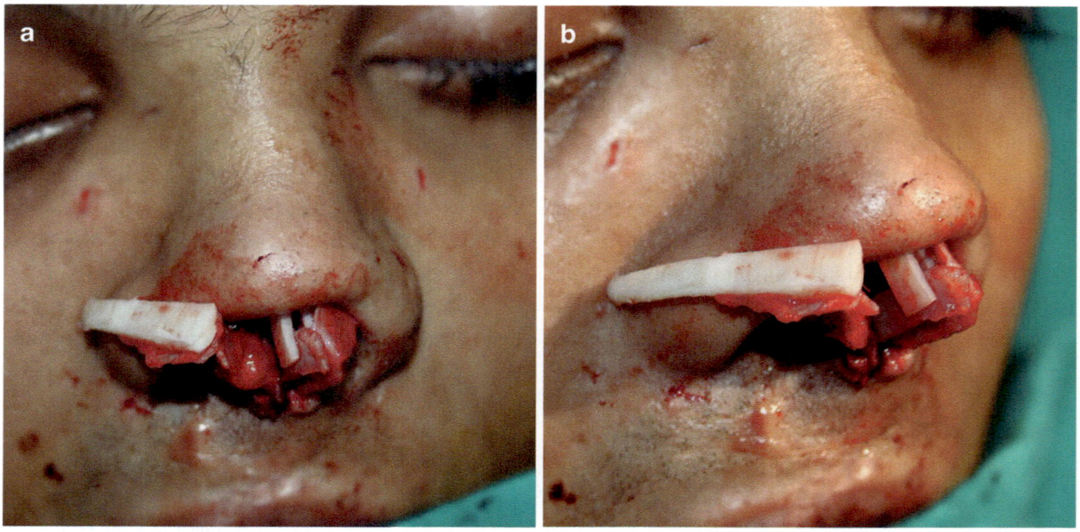

Fig. 11.11 (**a**, **b**) Lateral crural onlay graft placed on the right LLC

tic technique for pleasant aesthetic results. The nasal deformities like short columella, decreased nasal tip projection, hypoplastic premaxilla, etc. are quite similar to patients of Binder's syndrome; hence, the surgical management is similar.

11.3 Binder's Syndrome

Binder's syndrome or nasomaxillary hypoplasia is a congenital disorder of the face associated with underdeveloped maxilla and normal position of nasal bones, atrophic nasal mucosa and agenesis of frontal sinuses. This deformity is also known as fish face deformity, pertaining overall appearance of the retruded midface. The aetiology of this condition is attributed to the inhibition of ossification centre responsible for the growth of lateral and inferior borders of the pyriform aperture during the 5th–6th week of gestation. There is no sexual predominance, and most cases are sporadic. Few studies report familial propensity with Binder's syndrome, and inheritance may be as an autosomal recessive trait with incomplete penetrance or multifactorial.

Physical findings of Binder's syndrome are the result of hypoplasia (depression) of the anterior nasal floor (fossa prenasalis) and localised symmetric maxillary hypoplasia of the alar rim regions. On basal view, retracted columella-lip junction can be appreciated. Lack of normal triangular flare at the nasal base; a perpendicular alar-cheek junction; convex upper nasal tip with a wide, shallow philtrum; crescent-shaped nostrils without a sill; low-set and flat nasal tip; and stretched and shallow Cupid's bow are a few characteristic features. There is vertical shortening of the nose with lack of tip projection, perialar flattening and an acute nasolabial angle (Figs. 11.13, 11.14, 11.15, 11.16 and 11.17).

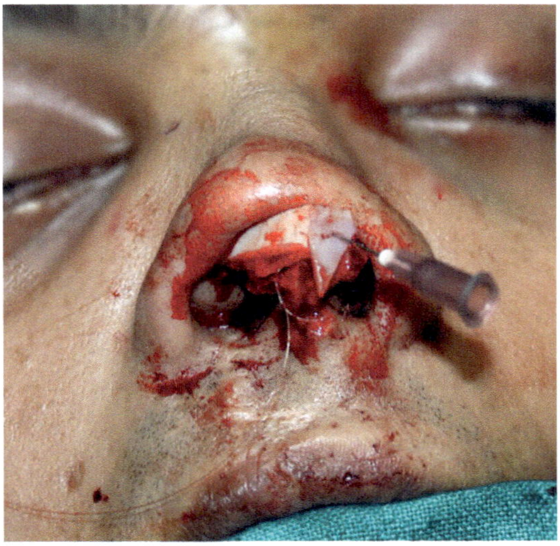

Fig. 11.12 Strong shield graft

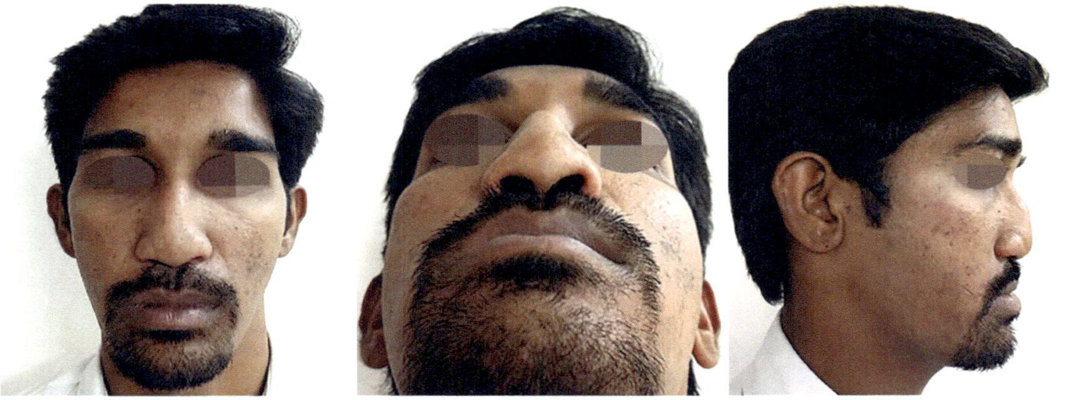

Fig. 11.13–11.15 (left: Fig. 11.13): Frontal view; (middle: Fig. 11.14): Basal view; (right: Fig. 11.15): Lateral view

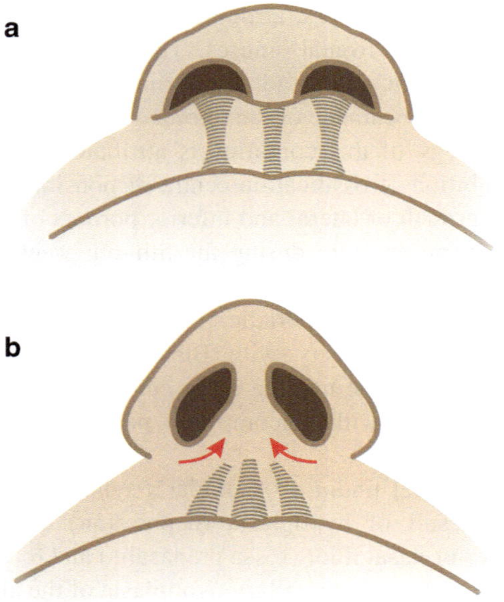

Fig. 11.16 (a, b) Pre- and post-op basal view picture of Binder's syndrome

11.3.1 Surgical Steps (Figs. 11.18, 11.19, 11.20, 11.21 and 11.22)

Other findings like cervical spine malformations, Down's syndrome, hearing loss, vitamin K deficiency, autonomic neuropathy and strabismus might also be found in a few patients.

11.3.2 Investigations

Apart from routine rhinoplasty workup, lateral cephalometry can be of adjunctive value to decide regarding maxillary advancement procedures. Cephalometry reveals absent anterior nasal spine and hypoplastic maxilla.

The CT PNS might reveal frontal sinus agenesis/hypoplasia in most of the cases.

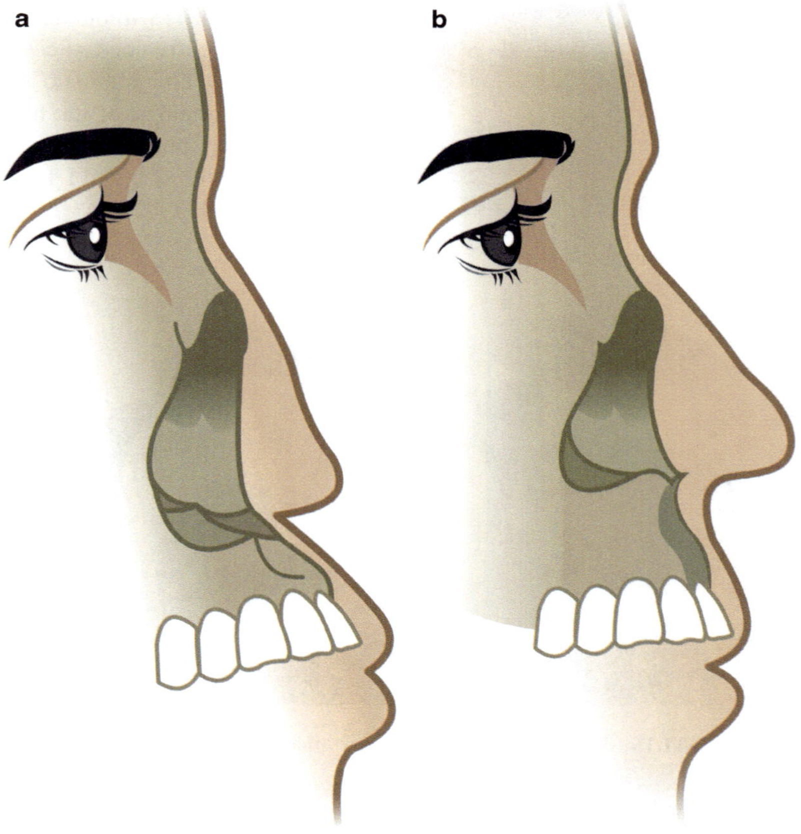

Fig. 11.17 (a, b) Pre- and post-op lateral view

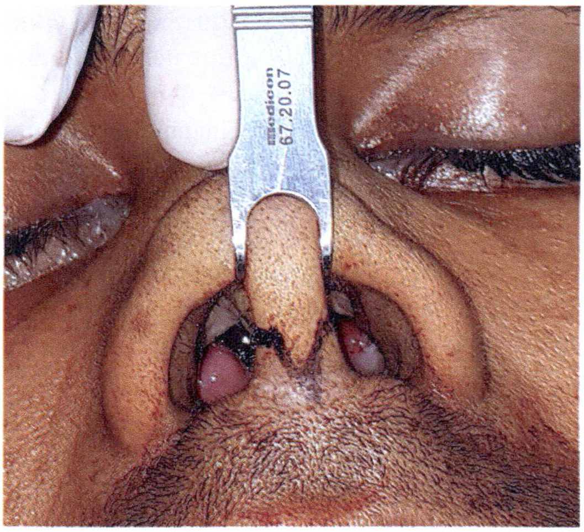

Fig. 11.18 Low columellar incision

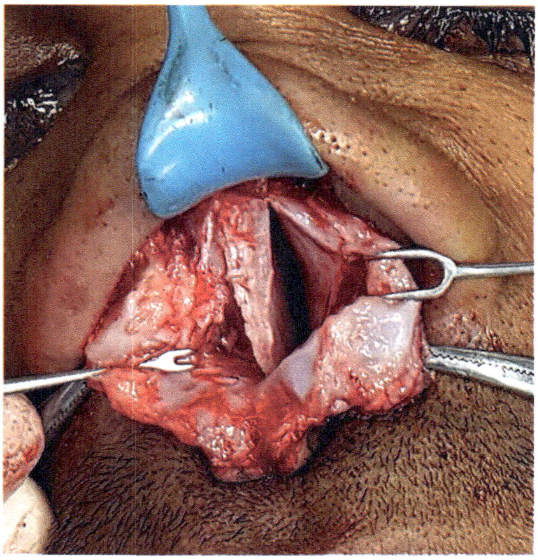

Fig. 11.19 Bilateral mucoperichondrial and mucoperiosteal elevation

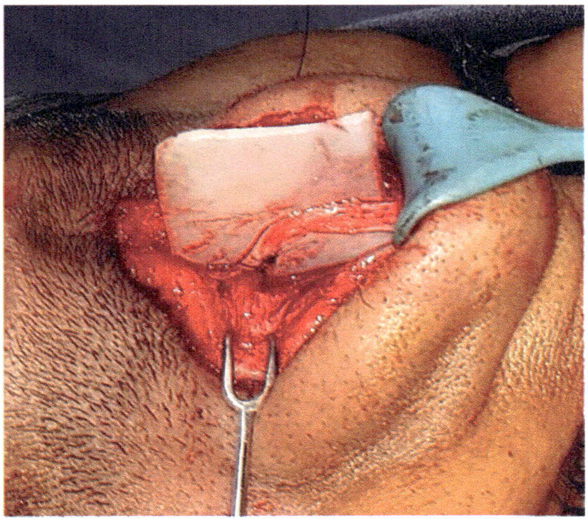

Fig. 11.20 Cartilaginous piece kept in between the septal flaps

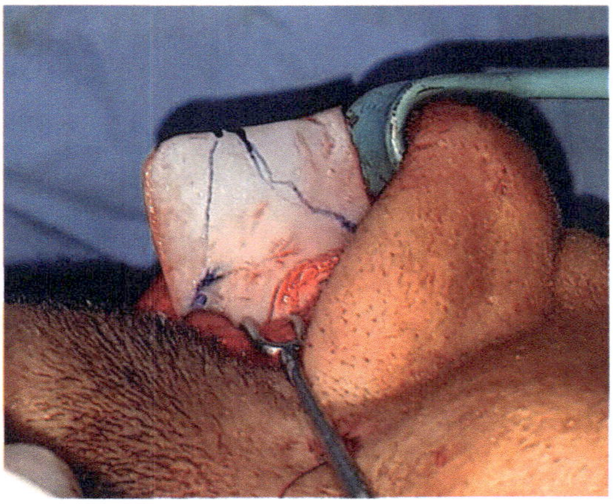

Fig. 11.21 The marked (blue) septum to be resected dorsally and caudally

11.3.3 Surgical Management

Adjuvant Procedures

Minor malocclusions if present can be treated by orthodontic treatment. In case of class 3 malocclusion, a Le Fort 1 osteotomy might seem necessary.

Definitive Rhinoplasty

Access to the nose is preferred via the open approach technique. In severe cases, a V-Y lengthening incision should be planned. Costal cartilage harvest along with rectus facia is a must owing to the multiple grafts required in these cases. The premaxilla is accessed subperi-

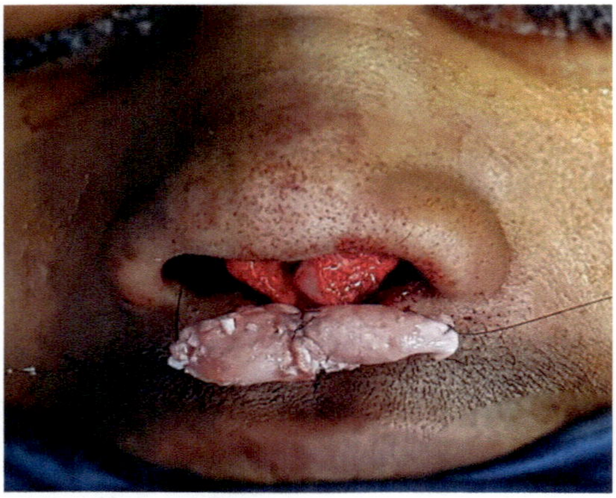

Fig. 11.22 DCF bag placed in the premaxillary area under the skin flap

osteally via the lateral limbs of the same columellar incision. A pocket is created bilaterally and premaxilla is augmented with a DCF of about 2–2.5 cm size. FIG 8 The anterior septum short and requires lengthening. FIG 9 This is achieved by using a septal extension graft, tailored according to the desired length of the nose. FIG 10,11 Bilateral extended spreader grafts articulating with the SEG give a strong foundation. The dorsum should be augmented using a solid dorsal onlay graft. Articulated alar rim grafts along with shield grafts give a good triangular configuration.

GPSR Compliance

The European Union's (EU) General Product Safety Regulation (GPSR) is a set of rules that requires consumer products to be safe and our obligations to ensure this.

If you have any concerns about our products, you can contact us on ProductSafety@springernature.com

In case Publisher is established outside the EU, the EU authorized representative is:

Springer Nature Customer Service Center GmbH
Europaplatz 3
69115 Heidelberg, Germany

Batch number: 10732809

Printed by Printforce, the Netherlands